PRIVATE GUNS
PUBLIC HEALTH

"In scholarly, sober analytic assessments, including rigorous critiques of NRA-popularized pseudoscience, David Hemenway constructs a convincing case that firearm availability is a critical and proximal cause of unparalleled carnage. By formulating such violence as a public health issue, he proposes workable policies analogous to ones that reduced injuries from tobacco, alcohol, and automobiles."
—JEROME P. KASSIRER, EDITOR-IN-CHIEF EMERITUS,
NEW ENGLAND JOURNAL OF MEDICINE,
AND DISTINGUISHED PROFESSOR,
TUFTS UNIVERSITY SCHOOL OF MEDICINE

"Much has been said in recent years about the 'public health approach to violence,' but it is unclear whether many well-intentioned people using that phrase understand what it means. Hemenway identifies problems in widely cited research and provides a clear and concise description of how public health approaches can be used to reduce firearm-related injuries and deaths. The book, which intersperses dispassionate critiques of population-based research with news bulletins about individuals, reads quickly and easily."
—SUSAN B. SORENSON,
UCLA SCHOOL OF PUBLIC HEALTH

"David Hemenway marshals solid empirical evidence to weave a forceful and persuasive argument for reasonable policies to minimize the harm from guns. He carefully constructs the argument for a regulatory structure that borrows from successful efforts to reduce injuries in everyday life. Every legislator should read this book."
—JEFFREY FAGAN,
PROFESSOR OF LAW AND PUBLIC HEALTH,
COLUMBIA UNIVERSITY

"As a former District Attorney and Attorney General, I know the urgency of providing safe homes, schools and neighborhoods for all. This remarkable tour-de-force is a powerful study of one promising solution: a data-rich, eminently readable demonstration of why we should treat gun violence as an American epidemic."
—SCOTT HARSHBARGER,
FORMER ATTORNEY GENERAL OF MASSACHUSETTS,
PRESIDENT AND CEO OF COMMON CAUSE

"Hemenway's book provides a comprehensive look at the epidemic of firearm injury in the United States. He writes that the experience of high-income nations shows that when there are reasonable restrictions on guns, gun injuries need not be such a large public health problem. This book is an important resource for educating politicians and the public who are looking to build safer communities. It is also an important reference for members of the public health and medical communities who see the results of firearm injuries and are struggling to find solutions to the gun wars waged both in our homes and on our streets."
—BARBARA BARLOW,
DIRECTOR OF SURGERY AT
HARLEM HOSPITAL CENTER

PRIVATE GUNS
PUBLIC HEALTH

David Hemenway

THE UNIVERSITY OF MICHIGAN PRESS
Ann Arbor

2007   2006   2005   2004   4   3   2   1

A CIP catalog record for this book is available from the British Library.

Library of Congress Cataloging-in-Publication Data

Hemenway, David, 1945–
Private guns, public health / David Hemenway.
p. ; cm.
Includes bibliographical references and index.
ISBN 0-472-11405-0 (cloth : alk. paper)
1. Gunshot wounds—United States—Prevention.   2. Firearms—Law and
legislation—United States.   3. Gun control—United States.   4. Public
policy—United States.   5. Medical policy—United States.   6. Firearms
ownership—United States.
[DNLM: 1. Firearm ownership—United States. 2. Wounds,
Gunshot—epidemiology—United States. 3. Public Health—United States.
4. Public Policy—United States.   WO 807 H498p   2004]   I. Title.

RD96.3.H45   2004
617.1'45'0973—dc22   2003024583

FOR MY FRIENDS IN
INJURY PREVENTION AND CONTROL

*Nothing is so powerful as an
idea whose time has come.
—Victor Hugo*

CONTENTS

CONTENTS

PREFACE

When I was growing up in the 1950s, cars did not have seat belts, shatterproof windows, collapsible steering columns, or air bags. In high school, when schoolmates of mine died in automobile accidents, people said they were driving too fast or too carelessly. Perhaps this was no surprise, it was thought, for, after all, they were teenagers.

In the late 1960s, I went to work for Ralph Nader, then at the height of his engagement with the automobile industry, and subsequently I became the Washington correspondent for Consumers Union. One of my first tasks was to interview the director of a new agency—now called the National Highway Traffic Safety Administration—that was responsible for improving the safety of motorists. Bill Haddon, M.D., M.P.H., one of the pioneers in the field of injury prevention, talked with me for hours about the science of injury prevention and the goals of his new bureau. After working with Nader and talking to Haddon, I began to realize that my schoolmates would probably still be alive if the cars in which they were riding were more forgiving of human error and bad judgment.

In 1975, after receiving a Ph.D. in economics, I took a job at the public health school that had trained Haddon. During the 1980s, inspired by both Haddon and Nader, I created a course that dealt with our scientific knowledge about injuries and its implications for public policy. Although injuries kill far more young people than do diseases, there were then only a couple of injury prevention classes in the entire country. Following a mid-1980s Institute of Medicine report that highlighted both the size of the U.S. injury problem and the lack of support for the field, an injury-control division was established at the Centers for Disease Control and Prevention (CDC). Only then did injury prevention start to become an integral part of public health practice.

Injuries include stairway falls, drownings, poisonings, child abuse, suicides, sports injuries, motor vehicle crashes, and firearm violence. Of these, motor vehicles and firearms are the leading agents of injury death in the

United States, with vehicles first and guns a close second. But while motor vehicles are used by almost everyone, every day, throughout the country and are crucial for our standard of living, the same is not true of firearms. And while a great deal of injury research deals with cars and trucks, until the late 1980s only a minuscule amount of research was devoted to firearm injuries.

Things have changed in the past decade. The public health community is now conducting a substantial amount of research on firearm injuries. This book seeks to provide a synopsis of this growing scientific literature, to describe the public health approach for reducing this injury problem, and to offer an overview of reasonable and feasible policies to reduce gun-related injury and death that such an approach suggests.

The mission of public health is the attainment for all peoples of the highest possible level of health—a state of complete physical, mental, and social well-being. Considering that each year tens of thousands of Americans die from gunshot wounds, the reduction of firearm injuries—and the reduction of the accompanying dread and fear of firearm violence—is clearly within the purview of public health.

Public health is prohealth; it is not anti-stairs, anti–swimming pools, anti-cars, or anti-guns. Unfortunately, many people who lobby for uncontrolled gun access dichotomize the world—into "progun" and "antigun," "us" and "them," "good guys" and "bad guys," "criminals" and "decent, law-abiding citizens." Dividing people into such categories is anathema to public health, whose mission is to unite diverse groups of people and to improve the health—and the conditions that promote health—for all peoples.

Public health is not anti–gun owner. A little more than one-third of American households currently contain working firearms, and the principal factor affecting whether someone becomes a gun owner is not any personality trait but simply whether the individual was raised in a gun-owning household. Polls show that the policies suggested in this book receive overwhelming support from gun owners and non–gun owners alike.

The text describes the public health approach to injury prevention. The effects of firearms on public health are broad and include both intentional and unintentional shootings, both self-inflicted and inflicted by others. The public health approach encompasses criminal justice (which focuses on homicide and other intentional other-inflicted gun uses), mental health (which focuses on suicide and some aspects of criminal gun use), and safety (which focuses on unintentional shootings). My interest is on the most important public health effects of firearms. Thus, this book does not examine some of the benefits of shooting, such as the social or recreational benefits, or all the costs, such as the loss of hearing of recreational shooters (Nondahl et al. 2000; Stewart, Konkle, and Simpson 2001) or the environmental lead poisoning caused by shooting ranges (Environmental Working Group 2001). The book also does not examine gun use in wars or by the police.

The book prescribes some specific policies that should reduce injuries from firearms. These policies would do little to affect the limited safety benefits derived from firearms but would substantially reduce the major health and human problems. It is shameful that tens of thousands of Americans die needlessly from guns each year while our gun policy is driven more by rhetoric than scientific information.

The book summarizes the scientific literature on the public health effects of firearm availability and firearm policies. It is important to recognize that no single piece of research is definitive. Only the cumulative effort of many studies leads to increased knowledge and understanding of the real world. Each study has limitations; journal articles in medicine and public health require that authors identify the main aspects of the study that limit the generalizability and validity of the findings. Articles in journals outside of public health do not always include such caveats.

A few articles are discussed in some depth in appendix A. These articles have typically been selected for more intensive analysis because (1) they have received a large amount of publicity, (2) the authors provide little if any discussion of the studies' limitations, and (3) the limitations are so substantial that they often tend to invalidate the authors' strong conclusions.

The Harvard Injury Control Research Center, which I direct, is funded in part by the CDC. One of the stipulations of our CDC grant is that "none of the funds made available for injury prevention and control may be used to advocate or promote gun control." No CDC money has been used to support any portion of this book. This book was funded entirely by grants to the author from two private foundations, the Robert Wood Johnson Foundation and the Open Society Institute. Portions of chapter 1 have been updated from my article, "Regulation of Firearms," *New England Journal of Medicine* 339 (1998): 843–45; portions of chapter 2 have been updated from my chapter, "Guns, Public Health, and Public Safety," in *Guns and the Constitution,* edited by D. Henigan, E. Nicholson, and D. Hemenway (Northampton, MA: Aletheia, 1995); portions of chapters 2 and 9 have been updated from my article, "The Public Health Approach to Motor Vehicles, Tobacco, and Alcohol, with Applications to Firearms Policy," *Journal of Public Health Policy* 22 (2001): 381–402.

PREFACE

The book emphasizes the need for better data. Unfortunately, when the book was completed in the spring of 2003, disaggregated data on firearm deaths were available only through 2000. Thus, much of the discussion here deals with the decade ending in 2000.

I had many reasons for writing this book. The most important were that there did not exist a good summary of the firearms literature from a public health perspective and that many public commentators did not appear to understand the public health approach. But what propelled me most was a 1995 *International Herald Tribune* article that had little to do with crime or injury:

MAMARONECK, NY: When the Canada geese were just passing through, in that lovely "V" formation, people here actually liked them. This was obviously before "Honk if you hate geese" bumper stickers, and way before village officials decided the birds should be shot.

It seems the geese just didn't know when to leave. All of Harbor Island Park—the beach, the docks, the fields—became saturated with their most unwelcome calling cards.

They had just about exhausted the public's good will and stumped village officials, who obtained a federal permit to allow hunters a crack at the problem. (Nieves 1995)

Fortunately, before the shooting started, the town tried an alternative approach. They hired a dog trainer with a couple of border collies, who successfully chased the birds away.

For me, the story illustrated an important point—the immediate reaction to a problem for many people in the United States is to get a gun. Yet it turns out that this response can often exacerbate the problem, while other actions may be far more effective.

Many people provided help with this book, including Deb Azrael, Matthew Roth, Michelle Schaffer, and Jon Vernick. Phil Cook, Rafe Ezekiel, Jens Ludwig, Matt Miller, Alix Smullin, Sara Solnick, Susan Sorenson, and Mary Vriniotis read the entire manuscript and made many useful suggestions and corrections. Many thanks to Matt Weiland for making the book more clear and readable.

David Hemenway
September 2003

CHAPTER 1 GUNS AND AMERICAN SOCIETY

The landmarks of political, economic and social history are the moments when some condition passed from the category of the given into the category of the intolerable. . . . I believe that the history of public health might well be written as a record of successive re-defining of the unacceptable.

—G. Vickers

On an average day during the 1990s in the United States, firearms were used to kill more than ninety people and to wound about three hundred more. Each day guns were also used in the commission of about three thousand crimes. The U.S. rates of death and injury due to firearms and the rate of crimes committed with firearms are far higher than those of any other industrialized country, yet our rates of crime and nonlethal violence are not exceptional. For example, the U.S. rates of rape, robbery, nonlethal assault, burglary, and larceny resemble those of other high-income countries (Van Kesteren et al. 2000); however, our homicide rate is far higher than that of other high-income nations (Krug, Powell, and Dahlberg 1998). This chapter discusses the nature and extent of the firearms injury problem in the United States (Hemenway 1995, 1998a) and describes the prevalence of firearms in contemporary America.

THE SCOPE OF THE GUN PROBLEM

Perhaps the most appropriate international comparisons are those between the United States and other developed "frontier" countries where English is spoken: Australia, Canada, and New Zealand. These four nations have roughly similar per capita incomes, cultures, and histories (including the violent displacement of indigenous populations). In 1992, the rates of property crime and violent crime were comparable across these four countries (Mayhew and van Dijk 1997); with the decline in U.S. crime, by the end of the century U.S. crime rates were actually lower than in these other countries (table 1.1). What distinguishes the United States is its high rate of lethal violence. In 1992 our murder rate was five times higher than the average of these three other countries (Krug, Powell, and Dahlberg 1998); in 1999–2000 it was still about three times higher (table 1.2). In contrast to these other nations, most of our murderers use guns. Comparisons with other high-income countries make our gun/lethal violence problem look even worse (Killias 1993; Hemenway and Miller 2000).

Canada, Australia, and New Zealand all have many guns, though not nearly as many handguns as the United States. The key difference is that these

TABLE 1.1. Percentage of People Victimized in 2000 (from comparable victimization surveys)

Nation	Car Theft	Burglary	Robbery	Sexual Incident	Assault or Threat	11 crimes
United States	0.5	1.8	0.6	1.5	3.4	21.1
Canada	1.4	2.3	0.9	2.1	5.3	23.8
Australia	1.9	3.9	1.2	4.0	6.4	30.0
New Zealand[a]	2.7	4.3	0.7	2.7	5.7	29.4
17 Industrialized Nations[b]	1.0	1.8	0.8	1.7	3.5	21.3

Source: Data from Van Kesteren et al. 2000.
[a]Data for 1992
[b]Australia, Belgium, Canada, Catalonia (Spain), Denmark, England and Wales, Finland, France, Japan, Netherlands, Northern Ireland, Poland, Portugal, Scotland, Sweden, Switzerland, United States.

TABLE 1.2. Firearm and Nonfirearm Homicide in the Frontier Countries, Rates per 100,000, 1999–2000

Nation	Firearm Homicide Rate	Nonfirearm Homicide Rate	Total Homicide Rate	Households with Guns (%)
United States	4.0	2.2	6.1	41
Canada	0.6	1.2	1.8	26
Australia	0.4	1.4	1.8	16
New Zealand (1997–98)	0.2	1.5	1.7	20

Source: Homicide data from CDC WISQARS (Note: U.S. Bureau of Justice Statistics give slightly lower homicide rates); Fedorowycz (Homicide in Canada 2000); Mouzos (Homicide in Australia 1999–2000); Injury Prevention Research Unit (New Zealand). Gun data from United Nations 1998.

other countries do a much better job of regulating their guns. Their experience and that of all high-income nations shows that when there are reasonable restrictions on guns, gun injuries need not be such a large public health problem. Their experience also shows that it is possible to live in a society with many guns yet one in which relatively few crimes are committed with guns.

A nation may be judged by how well it protects its children. In terms of lethal violence, the United States does very badly. For example, a comparison of violent deaths of five- to fourteen-year-olds in the United States and in the other twenty-five high-income countries during the 1990s shows that the United States has much higher suicide and homicide rates, almost entirely because of the higher gun death rates. The United States has ten times the firearm suicide rate and the same nonfirearm suicide rate as these other countries, and the United States has seventeen times the firearm homicide rate and only a somewhat higher nonfirearm homicide rate. Our unintentional firearm death rate is nine times higher (table 1.3).

Of particular concern was the rise in children's violent deaths in the early 1990s. For example, between 1950 and 1993, the overall death rate for U.S. children under age fifteen declined substantially (Singh and Yu 1996) because of decreases in deaths from both illness and unintentional injury. However,

TABLE 1.3. Homicide, Suicide, and Gun Deaths among Five- to Fourteen-Year Olds, United States versus Twenty-five Other Nations

	Gun Homicide	Nongun Homicide	Total
Homicide			
U.S.	1.22	0.53	1.75
Non-U.S.	0.07	0.23	0.30
Ratio	17:1	2:1	6:1
	Gun Suicide	Nongun Suicide	Total
Suicide			
U.S.	0.49	0.35	0.84
Non-U.S.	0.05	0.35	0.40
Ratio	10:1	1:1	2:1
Unintentional Gun Death			
U.S.	0.46		
Non-U.S.	0.05		
Ratio	9:1		

Source: Data from CDC, 1997b.

Note: The twenty-five other nations are the richest countries with a population greater than one million. Rates are per one hundred thousand (early 1990s).

3

during the same period, childhood homicide rates tripled and suicide rates quadrupled; these increases resulted almost entirely from gun violence.

Though gunshot wounds often result in death, even nonfatal wounds can be devastating, leading to permanent disability. Traumatic brain injury and spinal cord injuries are two of the more serious firearm-related injuries. For example, nonfatal gunshot injuries are currently the second-leading cause of spinal cord injury in the United States; it is estimated that each year, more than two thousand individuals who are shot suffer spinal cord injuries (DeVivo 1997; Cook and Ludwig 2000). Spinal cord injuries from gunshot wounds also tend to be quite serious—gunshot wounds are more likely than non-violence-related traumatic spinal cord injuries (e.g., from falls or motor vehicle collisions) to lead to paraplegia and complete spinal cord injury (McKinley, Johns, and Musgrove 1999).

The psychological ravages of firearm trauma can be especially long-lasting. For example, compared to other traumatic injuries, gunshot wounds are more likely to lead to the development of posttraumatic stress disorder (PTSD) in children (Gill 1999). Chronic PTSD following firearm injury is common: in one study, 80 percent of hospitalized gunshot-wound victims reported moderate or severe symptoms of posttraumatic stress eight months after the incident (Greenspan and Kellermann 2002); in another study, 58 percent of firearm assault victims met the full diagnostic criteria for PTSD-3 thirty-six months after the incident (Burnette 1998). Even witnessing firearm violence can have serious psychological consequences. In one study, high school students who witnessed firearms suicides were at higher risk than other demographically similar students to develop psychopathology—specifically, anxiety disorders and PTSD (Brent et al. 1993a).

The direct medical costs of gunshot wounds were estimated at six million dollars per day in the 1990s. The mean medical cost of a gunshot injury is about seventeen thousand dollars and would be higher except that the medical costs for deaths at the scene are low (Cook et al. 1999). Half of these costs are borne directly by U.S. taxpayers; gun injuries are the leading cause of uninsured hospital stays in the United States (Coben and Steiner 2003). The best estimate of the cost of gun violence in America, derived from asking people how much they would pay to reduce it, is about one hundred billion dollars per year (Cook and Ludwig 2000).

Fortunately, many reasonable policies can reduce this enormous and, among high-income nations, uniquely American public health problem—

without banning all guns or handguns and without preventing responsible citizens from keeping firearms.

THE FACTS ABOUT GUN OWNERSHIP

The United States "almost certainly has more firearms in civilian hands than any other nation in the world."

—Gary Kleck

The role of firearms in American history has been shrouded in myth and legend, none greater than the images of revolutionary militiamen with their trusty rifles defeating the world's most powerful nation and frontier cowboys— tough, brave, and independent— whose remarkable shooting made them memorable and heroic figures. Yet the key firearm in the Revolution was the inaccurate one-shot musket, and the regular army won the war. The militia had very limited success: George Washington considered it to be a "broken reed" (Emory 1904; Peterson 1956; Ropp 1959; Russell 1967; Kennett and Anderson 1975; Higginbotham 1988; Whisker 1997; Gruber 2002; Rakove 2002).

Long the subject of twentieth-century heroic myth, the realistic image of the nineteenth-century cowboy is "a hired hand with a borrowed horse, a mean streak, and syphilis." Cowboys were mostly young, single, itinerant, irreligious, southern-born men who lived, worked, and played in male company. Many were combat veterans, and almost all carried firearms. Youthful irresponsibility, intoxication, and firearms led to so many murders and unintentional injuries at the end of the trail that laws were enacted to force cowboys to check their guns before they entered towns (Courtwright 1996).

For today's gun enthusiasts, the citizen-soldier and the cowboy lawman remain two archetypes of American history (Kohn 2000). But what is not a myth is that America is currently awash with guns. It is estimated that there are more than two hundred million working firearms in private hands in the United States—as many guns as adults.

The total number of firearms in civilian hands has increased rapidly in the past forty years. Seventy percent of all new guns purchased in America during the twentieth century were bought after 1960. The type of gun purchased has also changed. In 1960, only 27 percent of the yearly additions to the gunstock were handguns; by 1994, that number had doubled to 54 percent (Blendon, Young, and Hemenway 1996; Cook and Ludwig 1996; Kleck 1997b).

While the number of guns has increased, the percentage of American households reporting that they own guns has declined markedly in recent years, from about 48 percent in 1973 to closer to 35 percent today (Blendon, Young, and Hemenway 1996; T. W. Smith 2001). This decline appears in part to result from the decreasing number of adults in each household and, since 1997, from a decline in the proportion of adults who personally own firearms (T. W. Smith 2001). However, current gun owners have been buying additional firearms; the average number of firearms owned by gun owners has been increasing in recent decades.

Currently, one in four adults owns a gun of some kind, but owners of four or more guns (about 10 percent of the adult population) are in possession of 77 percent of the total U.S. stock of firearms (Cook and Ludwig 1996). Many people, especially women, who live in households with a gun do not own any guns. Approximately 40 percent of adult males and 10 percent of adult females are gun owners (Cook and Ludwig 1996; T. W. Smith 2001). Even though we live in a land of firearms, the majority of males do not own guns, and only about one woman out of ten is a gun owner.

The percentage of households with long guns (rifles and shotguns) fell from 40 percent in 1973 to 32 percent in 1994, but household handgun ownership rose from 20 to 25 percent. Since the mid-1990s, even household handgun ownership has been declining (T. W. Smith 2001). Perhaps 16 percent of U.S. adults currently own handguns.

People report owning guns primarily for hunting, target shooting, and personal protection. The reasons for ownership differ for long guns and handguns. Handguns are owned primarily for protection, while long guns are used mainly for hunting and target shooting. While all guns pose risks for injury, compared to their prevalence in the gun stock, handguns are used disproportionately in crimes, homicides, suicides, and gun accidents. Thus, some proposed gun policies focus on handguns rather than long guns.

Gun ownership varies across geographic regions; it is highest among households in the South and in the Rocky Mountain region and lowest in the Northeast. It is higher in rural areas than urban areas; it is higher among conservatives than among moderates or liberals (Davis and Smith 1994; T. W. Smith 2001).

One of the most important predictors of gun ownership is whether one's parents had a gun in the home. Gun ownership is highest among those over forty years old and is more prevalent among those with higher incomes. While gun owners come from the entire spectrum of American society, people who admit to having been arrested for a nontraffic offense are more likely to own guns (37 percent versus 24 percent for those without an arrest) (Cook and Ludwig 1996); owners of semiautomatics are more likely than other gun owners to report that they binge drink (Hemenway and Richardson 1997); and combat veterans with PTSD appear more likely than other veterans to own firearms (and to engage in such potentially harmful behavior as aiming guns at family members, patrolling their property with loaded guns, and killing animals in fits of rage) (Freeman, Roca, and Kimbrell 2003).

A few fringe groups of gun owners may someday pose political problems for the United States. The militia movement made the front pages after the Oklahoma City bombing in April 1995 killed 170 innocent people. Armed paramilitary organizations, formed as a result of antigovernment sentiment, interpret the U.S. Constitution for themselves. In effect, they claim liberty as their exclusive right, which sometimes includes the right to attack violently the objects of their hate. The existence of independent armed militias, sometimes filled with white supremacist rhetoric, could threaten the peaceful conduct of government and public business. These militia often identify the government itself as the enemy. By contrast, the mission of state-sponsored militia of the colonial period was in part to subdue armed insurrections against the state (Halpern and Levin 1996).

SUMMARY

It is often claimed that the United States has a crime problem. We do, but our crime rates, as determined by victimization surveys, resemble those of other high-income countries. It is often claimed that the United States has a violence problem. We do, but our violence rates resemble those of other high-income countries. What is out of line is our lethal violence, and most of our lethal violence is gun violence (Zimring and Hawkins 1997b).

Over the past forty years, the increase in urbanization and the decline in hunting, combined with the fact that fewer adults live in each household, have resulted in a decreasing percentage of households with firearms. At the individual level, about 25 percent of adults currently own guns. On average, these individuals own more firearms than in the past, and the guns are increasingly likely to be handguns. Compared to other high-income nations, Americans own more guns, particularly handguns. And, as we shall see, these guns are readily available to virtually anyone who wants one.

CHAPTER 2   THE PUBLIC
HEALTH APPROACH

Assaultive injuries have been subjected to little prevention oriented research. Typically they have been regarded as a crime problem rather than as a health problem and blame and punishment of the perpetrators have been emphasized rather than measures to reduce the frequency and severity of such injuries.
                                                            —Institute of Medicine, 1985

During most of the twentieth century, gun assaults were seen almost exclusively as a criminal justice problem, gun suicides as a mental health problem, and unintentional gunshot wounds as a safety issue. Since the mid-1980s, it has become increasingly recognized that the most promising approach to reduce firearm injury is to emphasize prevention, focus on the community, use a broad array of policies, and bring together diverse interest groups. This approach is proactive rather than reactive, is pragmatic rather than doctrinaire, and has a distinguished history of success in addressing problems that affect the public's health—it is what I refer to throughout this book as the public health approach. This chapter describes the public health approach to reducing the firearm injury problem in the United States and the history and scientific basis of injury prevention and control as a public health field (Hemenway 1995). The chapter also contrasts the public health approach with the gun advocates' dichotomous view of a world inhabited solely by "good guys" and "bad guys" and explains why the public health perspective leads to more effective policy prescriptions.

WHAT PUBLIC HEALTH MEANS IN PRACTICE

The proactive, community-oriented approach of public health can be contrasted to the often reactive, individual focus of therapeutic medicine and traditional criminal justice. Medicine's principal focus is on curing the individual patient, one person at a time. Medical care providers across the country treat gunshot victims and their families on a daily basis, usually in humane and often heroic ways, but they do so one patient at a time.

Similarly, the law enforcement and criminal justice systems seek to apprehend and punish those committing crimes, one perpetrator at a time. Although deterrence is an important goal of the criminal justice and tort systems and prevention is increasingly seen as a police function, most of the activity still takes place after the fact. By contrast, the goal of public health is neither to determine fault nor to punish perpetrators. Instead, public health focuses directly on prevention—eliminating the problem before something bad happens.

The scientific core of public health is epidemiology, which identifies the risk factors, trends, and causes of health problems. But sound science is the starting point, not the end point, of the public health approach. Rallying political and social support around solutions is the way public health has achieved many of its goals.

Perhaps the most important public health advance of the nineteenth century was the "great sanitary awakening" (Winslow 1923), which identified filth as both a cause of disease and a vehicle of transmission. Sanitation changed the way society thought about health. Illness came to be seen as an indicator not of poor moral and spiritual conditions but of poor environmental conditions. Public health interventions began to emphasize the need to change the environment as well as individual behavior.

Early efforts to combat tuberculosis, for example, succeeded primarily because they addressed poor sanitation and overcrowding in urban neighborhoods rather than because of individual medical treatments (Haines 1997). The knowledge that social and environmental conditions could cause disease and the identification of societal actions that could dramatically reduce outbreaks meant that health could no longer be considered solely an individual responsibility. Public health came into its own.

In the United States, gun violence is a modern-day public health epidemic. Preventing gun violence requires not only individual (e.g., parental) accountability but also collective responsibility. Generating support for collective efforts to reduce gun violence is a current challenge for public health.

Although most of the improvement in the health of the American people (e.g., a rise in life expectancy from forty-seven years in 1900 to seventy-six years in 1990) has been accomplished through public health measures rather

9

than direct medical advances (Evans, Barer, and Marmor 1994), beneficiaries often do not recognize that they have been helped. This is one reason why public health, to succeed, must rally political and social support for collective as well as individual responsibility. While the medical and criminal justice communities deal with identifiable people in identifiable ways, the benefits of public health interventions usually involve only statistical lives. For example, a woman with appendicitis knows she is sick and is grateful to the medical providers who treat her. A victim of violence gains some satisfaction when the individual perpetrator is brought to justice. But the consumer who does not get poisoned because unsafe products are kept off the market does not even know that her life has been saved as a result of the efforts of the public health community.

Public health solutions, which rely on governmental and private sector actions, often meet with organized opposition. The "sanitary idea"—building a drainage network to remove sewage and waste—was quite controversial in the nineteenth century. In the twentieth century, campaigns to reduce public health burdens, such as those caused by tobacco or excessive alcohol use, riled powerful economic interests. For example, smokers resented attempts to raise tobacco taxes or to impose statutory limits on smoking in elevators, airplanes, and other public places, and the tobacco industry fiercely fought such measures.

Efforts to reduce the heavy U.S. injury toll have also met opposition, especially from product manufacturers. But the public health community recognizes that advocacy, based on sound scientific evidence, is essential for securing gains in social justice as well as health, well-being, and the quality of life.

THE SCIENTIFIC BASIS OF INJURY CONTROL

Often the best solutions to injury problems are passive ones. William Haddon Jr., MD, a founder of modern injury control research, urged public health professionals to focus on changing the product, rather than focusing exclusively on changing individual behavior.

—T. A. Karlson and S. W. Hargarten

More than half of all Americans who die before the age of forty die from injuries rather than disease. Injuries account for more lost years of productive life before the age of sixty-five than heart disease, cancer, and stroke combined. Not surprisingly, injury prevention is a public health priority in the United States.

For centuries, human injuries were regarded either as random or unavoidable events ("accidents" and "acts of God") or as the result of human evil or carelessness. From this perspective, the main strategies for prevention were prayer and human improvement (Institute of Medicine 1999), the latter often taking the form of moral education and punishment.

With industrialization in the nineteenth century and with the public health movement, environmental risk factors for injury became more discernible. Although research into industrial and home safety grew over the next hundred years, systematic scientific inquiry was rare, and ameliorative efforts were episodic and unconnected. The situation changed dramatically in the 1960s and early 1970s, spurred by a burst of federal regulatory action (e.g., the establishment of federal agencies to promote traffic safety, consumer product safety, environmental protection, and occupational safety) and the emergence of injury science as a distinct interdisciplinary field of research within the domain of public health (Institute of Medicine 1999).

An early pioneer in the injury field, Hugh DeHaven, survived an airplane crash during World War I. His experience led him to study survivors of falls from great heights. He concluded that the human body was less fragile than had generally been supposed, that the structural environment (such as the softness of the ground) often determined the extent of injury, and that the environment could be modified (DeHaven 1942).

William Haddon, a public health physician and first director of the federal National Highway Traffic Safety Administration, was a pioneer in establishing approaches to understanding and addressing injury. In the late 1960s and early 1970s he developed two conceptual frameworks to help physicians, researchers, and policymakers determine how best to prevent or ameliorate injury. The first, the "Haddon Matrix," emphasizes three temporal phases in relation to the injury event: (1) the preevent or preinjury phase; (2) the event or injury phase, when energy is transferred to the individual, resulting in an injury if the energy transfer exceeds the body's tolerance to absorb it; and (3) the postevent or postinjury phase, during which attempts can be made to restore homeostasis, repair the damage, and minimize its social importance (Haddon 1972). These temporal phases are then combined with the traditional public health categorization of risk factors (host, agent, physical, and social environment) to create a twelve-cell matrix.

A second framework lists ten methods of preventing and ameliorating injuries (Haddon 1970). Table 2.1 briefly describes the ten categories, broken down into the three temporal phases, and provides a few examples of interventions to reduce firearm fatalities in the appropriate categories. A key insight in both frameworks is that it may not be productive to search for a primary cause of injury. Most injuries result from a combination of many factors, and there are many opportunities to intervene to prevent injuries. An exclusive focus on the behavior of the individual product user means that many beneficial policies will be missed.

The reduction in motor vehicle injuries over the past forty years can be seen as a public health success story. Between 1920 and 1960, automotive policy in the United States was dominated financially and organizationally by the automobile industry. The manufacturers successfully promoted the view that they were responsible agents while drivers were irresponsible and unskilled. As historian C. A. MacLennan concluded, "From 1920 through the 1950s, the traffic safety establishment perpetuated the belief that drivers were responsible for accidents. . . . Drivers were suspect, while the actions of engineers and automakers were unquestioned. [The proposed remedies] dealt with eliminating driver fault. Federal policy reflected twin goals: punish the careless driver, and instill good driving habits in the general population" (1988, 237). But scientific crash research undertaken by engineers and physicians in the 1940s and 1950s slowly began to change this perception (MacLennan 1988).

DeHaven organized research on crash dynamics at the Cornell Aeronautical Laboratory. Funded by Liberty Mutual Insurance, the Cornell lab became the only center to carry out research on automobile crashes and to collect accident data continuously over several years.

A physician, Colonel John Stapp, started a second crash research operation at the University of California at Los Angeles with funding from the U.S. Air Force. That work survived only a few years; it has been suggested that auto manufacturers influenced Congress to cut off funding for Stapp's automobile work (Eastman 1981). Most manufacturers wanted safety efforts to focus on the driver, not on the car.

Detroit plastic surgeon Claire Straith directly lobbied automobile executives for specific safety features such as seat belts and padded dashboards. He had some success during the late 1940s with smaller companies such as Kaiser-Frazer and the Tucker Corporation.

Physician Fletcher Woodward's studies in the 1940s of automobile victims revealed the predominance of certain types of injuries that were directly asso-

TABLE 2.1. Examples of Options to Reduce Firearm Injuries (divided into Haddon's ten control strategies)

Primary Prevention (preinjury or preevent phase)
1. Prevent the initial creation of the hazard
   a. Require background checks before gun purchase
   b. Prohibit manufacture of certain types of firearms (e.g., plastic firearms)
2. Reduce the amount of the hazard created
   a. Encourage police to use less-lethal weapons
   b. Prohibit manufacture of specific types of ammunition
3. Prevent the release of a hazard that already exists
   a. Store firearms in locked boxes
   b. Ban firearms from bars
   c. Incarcerate firearm offenders

Secondary Prevention (injury or event phase)
4. Modify the rate of release or spatial distribution of the hazard
   a. Require registration of firearms
   b. Improve gun tracing through better firearm labeling
5. Separate, in time or space, the hazard from persons to be protected
   a. Require waiting periods for firearm purchases
   b. Install weapons detectors in some stadiums, high schools
   c. Arrest batterers; confiscate their firearms
6. Interpose a barrier between the hazard and person to be protected
   a. Provide bulletproof vests for police
   b. Offer bulletproof barriers for convenience store clerks, taxi drivers
7. Modify contact surfaces and structures to reduce injury
   a. Redesign bullets to reduce injury severity
   b. Redesign firearms to reduce rate of fire, muzzle velocity
8. Strengthen the resistance of persons who might be injured
   a. Provide training and counseling for persons with repeated victimizations
   b. Train people in nonlethal means of self-defense
   c. Promote nonlethal measures for self-defense, home security

Tertiary Prevention (postinjury or postevent phase)
9. Rapidly detect and limit the damage
   a. Improve emergency medical and law enforcement response
   b. Provide air transport for victims in rural areas
   c. Assure prompt incarceration of firearm offenders
10. Initiate immediate and long-term reparative actions
    a. Improve physical rehabilitation
    b. Improve counseling for victims of violence
    c. Assure accessibility of workplaces and other areas to those disabled by firearms

Source: Adapted from Kellermann et al. 1991.

ciated with specific features of vehicle design. He argued that it was time to shift the emphasis of safety efforts from the driver to the vehicle itself. He unsuccessfully advocated cooperation between engineering and medicine in reducing injuries, as had occurred for airplane safety during World War II (Eastman 1981).

William Harper, a physician who served as an automobile-accident consultant to insurance companies and police departments, concluded, in 1952, after fifteen years of work and the study of three thousand accidents that too much emphasis was being placed on driver error and not enough on ways to make the vehicle and the highways more survivable: "We have spent too damn much time worrying about the cause of accidents. It's time we started worrying about the cause of injuries." Harper recommended the installation of seat belts, the padding of the dashboard, and the removal of knobs that inflicted severe eye and facial injuries during collisions (Eastman 1981, 419).

As a result of the work of physicians such as Straith, Woodward, Stapp, and Harper, the American Medical Association (AMA) passed a resolution in 1953 recommending that auto manufacturers "consider equipping all automobiles with safety belts," and the AMA and the American College of Surgeons established subcommittees on automobile safety (Eastman 1981, 421).

One of the speakers at the 1954 American College of Surgeons meeting was Dr. Horace Campbell. He pointed out that 38,000 people each year were killed in automobile accidents, and 1.5 million were injured.

> These deaths, for the most part, occur because the motorcar manufacturer makes no provision whatsoever for the control of the occupants when they must decelerate rapidly. What happens to the motorcar rider under conditions of rapid deceleration is left entirely to chance. (Eastman 1981, 421)

Campbell argued that physicians should lead the public in the demand for and use of safety belts and safer automobile design.

Physicians who studied automotive injury knew that the sources of injury—the steering column, windshield, dashboard, and passenger compartments—could be modified through obvious technical improvements, such as collapsible steering columns, padded interiors, shatterproof windshields, crush-resistant passenger compartments, and anchored seat belts. Physicians found it appalling that manufacturers did so little to prevent the large numbers of deaths and injuries.

14

One of many steps in the long struggle for automotive safety was Dr. C. Hunter Shelden's comprehensive 1955 *Journal of the American Medical Association* article, which stated that no aspect of the automobile interior was designed from a safety standpoint and that proper motor vehicle design could prevent 75 percent of fatalities. He pointed out that if an epidemic disease claimed thirty-eight thousand lives in one year and the medical profession did nothing to halt it, there would be a congressional investigation, and he concluded, "Possibly that is the only solution to the problem of auto deaths" (Eastman 1981, 424).

Shelden discussed automobile safety with Senator Paul Douglas (D-Ill.), on whom Shelden had operated, and Campbell, the personal physician to Mamie Eisenhower's family, lobbied for attention to the problem. Shelden's efforts paid off: Douglas cosponsored a U.S. Senate resolution calling for a comprehensive study of highway safety by the Department of Commerce. Furthermore, in December 1955, the AMA passed a resolution urging the president "to request legislation from Congress authorizing the appointment of a national body to approve and regulate standards of automobile construction" (Eastman 1981, 424). At 1956 congressional committee hearings, physicians were among the most important witnesses. The hearings highlighted, for both Congress and the general public, effective solutions to the highway traffic safety problem.

In his best-selling 1965 book, *Unsafe at Any Speed*, lawyer Ralph Nader popularized the concept of occupant protection, or "crashworthiness," that physicians and engineers had been describing in professional journals in the 1950s. He also argued for the regulation of the industry:

> A great problem of contemporary life is how to control the power of economic interests which ignore the harmful effects of their applied science and technology. The automobile tragedy is one of the most serious of these man-made assaults on the human body. The history of that tragedy reveals many obstacles which must be overcome in the taming of any mechanical or biological hazard which is a by-product of industry or commerce. (ix)

Further congressional hearings in the mid-1960s led to the landmark Motor Vehicle Act of 1966, which created a federal agency to ensure the safety of highways and automobiles. The first administrator of the new agency was Haddon, the physician and public health expert. During his tenure, the systematic surveillance system (data system) on motor vehicle injuries was started and many federal safety standards were mandated, reducing the likelihood of collision and markedly improving motorists' survival in crashes.

Other physicians have also participated actively in the struggle for automotive safety. The work of Robert Sanders, a Tennessee health officer and pediatrician, led to the passage of the first mandatory child safety seat law in 1978. Within eight years, all fifty states passed such legislation, and child safety seat use rose to more than 80 percent. Children not in restraint devices have been shown to be eleven times more likely to die in a crash than those who are restrained (Kalbfleisch and Rivara 1989).

The key to reducing motor vehicle injuries in the second half of the twentieth century was a change in approach. Rather than focusing on educating drivers, injury-control experts recognized that there were better ways to reduce the likelihood of collision—improving the vehicle and the highway environment. It is, after all, often easier to change the behavior of a few corporate executives at one point in time than that of two hundred million drivers on a daily basis.

Better braking and the third brake light on the back of cars are two of the many ways in which the automobile has been improved to reduce collisions. Divided highways, limited-access roads, and better lighting and signage are a few of the ways in which highways have been made safer. Methods were also sought to reduce the chance of serious injury once collisions occurred. People make mistakes, and sometimes they behave recklessly and inappropriately. But when they do, should they or others die? The goal was to build a system that not only made it less likely for people to make errors but also was more forgiving when errors were made or people behaved illegally or improperly.

Probably the most important traffic safety advances over the past forty years involved making the motor vehicle safer for human occupants (Crandall et al. 1986). For example, we now have steering wheels that collapse on impact rather than spear the driver, air bags that cushion occupants in head-on collisions, windshields that do not shatter and rip car occupants' faces, seat belts that prevent occupants from flying around the car's interior, and gas tanks that do not rupture and explode.

The roads on which we drive are also much safer. For example, many human-created roadside hazards have been removed or modified: telephone poles have been removed from the sides of highways, and signs often break away on impact. Finally, advances in emergency medical services have reduced the disabilities caused by crashes. Helicopters now race the seriously injured to trauma centers to receive immediate medical attention.

No one believes that today's drivers are more careful than those of the 1950s—indeed, many people believe that road rage has increased along with traffic. Yet the number of motor vehicle fatalities per mile driven has been reduced by more than 80 percent. The United States has one of the lowest rates of death per vehicle mile in the world. The key was reframing the policy question from the fatalistic "How can you change human nature?" to the realistic "What are the most cost-effective ways to reduce injury?" (Hemenway 1995).

The improvements in motor vehicle safety in the United States have been deemed a "twentieth century public health achievement" by the Centers for Disease Control and Prevention (CDC 1999a). The National Highway Traffic Safety Administration's creation of an excellent surveillance (i.e., data) system has enabled us to determine the key factors that change the traffic fatality rate, which policies work, and which do not (P. F. Waller 2002). Areas for continued improvement of course exist, particularly the area of reducing injuries to pedestrians, teens, and elderly drivers.

The struggle for motor vehicle safety has many lessons for the firearms field. One is that the industry often tries to place the entire blame on individual users. The automobile industry from the 1920s to the 1960s used the gun lobby mantra, arguing in effect that "motor vehicles don't kill people—people kill people." And like gun advocates today (Foster 2000), motor vehicle manufacturers argued exclusively for better education of automobile users and increased punishment of automobile misusers. Public health practitioners know that the effort to find fault and place blame is often counterproductive, that the most effective approach to safety is a multifaceted one, and that the most cost-effective interventions are often those that improve the product and the environment.

A second lesson for firearms safety is the important role played by physicians in reducing the toll of motor vehicle injuries. Like motor vehicle safety, firearm safety should be a concern for physicians and public health officials. It is also important to realize that the work of a single individual (for example, Sanders's work concerning child safety seats) can make an enormous difference. Note too that few people have ever heard of Sanders or other public health scientists.

Physicians who study the circumstances of gun injuries—such as young children finding improperly stored firearms and shooting themselves or other people or adolescents shooting each other when they believe guns to be unloaded—know that there are readily available technological solutions, such as childproof firearms, smart guns, and magazine safeties. In the firearms field, numerous public health physicians and academics—including Steve Teret, Arthur Kellermann, Garen Wintemute, and Steve Hargarten—advocate for safer guns and a firearms injury surveillance system.

A third lesson is that public health success in the motor vehicle area has largely resulted from the availability of good data, which permits good science, combined with the existence of a regulatory authority with some power over the industry. As with firearms, the product is constantly changing, and continual oversight is necessary to protect the public health.

The multifaceted yet simple and straightforward scientific approach that has been applied by injury control experts to auto safety and many other areas is beginning to be applied to reducing firearm violence. Recognition of the enormous health consequences of violence led the public health community in the 1980s to consider violence a public health problem (National Committee 1989). In 1985 the surgeon general conducted a workshop on violence and public health, signaling public health's entry into what had largely been the sole domain of criminal justice (U.S. Department of Health and Human Services 1986).

In 1992, Surgeon General Antonia Novello wrote a stirring editorial that appeared in the *Journal of the American Medical Association.* She declared, "Violence in the United States is a public health emergency. . . . Just as we health professionals have done for other health problems, we have a clear duty to take a leadership role in the antiviolence movement" (Novello, Shosky, and Froehlke 1992, 3007). The editorial was a call for action—public health action. Novello urged physicians to "establish coalitions with parents, educators, law enforcement personnel, social service workers, clergy, community leaders, government officials, and other health care professionals" to "fight this plague" (3007). In the public health tradition, she exhorted,

> We must offer a strong sense of community. . . . We must encourage recognition of the importance of each individual and teach the politics of inclusion not exclusion. We must offer hope and take the necessary steps to make that hope a reality. As health professionals, the prevention of violence by using public health methods in our communities is as much our responsibility as is the treatment of its victims. (3007)

Given that a majority of both suicides and homicides in the United States are firearm deaths, it was a small step to reframe the issue of gun violence as a public health problem. Editorials in leading medical journals urged physicians to take action. The *New England Journal of Medicine* asked and then answered the question, "What can physicians do?"

> They can look on gun-related deaths not only as a social problem but also as a medical problem. They should acknowledge that the epidemic of injuries and deaths from firearms consumes their time and expertise . . . and drains resources from other critical health needs. . . . They should speak out and be counted as they did in the campaign against cigarettes. (Kassirer 1991, 1649)

Doctors have increasingly heard the message. A national survey of internists and surgeons found that most were no longer comfortable in a passive, peripheral role. The overwhelming majority agree that gun violence is a major public health problem and that various actions, including legislation, regulation, and direct clinician involvement, should be taken to help break the cycle of gun violence (Cassel et al. 1998).

Physicians' groups, including the American Academy of Pediatrics, the Society for Adolescent Medicine, and the American College of Physicians, have endorsed position papers concerning firearms. For example, the American College of Physicians urges doctors to inform patients about the dangers of keeping firearms, particularly handguns, in homes; if guns are kept in homes, physicians should counsel adults to keep guns away from children. Wrote physician Frank Davidoff

> Our patients looked at us strangely in the 1970s when we began asking them whether they used seat belts. "What's that got to do with my medical condition?" But clinicians kept at it, and seat-belt counseling, along with improved seat-belt technology and mandatory seat-belt laws, is now seen as part of good preventive practice. (1998, 235)

As with smoking and sexually transmitted diseases, preventive clinical practice and rational public policy can work together, and they seem to work synergistically. Public health physicians believe the same synergy can be found when it comes to preventing firearm violence.

PRIVATE GUNS, PUBLIC HEALTH

THE WRONG MEDICINE:
"GOOD GUYS" AND "BAD GUYS"

> Among the devices that we use to impose order upon a complicated world, classification must rank as the most general and pervasive of all. And no strategy of classification cuts deeper than our propensity for division by two, or dichotomy.
>
> Some basic attributes of surrounding nature do exist as complementary pairings so we might argue that dichotomization amounts to little more than good observation of the external world. But far more often than not, dichotomization leads to misleading or even dangerous oversimplification. People and beliefs are not either good or evil (with the second category ripe for burning).
>
> —Stephen Jay Gould

A wag once said that there are two kinds of people in the world, those who divide the world into two kinds of people and those who do not. Among the former are many gun advocates. They talk as if there were only two types of individuals: criminals and decent, law-abiding citizens. This dichotomous worldview is both incorrect and dysfunctional. It tends to narrow the perceived range of policy options to two: strengthen the good guys, and weaken or punish the bad guys. The gun lobby argues almost exclusively for (1) virtually no firearm restrictions on law-abiding citizens and (2) increased punishment for bad guys.

The good guy–bad guy view of people permeates not only the arguments of the gun lobby but also the analyses of the few firearm researchers and many firearm advocates who see a virtue in a heavily armed citizenry. The quotes that follow are representative: "[Gun control] focuses on restricting the behavior of the law-abiding rather than apprehending and punishing the guilty" (Snyder 1993, 46). "No matter what laws we enact, they will be obeyed only by the law-abiding—this follows by definition" (J. D. Wright 1988, 30). "The proponents of adding to the twenty thousand gun laws on the books have yet to explain how 'passing a law' will disarm violent sociopathic predators who already ignore laws against murder and drug trafficking" (Suter 1994, 145).

The bad guys in this world are like the violent sociopathic predators from the *Lethal Weapon* and *Die Hard* movies. They are so bad that they obey no laws; almost no murders would be prevented if guns were unavailable to these individuals since they would merely select some other method of killing. The good guys, in stark contrast, would never use a gun inappropriately. Almost by definition, gun crime cannot be committed by one's friends or associates. "Unless the gun owner is already a violent thug, he is very unlikely to kill a relative in a moment of passion" (Kopel 1988, 8).

The dichotomous view of people extends to suicide. There are those who really want to kill themselves and those who don't. Those who want to die will invariably succeed. "If someone in the house is intent on suicide, he will kill himself by whatever means are at hand" (Kopel 1988, 8). In this mind-set, no deaths can be prevented by any type of gun policy.

Adding unintentional injuries to the equation does not change the "us versus them" mentality. "Gun accidents involve a rare and atypical subset of the population" (Kleck 1991, 304). These are "self-destructive individuals. . . . Without guns they would likely find some other way to kill themselves accidentally" (Kopel 1992, 415). These people are not like us, and no gun policy can be effective—"They will likely find some other way to kill themselves."

The real world is far more complex and more interesting than the one described by the advocates of the good/bad or us/them approach. People are multidimensional, and along any of the dimensions there are a few blacks and whites and many more grays. Of course, some people are at higher risk for homicide, suicide, or unintentional gun injury. Indeed, one of the aims of epidemiology is to determine risk factors for illness and injury and thereby to better target interventions. However, the purpose is not to marginalize individuals or groups but to develop constructive solutions for reducing injury.

As subsequent chapters will show, the scientific evidence demonstrates that a substantial number of murders, suicides, and unintentional firearm fatalities can be prevented with reasonable gun policies. However, it is instructive here to discuss the assertions that criminals, by definition, will not obey laws and that unintentional injuries occur only to a narrow group of self-destructive individuals.

Sociologist J. D. Wright claims that "everything the bad guys do with their guns is already against the law," so gun control is futile because criminals are "indifferent to our laws" (1995, 266). "It is more than a little bizarre to assume that people who routinely violate laws against murder, robbery or assault would somehow find themselves compelled to obey gun laws" (267) .

However, as Cook (1996) explains, the fact that someone is not always law-abiding does not imply that s/he obeys no laws. Most "bad guys" do not routinely murder and steal; even the worst do not kill everyone who irritates them or steal everything they want. Will they all feel compelled to obey gun laws? No. Will they be influenced by these laws and in some cases dissuaded from obtaining or carrying a gun? Yes. Raising the price or increasing the difficulty of and punishment for obtaining and using firearms can have a deterrent effect. One survey asked incarcerated felons who did not carry weapons during the commission of their crimes for the various reasons why they did not. Seventy-nine percent chose "Get a stiffer sentence," and 59 percent chose "Against the law" (J. D. Wright and Rossi 1986).

The differences between a dichotomous mind-set and the public health approach are most starkly demonstrated in discussions of unintentional firearm injuries (Hemenway 1995). Criminologist Gary Kleck (1991, 1997a) used three data sets: one on the demographics of unintentional gunshot victims, one from 1946–66 claims files of the Metropolitan Life Insurance Company, and one from a study of unintentional gun injuries in Vermont in 1967 that contrasts thirty-four shooters with a comparison sample of licensed drivers (J. A. Waller and Whorton 1973). The Vermont data (described by Kleck as "one of the most important studies of gun accidents" [286]) found that 21 percent of the shooters but only 5 percent of the controls had had arrests involving alcohol (including driving while intoxicated), that 32 percent of the shooters but only 5 percent of the controls had nonhighway police investigations or arrests for violence, and that 62 percent of the shooters but only 39 percent of the controls had been the driver in a highway collision (J. A. Waller and Whorton 1973).

The world becomes more and more polarized into *us* versus *them* as Kleck proceeds in his conclusions:

> Males, blacks and persons aged 15–24 all are far more likely to be involved in fatal gun accidents than other groups. . . . These are the same groups that show the highest rates of intentional violence such as homicide. . . . Accidental and intentional killers may share some underlying personality traits, such as poor aggression control, impulsiveness, alcoholism, willingness to take risks, and sensation seeking. . . . Gun accidents are not an inevitable by-product of routine gun ownership by ordinary people. . . . At minimum, a third of the deaths in these samples of fatal gun accidents involved obviously reckless conduct. . . . They appear to most commonly be the result of reckless or aggressive behavior by the same kind of individuals responsible both for intentional violence and other types of accidents. . . . Many gun accidents, perhaps the majority of them, involve chronically reckless people whose impulsiveness, emotional immaturity, or alcoholism cannot be eliminated by a

few hours of safety training. . . . Gun accidents are generally committed by unusually reckless people with records of heavy drinking, repeated involvement in automobile crashes, many traffic citations, and prior arrests for assault. Gun accidents, then, involve a rare and atypical subset of the population. (Kleck 1991, 282–304)

According to Kleck, gun accidents are clearly perpetrated by the bad guys. Alcohol and aggressive behavior certainly are risk factors for unintentional shootings, but consider what the Vermont data actually say: 79 percent of the unintentional shooters had no evidence of alcohol problems, 68 percent had no evidence of violence, and 38 percent had never even been involved as a driver in any type of traffic accident. Yet the whole group is basically written off—they are a "rare and atypical subset of the population," not like you and me.

Kleck's position clearly misrepresents the data. The bulk of unintended shooters are not different from us. But even if 100 percent of the shooters had been involved in previous violent incidents or motor vehicle collisions, should that mitigate our efforts to prevent them from accidentally shooting themselves and others? Drivers involved in motor vehicle collisions are more likely than other motorists to have alcohol problems, traffic violations, and arrests for violence (Evans 1991). These facts have not prevented rational policy from achieving a dramatic reduction in motor vehicle injuries.

One problem with the bipolar view of the world is that it often extends to discussions of public policy. Gun control is a contentious policy issue, in part because of the tendency of the gun lobby to rigidly classify all people as either progun or antigun and to classify all policy initiatives as attempts to take away the guns of all citizens. But public health professionals seek only to reduce injuries and death. Promoting reasonable gun policies does not make them "antigun" any more than the Insurance Institute for Highway Safety is "anticar." Public health advocates could as easily label themselves "prosafety" or "prohealth" and anyone who disagreed with their policy prescriptions "antihealth," yet this polarization would be anathema to the entire public health approach.

Another problem with an "us versus them" mind-set is the tendency to focus on blame. For intentional assaults, this approach emphasizes blaming the perpetrator; hence, most of public policy discussion concerns capturing and punishing the criminal. For unintentional injury and suicide, the approach tends to blame the victim. In previous centuries, those afflicted with disease were sometimes considered to have a moral failing; currently, the dichotomous way of thinking often suggests that the victims got what they deserved.

By examining the role of the gun in firearm injuries, public health professionals are often accused of "blaming the gun." "Blaming a gun for misuse is animism" (Weiss 1994, 66). By "blaming objects, a person can avoid having to blame individuals for their moral choices and lack of self-control" (Kopel 1992, 388). Yet the public health approach is not interested in blaming anything or anyone but instead looks to prevent. The public health approach broadens the policy options from an exclusive focus on holding individual citizens responsible for their actions (which they should be) to also considering ways to improve the physical and social environment (1) to reduce the likelihood of impulsive, imprudent, improper, and immoral behavior and (2) to reduce the harm done by such conduct.

Consider an example that involves neither guns nor motor vehicles. A seventeen-year-old, home alone, drinks to excess, begins smoking a cigarette, falls asleep on the couch, and dies in the resulting fire. Whose fault is it? His fault alone? Or also the fault of his parents, the outlets that unlawfully sold him the alcohol and the cigarettes, or the couch manufacturer whose fabric did not meet federal standards for flammability?

The question may be important for legal liability, but for the injury-control community, the question is largely irrelevant and may be counterproductive. Rather, the question is what is the most fair and cost-effective way of preventing such tragedies? Education? Liability for the retail outlets? Improved flammability standards? Or maybe fire-safe cigarettes that do not burn hot enough to ignite upholstery? (McGuire 1992)

Public health neither marginalizes nor stigmatizes any group of people. "Reframing gun violence as a medical issue obviously seizes on the destructive side of gun use, but reframing does not automatically make all gun owners and use pathological any more than considering alcoholism a disease automatically makes all alcohol use suspect" (Davidoff 1998, 234).

In sharp contrast to the us-them division, public health rests on notions of community, of shared fate. Public health aggregates rather than segregates the population (Morone 1997). Most important, public health brings the American spirit of pragmatism and hope. Public health has a history of success, and in the firearms policy arena, it can point to the experience of every other developed country to show that it is possible for the United States to do much better.

THE PUBLIC HEALTH APPROACH

SUMMARY

A key step in the public health approach is to change social norms—not only norms of behavior but also norms of attitude about what conditions are acceptable. In the nineteenth century, the goal was to change the fatalistic beliefs that childhood disease would always be with us. For example, in 1762, philosopher Jean-Jacques Rousseau wrote, "Half of all children will die by their eighth birthday. This is nature's law. Do not try to contradict it" (Foege 1996a, 176).

In the early twentieth century, spitting in public places changed from a normal to an unacceptable practice. More recently, the norm of cigarette smoking changed; smoking is now viewed less often as a mature, sophisticated, and attractive activity and more often as a harmful addiction. In the case of firearms, we need to change the norm that accepts lethal violence as a normal part of everyday American life (Hemenway 1998a).

The public health approach is ideally suited to deal with our gun problem. Public health emphasizes prevention rather than fault-finding, blame, or revenge. It uses science rather than belief as its basis and relies on accurate data collection and scientific analysis. It promotes a wide variety of interventions—environmental as well as individual—and integrates the activities of a wide variety of disciplines and institutions. Most important, public health brings a pragmatic attitude to problems—finding innovative solutions and eliminating the fatalistic and complacent beliefs that little can be done to reduce the problem.

Public health involvement has many beneficial consequences. It broadens the issue from an exclusive focus on crime to a focus on all firearm injuries—unintentional as well as intentional, self-inflicted as well as other-inflicted. After all, from the surgeon's perspective, treating a bullet in the head is the same whether the wound occurred during a robbery, a suicide attempt, or adolescent horseplay. All firearm injuries should be prevented. Optimal gun policies should be concerned with reducing suicides and gun accidents as well as firearm assaults and other crimes.

Public health also adds new data sources (e.g., the National Center for Health Statistics, the National Health Interview survey), new analytic tools (e.g., an emphasis on surveillance data, epidemiological analysis of risk factors, cohort and case-control analyses), and new research professionals from the public health and medical communities. Much of our current scientific knowledge about guns and gun injuries has come from this research.

In addition, public health attracts new practitioners and organizations into the arena. Physicians, for example, have firsthand experience concerning the human and medical implications of gunshot wounds and the long-run sequelae of injury, and this medical testimony carries much weight; politically, physicians have authority and clout. Public health offers a wide-angle lens to supplement physicians' individual patient focus. In addition, public health can attract and mobilize the efforts of such disparate groups as physicians, women's and youth organizations, civil rights groups, and consumer organizations.

Public health is not merely an academic specialty but also a government sector. Agencies from the Centers for Disease Control, the National Institutes of Health, and the U.S. Public Health Service down to state and local health departments have the potential to work to reduce gun violence (Haines 1997).

Finally, and perhaps most importantly, the injury control/public health approach emphasizes that many reasonable and beneficial interventions can reduce the gun carnage, showing a way past the old sterile debates about guns and gun control. Contrasted against the pessimism of others (e.g., Jacobs 2002), the can-do attitude of public health, combined with its past successes, brings hope and inspiration to those who seek to solve the problem.

CHAPTER 3   GUN-RELATED
INJURY AND DEATH

Environmental modifications are premised on the assumption that humans can alter and control their surroundings to make them less hazardous. This is hardly a startling insight, although it is too frequently ignored (as, for example, in the case of firearm design and accessibility).

—T. Christoffel and S. S. Gallagher

The Centers for Disease Control and Prevention divides injury deaths into accidents (unintentional injuries), suicides, and homicides. This chapter discusses the extent to which firearms contribute to deaths in each of these categories, including scientific evidence regarding the problem, and examines gun use in robberies, assaults, and other crimes. The chapter also briefly describes some specific policies that could prevent many of these incidents.

GUN ACCIDENTS

Between 1965 and 2000, more than sixty thousand Americans died from unintentional firearm shootings. That is more Americans than were killed in our wars or from coal mine injuries during the same period. In the 1990s, an average of twelve hundred Americans died each year from gun "accidents"—an average of more than three people per day (table 3.1). In addition, about four hundred people each year (one person a day) were killed in situations where the intent was undetermined.

Young people are the primary victims. More than half of all unintentional firearm fatalities are individuals under twenty-five years of age. Although relatively few adolescents own guns, the fifteen- to-nineteen-year-old age group has by far the highest rate of unintentional firearm fatalities; second is the twenty-to-twenty-four age group, followed by the ten-to-fourteen age group.

Children under age fifteen in the United States are nine times as likely to die as a result of a fatal gun accident as similarly aged children in the rest of the developed world (CDC 1997b). Between 1991 and 2000, unintentional firearm fatalities per year averaged 23 for children aged zero to four, 31 for children aged five to nine, and 105 for children between ages ten and fourteen. As with almost all injuries, males are at highest risk (CDC 2003b).

According to criminologist Gary Kleck, "Most surprisingly, general gun ownership levels . . . appear to be unrelated to rates of fatal gun accidents" (1997b, 384). This claim is indeed surprising, and it is incorrect. Where there are more guns, there are more accidental gun deaths. One study examined data from 1979 to 1997 and found that for every age group, for men and for women, for blacks and for whites, people living in states with more guns were far more likely to die in gun accidents. Even after accounting for poverty, urbanization, and region, the differences were enormous (Miller, Azrael, and Hemenway 2001).

To help illustrate the size of these differences, table 3.2 contrasts the number of accidental gun deaths in states at the extremes in terms of gun prevalence. The five lowest gun states were selected, as determined by the percentage of the population living in households with firearms, with the data coming from the CDC's 2001 Behavioral Risk Factor Surveys conducted in all fifty states. These five low gun states were Hawaii, Massachusetts, Rhode Island, New Jersey, and Connecticut. Since many of the high gun states have

TABLE 3.1. Unintentional Firearm Deaths in the United States, 1965–2000

Year	Number of Deaths	Rate per 100,000[a]
1965	2,344	1.3
1970	2,406	1.2
1975	2,380	1.1
1980	1,955	0.9
1985	1,649	0.7
1990	1,416	0.6
1995	1,225	0.5
2000	776	0.3
1965–2000	62,213	0.8

Source: Data from CDC 1997a, 2000, 2003c (accessed January 23, 2003).

[a]Age-adjusted.

small populations, to get an equivalent population at risk among high gun states required taking the eleven states with the most people living in households with firearms (Wyoming, Montana, Alaska, South Dakota, Arkansas, West Virginia, Alabama, Idaho, Mississippi, North Dakota, and Kentucky). Between 1991 and 2000, a typical resident from a high gun state was over ten times more likely to die in a gun accident than someone from a low gun state. For example, although there were virtually the same number of children aged zero to four in both groups of states, 38 died from accidental gunshot wounds in the high gun states, compared to none in the low gun states (table 3.2).

Two studies of adults created by pooling two national surveys also found that a gun in the home was a risk factor for accidental firearm death. Factors controlled for included gender, race, region, income, marital status, and education (Merrill 2002; Wiebe 2003a).

TABLE 3.2.   Unintentional Firearm Deaths
Numbers of Deaths in the Eleven U.S. States with the Most Guns and the Five States with the Fewest Guns, 1991–2000

Age Group	Number of Accidental Gun Deaths in the High-Gun States	Number of Accidental Gun Deaths in the Low-Gun States	Ratio of Mortality Rates
Total Population (person years) at Risk: 1991–2000	195.8 million	195.1 million	
0–4	38	0	Infinite
5–14	261	10	24.0
15–19	407	38	8.5
20–24	341	32	9.3
25–34	383	48	9.0
35–44	328	23	15.3
45–54	182	24	7.7
55–64	113	12	8.9
65+	184	20	9.8
All Ages	2,237	207	10.8

Source: Mortality data from CDC WISQARS 2003.

Note: Gun prevalence determined by the percentage of people in each state residing in households with firearms. Gun prevalence data come from the 2001 CDC Behavioral Risk Factor Surveys for each state. Similar results are obtained if gun prevalence is either the percentage of suicides with guns, or "Cook's Index."

The eleven high-gun states are, in order, Wyoming, Montana, Alaska, South Dakota, Arkansas, West Virginia, Alabama, Idaho, Mississippi, North Dakota, and Kentucky; the five low-gun states are, in order, Hawaii, Massachusetts, Rhode Island, New Jersey, and Connecticut.

There are currently (1999–2000) two to three accidental firearm deaths each day, but this is, of course, only the tip of the iceberg. For every unintentional firearm fatality, it is estimated that approximately thirteen victims are injured seriously enough to be treated in hospital emergency departments (Annest et al. 1995). In other words, more than thirty people a day are shot unintentionally but do not die. This number does not include any of the more than eighty people each day who are treated in emergency rooms for BB/pellet gun wounds or the more than fifty people injured by firearms in other ways (e.g., powder burns, struck with firearms, injured by firearms' recoil), many unintentionally. These figures also do not include other unintended health effects of shooting, such as lead poisoning or hearing loss.

As with fatal firearm accidents, young males aged fifteen to twenty-four are at highest risk for nonfatal accidental firearm injuries. More than one-third of unintended firearm wounds require hospitalization. The large majority of wounds are self-inflicted, and most are caused by handguns. Injuries generally occur during fairly routine gun handling—cleaning a gun, loading and unloading, hunting, target shooting, and so forth (Sinauer, Annest, and Mercy 1996).

For other products, our society takes many reasonable actions to reduce injuries. Government has helped to create safety standards for chainsaws and lawn mowers, which never caused as many unintentional fatalities as guns. We are especially concerned if children may be hurt, and thus we mandate safety standards for such relatively safe products as teddy bears and toy guns. By contrast, there are no federal safety standards for firearms. When airbags were shown to have been responsible for an average of six child deaths per year in the 1990s, intense media attention, myriad studies and conferences, and manufacturer and governmental responses ensued. The deaths of these children were deemed unacceptable.

Over the past twenty years, an average of one child per year has died from injuries caused when soccer goals tip over and crush children climbing on the goals or hanging from crossbars. The Consumer Product Safety Commission and the soccer goal industry moved quickly to help develop a new safety standard to reduce the risk of tipping. "We want kids to have fun, be active, and play soccer with goals that are safely anchored into the ground," said commission chair Ann Brown, introducing the standard that was approved in 1999 (Injury Prevention 1999).

Similarly, during the 1990s an annual average of two children per year under age fifteen died by locking themselves in automobile trunks. The

National Highway Traffic Safety Administration appointed a panel to study how to reduce trunk entrapment. Manufacturers were rightfully concerned, and in 1999, General Motors and Ford began offering an escape handle and a trunk latch mechanism to prevent the trunk from shutting unless an adult manually resets the latch. It is certainly reasonable to expect a response to the far greater problem of accidental gunshot injuries, which were killing eighty times more children under age fifteen each year.

The causes and circumstances of firearm accidents are myriad. For example, at a restaurant during the annual American Public Health Association conference held in Indianapolis in 1997, a patron bent over and a derringer fell from his pocket. The gun hit the ground, discharged, and wounded two convention delegates. The patron had a permit to carry the gun, and the firearm met all relevant safety standards—of which there were none (Bijur 1998). Mandatory safety standards are needed to prohibit the manufacture of firearms that cannot pass a simple drop test.

Recreational hunting frequently leads to accidental shootings. Tour de France winner Greg LeMond was unintentionally shot in the chest by a close relative when they were hunting. Basketball coach Bobby Knight accidentally shot a friend in 1999 while hunting grouse without a license—and failed to report the mishap (*Beloit Daily News* 1999). During the first fifteen days of Michigan's 2000 hunting season, six people were killed and a dozen more injured. One victim just happened to be out for a walk in the woods; one hunter mistook another hunter for a deer (Waldmeir 2000). It is estimated that there were approximately one thousand hunter-related casualties in 1997–98 in the United States and parts of Canada (International Hunter Education Association 2003).

Hunting accidents can be reduced by a variety of methods. For example, since the 1987 hunting season, hunters in North Carolina have been required to wear a bright orange ("hunter orange") article of clothing while in the woods. Comparing the four years before the law with the four years after, gunshot deaths of hunters "mistaken for game" fell from twelve to two, while hunters accidentally shot and killed for other causes remained constant at twenty-two (Cina et al. 1996). In Pennsylvania between 1987 and 1999, there were 1,382 hunting-related injuries and 77 fatalities; fall turkey hunters had the highest injury rates. With the implementation and subsequent relaxation of hunter orange clothing regulations, turkey hunter injury rates due to poor judgment decreased and then increased substantially (J. L. Smith et al. 2002).

Accidental firearm injuries also occur when guns are fired into the air in celebration. A Houston man accidentally shot and killed his seven-year-old daughter when he fired a gun to celebrate the new year (*Boston Globe* 1997b). One study examined patients at a California medical center who had been hit by spent bullets—the result of firing weapons into the sky. More than three-quarters were hit in the head, and 32 percent died (Ordog et al. 1994). Laws have since been enacted to help prevent this terrible waste of life, but increased education and enforcement seem essential (Frolik 1999; CBS 2000).

Whatever their cause, accidental firearm injuries disproportionately affect children. The Violence Policy Center used a national news clipping service to look for articles on a very narrow range of accidental shootings—incidents in which both the victim and the shooter were under age eighteen. During a ten-month period, more than 220 such shootings occurred, and a number involved very young children (Violence Policy Center 1997). Children as young as three and four years old are strong enough to fire most commercially available handguns (Naureckas 1995). An easy remedy is to require minimum trigger-pull standards to help prevent very young children from being able to pull a gun's trigger.

Another set of incidents involve young children and adolescents who are unaware that firearms are loaded. One analysis of unintentional injury deaths among children found that in at least 20 percent of cases, the child shooting the gun did not know it was loaded (Wintemute, Teret, and Kraus 1987). Injuries to all age groups have occurred because shooters did not know guns were loaded. A national survey found that 20 percent of adults incorrectly believe that a pistol with its magazine removed cannot be shot, and 14 percent do not know whether it can be shot; 28 percent of these adults who answered incorrectly or did not know lived in gun-owning households (Vernick et al. 1999). The percentages would undoubtedly be higher for children. These are tragedies waiting to happen—and many are easy to avert.

A government study (U.S. General Accounting Office 1991) of accidental firearm fatalities in ten cities concluded that 8 percent of the deaths could have been prevented by childproof safety devices. An additional 23 percent of the deaths might have been prevented by loaded-chamber indicators that alert the user that the gun's chamber contains a bullet and by magazine disconnect devices (magazine safeties) that prevent a gun from firing once the ammunition magazine has been removed, even when a bullet remains in the chamber. A study of accidental firearm deaths in Maryland and Milwaukee concluded that there was strong evidence that 20 percent of fatalities could have been prevented by loaded-chamber indicators (Vernick et al. 2002). A study of unintentional firearm injuries in the Atlanta area found that loaded-chamber indicators, magazine safeties, and firing pin blocks might have prevented as many as 32 percent of the shootings (Ismach et al. 2003).

It is difficult to understand why a person using a camera can tell whether it is loaded without opening it up, but a person with a firearm often cannot. Given that child-resistant packaging of aspirin and prescription drugs has prevented hundreds of child deaths (Rodgers 1996), why can't we also try to childproof firearms?

Most shootings of younger children involve firearms belonging to parents or grandparents. Here, too, many tragedies could be prevented—for example, if guns were "personalized," or designed so that only authorized users could fire them. To this end, manufacturers could incorporate current technology—such as magnetic devices, radio frequency transponders, and combination locks—into guns. A personalized gun would be inoperable not only by a curious child but also by a depressed teenager or a thief (Robinson et al. 1996).

Proper gun storage can also make a difference. Pediatric morbidity and mortality due to accidental gunshot wounds are typically the result of spontaneous events when children find and play with loaded guns (Heins, Kahn, and Bjordnal 1974; Keck et al. 1988). For example, a California study of incidents in which young children fatally shot themselves or their playmates found that in almost half of the residential shootings, the gun had been left loaded and unlocked in the house where the shooting occurred (Wintemute, Teret, and Kraus 1987). Increased education about the dangers of guns to children and state-level child access prevention liability laws—which hold guardians liable for injuries if improper gun storage allowed children access to firearms—may help.

While some people are at higher risk than others for unintentional shootings, accidents can happen to anyone. In just the past few years there have been many newspaper reports of accidental shootings involving firearms instructors, county sheriffs, security guards, and other experienced gun handlers (*Red Deer Advocate* 1996; *San Antonio Express-News* 1999; B. Anderson 2002; Galloway 2002; Holien 2002; Schrade 2003; Canham 2003). An improved product can help safeguard even the most experienced shooters.

It is important to note that the reported rate of accidental firearm fatalities has more than halved since 1965 (table 3.1). In general, this decline matches that found with other products and risks—the rate of accidental fatalities has been steadily declining as we have become a "safer" society through product and environmental improvements and better and faster medical care. Yet some part of the decline in fatal gun accidents is a statistical artifact. For example, in 1968 a new "undetermined intention" category for firearm fatalities was created; many deaths previously reported as unintentional now appear in that category. The number of accidental gun deaths would probably be about 20 percent higher today if that and other classification changes had not been made (Ikeda et al. 1997).

In addition, improvements in the classification of suicides and homicides probably mean that a smaller percentage of such fatalities are now miscategorized as accidents. For example, suicides in the 1950s and 1960s were underreported as a result of social and cultural pressures against the finding of suicide (Gist and Welch 1989; Males 1991). Older studies on suicide classification found that some medical examiners were unwilling to classify deaths as suicides when no suicide note was present (Litman et al. 1963), which is the majority of the time. By contrast, evidence indicates that there is currently an undercounting of accidental gun deaths, which are being incorrectly classified as suicides or homicides (Barber et al. 2002; Schaechter et al. 2003). For example, a study of pediatric firearm fatalities in the Miami area discovered more than six times more unintended gun deaths than reported by medical examiners, who classified any death when the shooter intentionally pulled the trigger as a homicide or suicide, independent of whether there was intent to harm (e.g., the child thought the gun was unloaded) (Schaechter et al. 2003).

But a good part of the decrease in accidental firearm deaths per capita in the past decades is certainly real (Frattaroli, Webster, and Teret 2002). The unintentional firearm fatality rate has been falling in other countries as well; for example, while our reported rate fell 44 percent between 1970 and 1994, the Canadian rate fell 64 percent (Canadian Department of Justice 1999). In addition, U.S. death rates from most other types of unintentional injuries have been decreasing during this period. Unintentional injuries from most causes have been decreasing in other industrialized countries as well (Morrison and Stone 1999). A higher standard of living should probably take part of the credit—fatality rates for many types of injuries, including unintentional gun injuries, are lower among higher-income populations (Baker et al. 1992).

Improvements in emergency medicine have also been responsible for reducing trauma fatality. Studies indicate that response time—the time between a firearm discharge and the initial provision of care—has declined (Mayer 1979; Mayron, Long, and Ruiz 1984) and that further improvements are possible (Dodge et al. 1994). The advent of the 911 emergency number, helicopter transport services, prehospital advanced life support, the designation of trauma centers, and twenty-four-hour emergency hospital services reduce the risk of death among injured patients (Ornato et al. 1985; Pons et al. 1985; Rutledge et al. 1992; O'Keefe et al. 1999).

Another potential explanation for the decline in unintentional gun fatality rates is reduced exposure to firearms. For example, the percentage of households with guns has dropped from approximately 48 percent in 1973 to 35 percent in 2001 (T. W. Smith 2001). The number of hunters is declining, and the age profile of shooters is also changing. The biggest drop in hunters has been among young people, who are at highest risk for accidental shootings. A 1995 survey by the National Shooting Sports Foundation found that only 25 percent of hunters were under the age of thirty-five, down from 48 percent a decade earlier (S. Simon 1999). These trends are continuing (Dahl 2003).

Increased urbanization of the population also explains part of the reduced exposure to firearms. The percentage of the population in rural areas decreased from 30 percent in 1960 to 21 percent in 2000. A higher percentage of rural households have guns, and the evidence suggests that unintentional firearm fatalities are at least twice as high in rural areas as in nonrural areas (Patterson and Holguin 1990; Baker et al. 1992; CDC 1992; Zwerling et al. 1993).

It seems axiomatic that reduced exposure to firearms should reduce unintentional firearm injuries, all other things being equal. At the extreme, if there are no guns, there certainly can be no gun accidents. States with more guns per capita and less strict handgun control laws appear to have more accident gun fatalities; similarly, high-income nations with more guns seem to have more accidental gun deaths (Lester and Murrell 1981; Lester 1993; Miller, Azrael, and Hemenway 2001).

The decrease in unintentional firearm fatalities has been a welcome trend. Still, with some thirty accidental shootings per day resulting in injury or death, much more can be done to reduce this totally unacceptable level of morbidity and mortality.

SUICIDES

Morrilton, Ark.: A third-grader shot and killed himself while his mother was outside getting a switch to whip him because of a bad report card. Christopher Parks,

8, apparently climbed onto a dresser to get a gun that was hanging from a nail on the wall, then shot himself in the head.

—*Boston Globe* 1998b

Almost fifty people a day kill themselves with guns in the United States. These numbers increased 75 percent between 1965 and 1985 and have stayed reasonably constant since then (table 3.3). Since 1965, more than half a million Americans have committed suicide with a firearm, nearly ten times as many as have died from gun-related accidents.

In the United States, more people kill themselves with guns than by all other methods combined. Males are at high risk for suicide and for gun suicide in particular. Guns accounted for 61 percent of male suicides in 2000 but only 37 percent of female suicides. Still, guns are also the single most common means by which women kill themselves (CDC 2003b).

Among methods of suicide, firearms are typically the most lethal. For example, a study in Canada found that 92 percent of gun attempts result in death, compared to 78 percent of attempts using carbon monoxide or hanging, 67 percent of drowning attempts, and 23 percent of intentional drug overdoses (Chapdelaine, Samson, and Kimberly 1991). A study from Dallas found that of those attempting suicide with a gun, 76 percent died, while only 4 percent of those who attempted suicide by other means died (Cook 1991). An eight-state study found that 82 percent of firearm suicide attempts resulted in death, compared to 61 percent for hanging/suffocation, 34 percent

TABLE 3.3.   Suicide Deaths by Firearm in the
United States, 1965–2000

Year	Number Deaths	Rate per 100,000[a]
1965	9,898	5.2
1970	11,772	5.9
1975	14,873	6.9
1980	15,396	6.4
1985	17,363	6.7
1990	18,885	7.0
1995	18,503	6.6
2000	17,424	5.8
1965–2000	558,825	6.3

Source: Data from CDC 1997a, 2000, 2003c (accessed January 23, 2003).

[a]Age-adjusted

for jumping, 1.5 percent for drug poisoning, and 1.2 percent for cutting/piercing (Spicer and Miller 2000). A Chicago study found that more than 95 percent of attempted firearm suicides resulted in death (Shenassa, Catlin, and Buka 2003). A recent study of northeast states examined suicidal acts serious enough to result in hospitalization or death. Over 90 percent of suicidal acts with a gun resulted in death, compared to 2 percent of drug overdoses and 3 percent of attempts by cutting or piercing. Drugs and cutting or piercing accounted for 94 percent of all nonfatal suicidal hospitalizations (Miller, Azrael, and Hemenway 2003).

Among industrialized nations, the overall suicide rate in the United States falls roughly in the middle (Moscicki 1995). However, our suicide rate for children five to fourteen years of age is twice the average of that in other developed countries because of our firearms-related suicide rate, which is ten times that of the average of the other nations (CDC 1997b) (table 1.3). For fifteen- to twenty-four-year-olds, our firearm suicide rate is second only to Finland, but our overall suicide rate for this age group is only slightly above the average of other developed nations (G. R. Johnson, Krug, and Potter 2000).

Although the risk of suicide increases for the elderly, in comparison to most life-threatening diseases, suicide disproportionately affects younger people. Suicide accounts for 12 percent of all deaths among five- to twenty-four-year-olds, the third-leading cause of death behind only motor vehicle crashes (28 percent) and homicides (21 percent) (CDC 1996). In terms of the number of people dying, suicide is a young adult/middle age problem. In 2000, 57 percent of all suicide deaths were to individuals 25–54 years old (CDC 2003b).

Women attempt suicide roughly three times as often as men, yet more than four times as many men die (CDC 1996). The gun suicide rate in 2000 was almost 7 times higher for men than for women; the nongun suicide rate was 2.5 times higher. Suicide rates are higher for whites than for nonwhites: in 2000, whites had twice the suicide rate of African Americans.

In addition to age, gender, and race, many other variables—including marital status, income, unemployment, and cigarette consumption—are associated with suicide rates. The strongest individual risk factor for attempting suicide is a psychiatric or substance abuse disorder. Although more than 90 percent of suicides are associated with a mental or addictive disorder (Rich, Young, and Fowler 1986; Brent, Perper, and Allman 1987), the parameters of what constitutes such a disorder are so broad that it is estimated that perhaps

30 percent of the U.S. population, or eighty million people, has one (Gold-smith et al. 2002). Not surprisingly, this makes identifying individuals likely to commit suicide difficult indeed (Goldstein et al. 1991). As noted in one report, "There is no single, readily identifiable, high-risk population that constitutes a sizeable portion of overall suicides and yet represents a small, easily targeted group" (Gunnell and Frankel 1994, 1231).

The problem of identifying those likely to commit suicide is particularly difficult among teenagers. A study of students in Massachusetts high schools found that 26 percent reported that they had seriously considered suicide, 18 percent had made plans, 10 percent had attempted suicide in the previous twelve months, and almost 4 percent needed medical attention (Overlan 1996). Studies show that more than 75 percent of all U.S. suicides are not in psychiatric treatment at the time of their death, and half do not appear to have had any prior treatment (Rich, Young, and Fowler 1986).

Many suicides appear to be impulsive acts. Individuals who take their own lives often do so when confronting a severe but temporary crisis (Seiden 1977). In one small study of men who survived self-inflicted intentional gun-shot wounds to the face, few attempted suicide again (Shuck, Orgel, and Vogel 1980). In another study of nearly lethal suicide attempts, 24 percent of attempters reported spending less than five minutes between the decision to attempt suicide and the actual attempt (T. R. Simon et al. 2001). In yet another study of self-inflicted gunshot wounds that would have been fatal without emergency treatment, none of the thirty attempters had written a suicide note, and more than half reported having suicidal thoughts for less than twenty-four hours. In two years of follow-up, none of the thirty attempted suicide again. As the lead researcher put it, "Many patients in our sample admitted that while they had originally expected to die, they were glad to be alive, and would not repeat the self-destructive behavior, despite the continued presence of significant medical, psychological and social problems" (L. G. Peterson et al. 1985, 230).

Suicidal individuals are often ambivalent about killing themselves. K. R. Jamison (1999, 47) estimates that no more than 10 to 15 percent of suicides display an unbreakable determination to kill themselves. For the rest, the risk period is transient: "Most suicidal people do not want death; they want the pain to stop" (NAMI Advocate 1999). Reducing the availability of firearms—the most common, lethal, and symbolically resonant instruments—during this period may prevent suicide attempts and would certainly reduce the rate of suicide completion. A summary of suicide prevention for young adults (age 18–30) concludes:

> Impulsivity is a strong suicide risk factor in many conditions, and a major impact could be produced by interventions that reduce impulsivity and that render impulsive acts less lethal. In this young adult cohort, notorious for its impetuosity, . . . protection could be obtained by restricting firearms: this would be an effective tool for reducing the lethality of the suicide attempts that occur. (Lipschitz 1995, 167)

Psychiatric and penal institutions have long recognized the importance, in all age groups, of restricting access to lethal means of suicide for newly admitted and potentially suicidal inmates; we ought to make it a priority to restrict access to other individuals at high risk for suicide.

There has long been agreement that increased firearm availability increases the firearm suicide rate. However, a point of debate was whether gun availability increases the overall rate of suicide or whether suicidal individuals merely substitute other lethal means if guns are not available. Kleck claims that "general gun ownership levels . . . appear to have no net effect on total suicide rates" (1997b, 384). This conclusion is contrary to the available evidence.

Three recent review articles conclude that the evidence shows that gun availability is a risk factor for suicide (Miller and Hemenway 1999; Brent 2001; Brent and Bridge 2003). For example, in the past twenty years, ten individual-level studies (case-control and cohort studies) have examined the relationship between gun ownership and suicide in the United States, and all find that firearms in the home are associated with substantially and significantly higher rates of suicide (Brent et al. 1988, 1991, 1993b, 1994; Kellermann et al. 1992; Bukstein et al. 1993; Cummings, Koepsell et al. 1997; Conwell et al. 2002). (See appendix A for a discussion of the case-control method and ecological study designs.)

Five overlapping studies by one research team have focused on adolescent suicides (Brent et al. 1988, 1991, 1993b, 1994; Bukstein et al. 1993). One study found that guns were in the homes of 72 percent of the suicide victims but only 37 percent of the controls (Brent et al. 1991). Cases and controls were matched on age, gender, and county of origin. Even after matching and statistically accounting for other risk factors—such as psychiatric diagnosis, sui-

39

cide intent, or presence of a male in the home—guns were significantly more likely to be found in the homes of suicide victims. Another in this series of case-control studies found that for adolescents with no apparent psychiatric disorders, handguns and loaded guns in the home present a particularly large relative risk of suicide (Brent et al. 1993b). This finding suggests that the danger of having a gun in the home applies to all adolescents and not just to adolescents with known psychiatric or substance abuse problems.

Two large case-control studies have included both adults and adolescents. One focused on suicides that occurred at home in two urban areas: Shelby County, Tennessee, a predominantly poor black community, and King County, Washington, a predominantly upper-middle-class white community (Kellermann et al. 1992). This study found that 65 percent of the victims had firearms in the home, compared to 41 percent of the controls. After matching for age, gender, race, and neighborhood and statistically controlling for six variables—education, living alone, consumption of alcohol, previous hospitalization due to drinking, current use of prescription medication for depression or mental illness, and use of illicit drugs—the presence of a gun in the home was associated with a fivefold increase in the risk of suicide. Restricting the analysis to those suicides without a history of mental illness or depression revealed that guns were even more strongly associated with suicide. Individuals in homes with handguns, loaded guns, and unlocked guns all had higher risks of suicide than other individuals. Having any gun in the home was a risk factor for suicide for women as well as men, for whites, and for all age groups, but especially for adolescents and young adults. The major limitations of the study were that it examined only suicides that occurred in the home and relied on self-reports of household gun ownership.

Another large case-control study eliminated these problems by analyzing whether the purchase of a handgun from a licensed dealer (using information compiled by the dealers) was associated with an increased risk of suicide, whether or not the suicide took place in the home (Cummings, Koepsell et al. 1997). Results showed that individuals who committed suicide were more likely than controls to have a family history of handgun purchase (25 versus 15 percent). The most serious limitations of this study were its inability to account for psychological risk factors such as a history of psychiatric disorders, previous suicide attempts, or substance abuse. However, it did seem to show that the higher risk for gun purchasers could not be fully explained by victims buying guns to commit suicide. While the relative risk for suicide was greatest within the first year after purchase, it remained elevated even after five years; the median interval between the first handgun purchase and any suicide with a gun was eleven years. The risk for suicide was higher for individuals with a family handgun purchase even if a family member other than the victim had purchased the gun. In other words, it appears that the association between guns in the home and suicide did not result from some individuals obtaining guns to commit suicide.

A recent case-control study found that among middle-aged and elderly adults, those with a gun in the home had higher rates of suicide. Presence of a firearm in the home was associated with an increased risk for suicide even after controlling for psychiatric illness. Among subjects who kept guns in the home, storing the weapon loaded and unlocked were independent predictors of suicide. Only 10 percent of firearm suicides had recently purchased the firearm (Conwell et al. 2002). The results suggest that poor gun storage may increase the likelihood of suicide.

A national case-control study of U.S. adults for 1993/94, created by pooling two national surveys, found that a gun in the home was associated with a tripling of the likelihood of suicide; a handgun in the home posed a higher risk than a long gun. Fifty-three percent of case households had a handgun in the home compared to 20 percent of controls. The study controlled for age, gender, race, income, marital status, education, living alone, region, and population size (Wiebe 2003b). An analysis using similar data reached similar conclusions (Merrill 2002). A limitation of these large national studies was that data on gun presence was missing for 30 percent of case subjects.

Finally, a longitudinal cohort study found that during the first week after a handgun purchase, the rate of suicide was fifty-seven times higher than the age-adjusted rate for the general population. That finding suggests that individuals sometimes purchase guns with the immediate intention of killing themselves, but the study also found that the higher risk for suicide persisted for at least six years (Wintemute, Parham et al. 1999). Again the indication is that the gun-suicide connection does not result from depressed individuals purposely buying guns as a means to commit suicide.

Many studies have examined whether areas with higher levels of gun ownership have higher rates of suicide. The unit of analysis in these studies has been nations (Lester 1990b; Sloan et al. 1990; Killias 1993; Hemenway and Miller 2000), U.S. regions (Markush and Bartolucci 1984; Lester 1988; Birckmayer and Hemenway 2001; Miller, Azrael, and Hemenway 2002a, 2002b, 2002d; Hemenway and Miller 2002), U.S. states (Lester 1987, 1989; Miller, Azrael, and Hemenway 2002a, 2002b, 2002d), and urban areas (Kleck and

Patterson 1993; Hellsten 1995). A limitation of international and regional studies is the relatively small number of high-income countries (twenty-six with more than one million population) and U.S. regions (nine). A limitation of past U.S. state and city studies has been the lack of reliable data on gun ownership at either the city or state level (until the 2001–2002 state Behavioral Risk Factor Surveys). Proxies have been used, such as the percentage of homicide and suicide deaths with a gun (Cook's index) (Hemenway and Miller 2000), the accidental death rate from firearms (Lester 1987), and subscriptions to gun magazines (Lester 1989). The limited number of observations and the use of proxy measures substantially reduce the likelihood of finding a significant relationship between gun prevalence and suicide.

The one area where the gun-suicide connection is not apparent is in cross-national studies. For example, among high-income countries, the United States has the most guns but only average suicide rates. While one study of fourteen countries found that national rates of suicide were significantly associated with gun ownership rates (Killias 1993), another study by the same author that included more countries did not find this effect (Killias, Van Kesteren, and Rindlisbacher 2001). Unfortunately, it does not appear that anyone has done a study that explains the differences in suicide rates across nations.

However, firearm availability may explain national differences in suicide rates of young people. For example, the United States has high rates of suicide among five- to fourteen-year-olds, and a study with data from seventeen nations found a significant positive association between gun levels and suicides among males aged fifteen to twenty-four (G. R. Johnson, Krug, and Potter 2000).

In the United States, some regional-level analyses (e.g., Markush and Bartolucci 1984), state-level analyses (e.g., Lester 1989), and city-level analyses (e.g., Kleck and Patterson 1993) have shown a statistically significant relationship between gun prevalence and suicide rates. No study has found a negative relationship between firearm availability and suicide rates.

One study examined the 169 largest urban counties in the United States for 1970, 1980, and 1990. Holding many potential factors constant, including divorce, unemployment, and migration, the study found that in each of these three years, a proxy for firearm availability (the death rate by firearms [accidents plus homicides] per one hundred thousand population) was significantly associated with male suicide rates. Indeed, firearm availability was the one factor significantly affecting male suicides in all three time periods (Hellsten 1995).

One study examined regional suicide data for sixteen years, from 1979 to 1994, using estimates of gun ownership levels collected by the National Opinion Research Center's General Social Surveys. A strong association existed between household gun ownership levels and suicide rates for every age group. Even after accounting for divorce levels, education, unemployment, poverty, and urbanization, suicide rates for young people and the elderly were significantly higher in regions with a higher level of household gun ownership (Birckmayer and Hemenway 2001). Another study discovered that the regional association between levels of household handgun ownership and suicide rates could not be explained by differences in regional levels of major depression or serious suicidal thoughts (Hemenway and Miller 2002).

A series of studies examined suicide rates across U.S. states for the ten-year period 1988–97. Suicide rates were significantly higher in states with higher levels of household gun ownership; this relationship held true for every age group, even after accounting for differences in poverty, urbanization, divorce, unemployment, alcohol consumption, and education (Miller, Azrael, and Hemenway 2002a, 2002b, 2002d). Comparing the five states with the highest levels of household gun ownership with the five states with the lowest levels, gun suicide rates were 3.8 times higher in the high-gun states, and overall suicide rates were 60 percent higher. One of the compelling aspects of this series of studies is that the findings tell the same story whatever measure of gun prevalence is used. The authors used two validated proxies (the percentage of suicides with guns and Cook's index) and subsequently checked their findings with data available for 2001 from surveys of household gun ownership for each state from the Behavioral Risk Factor Surveys.

A 2003 study gathered data from the Northeast on suicide attempts serious enough to require hospitalization. Deaths from suicides were significantly higher in states with higher levels of firearm ownership (due to higher levels of firearm suicide); there was no significant association between gun ownership levels and nonfirearm suicidal deaths. Firearm suicide *attempts* were higher in states with more firearms; there was no significant association between levels of household gun ownership and suicide *attempts* by other means. The relationship between firearm levels and suicide across these states could not be explained by differences in the overall rate of suicidal attempts (Miller, Hemenway, and Azrael 2003).

A variety of studies have examined the relationship between the strictness of gun control laws and suicide rates. Many cross-sectional studies find that strict state gun control laws are significantly associated with lower levels of suicide (Lester and Murrell 1982, 1986; Medoff and Magaddino 1983; Boor and Bair 1990; Yang and Lester 1991). Time-series studies in the United States and Canada also find a significant reduction in suicide rates after the enactment of stringent gun control laws (Loftin et al. 1991; Carrington and Moyer 1994).

Overall, the evidence summarized here on the gun-suicide connection within the United States is quite compelling—firearm availability appears to increase the rate of suicide. Perhaps the best evidence concerning the connection between gun availability and suicide comes from the case-control studies. The results are persuasive in part because these studies account for many other important factors associated with suicide. The recent cross-sectional evidence—within the United States—showing a strong association between guns and suicides across states and regions is also quite persuasive, again because many other explanatory variables are taken into account. The studies linking gun control laws and suicide are suggestive.

The American Association of Suicidology consensus statement on youth suicide concludes,

> There is a positive association between the accessibility and availability of firearms in the home and the risk of youth suicide; guns in the home, particularly loaded guns, are associated with increased risk for suicide by youth, both with and without identifiable mental health problems or suicidal risk factors. (Berman et al. 1998, 90)

Many strategies can and should be used to reduce suicide, including school-dropout prevention and role modeling, suicide awareness among health professionals, substance abuse treatment, and training high-risk individuals in depression management and anger control. Educational campaigns are needed to help remove the stigma surrounding mental illness and increase awareness that clinical depression can often be effectively treated with antidepressant medications and talk therapy.

But based on all available data, one of the best strategies for reducing suicide appears to be the removal of firearms from the home, particularly where there are adolescents or young adults. The evidence supporting the effectiveness of removing guns is probably stronger than that for almost any other single suicide-prevention policy. Removing guns will not eliminate all or probably even most suicides. Some determined individuals will find ways to get guns or will choose alternative lethal methods. But many others will choose less lethal methods or may not even try at all.

HOMICIDES

No large industrial democracy other than the United States reports firearms as the cause of a majority of its homicides. Scholars engaging in international comparisons are confronted with two extraordinary distinctions between homicide in the United States and in the rest of the developed Western world: very much higher rates of homicide in the United States, and a uniquely high percentage of gun use in U.S. violence.

—F. E. Zimring and G. Hawkins

Since 1960, approximately five hundred thousand Americans have been murdered with guns. To put that number in perspective, more Americans have been murdered with guns in the past forty years than were killed by all methods in all wars in the twentieth century—in World War I, World War II, the Korean War, the Vietnam War, and the Gulf War. Between 1991 and 2000, forty Americans were murdered with guns on an average day. Gun murders account for more than two-thirds of all murders, and our overall murder rate for this period was five times higher than the average rate for other developed nations (table 3.4).

The easy availability of firearms in the United States makes committing homicide easy. Guns are one of the most effective tools for committing murder and many other offenses. Among other things, guns facilitate violent attacks against powerful targets. All four U.S. presidential assassinations (Lincoln, Garfield, McKinley, Kennedy) have been committed with firearms, as have most presidential assassination attempts (T. Roosevelt, F. Roosevelt, Ford [twice], and Reagan). Nearly all murders of police officers have been committed with firearms (Cook 1991). Few armored truck robberies or bank robberies could occur without criminal access to guns.

Guns allow the killing of people at a distance and in an impersonal way (Kleck and McElrath 1991). A gun is not necessary to kill another person, but at fifty yards, a gun is the most efficient and effective means. It is also a help at a distance of five yards, five feet, or five inches; we have many drive-by shootings in the United States but few drive-by knifings or drive-by punchings. As researcher S. P. Baker put it, "People without guns INJURE people; guns KILL them" (1985, 588).

The presence of a gun makes quarrels, disputes, assaults, and robberies more deadly. For example, the overwhelming majority of robberies are spontaneous, often committed by addicts who engage in only the most cursory planning (Gabor 1994). While there is no evidence that gun robbers have any greater intent to kill than other robbers—indeed, robbers often report that they carry guns to avoid unnecessary physical confrontations with victims and bystanders—the likelihood of a victim death in a firearm robbery is three times higher than in a knife robbery, which in turn is seven times higher than the likelihood of victim death in an unarmed robbery (R. Block 1977; Cook 1987).

Three-quarters of felons who fire guns in criminal situations claim to have had no prior intention of doing so. And about half who fire guns while committing crimes claim to have done so in self-defense (J. D. Wright, Rossi, and Daly 1983).

TABLE 3.4.   Age-Adjusted Homicide Rates in
High-Income Nations (1995–98)

Nation	Homicide Rate per 100,000
United States ('95–'97)	8.2
Finland ('96)	3.3
Northern Ireland ('96–'97)	2.3
Scotland ('96–'97)	2.2
Belgium ('93–'94)	1.8
New Zealand ('94–'96)	1.7
Australia ('95)	1.6
Canada ('96–'97)	1.6
Italy ('94–'95)	1.4
Netherlands ('96–'97)	1.3
Singapore ('96–'97)	1.2
Denmark ('94–'96)	1.2
Sweden ('96)	1.2
Norway ('95)	1.0
Israel ('96)	1.0
France ('95–'96)	1.0
Austria ('96–'98)	1.0
Germany ('96–'97)	1.0
Ireland ('94–'96)	0.8
Spain ('95)	0.8
Luxembourg ('96–'97)	0.6
England/Wales ('96–'97)	0.6

Source: Data from World Health Organization.

More people are murdered during arguments with someone they know than during the commission of a robbery (fig. 3.1). Many murders are committed in moments of rage. For example, a large percentage of homicides occur during altercations over such matters as love, money, and domestic problems involving acquaintances, neighbors, lovers, and family members. Furthermore, in many cases, the assailant, the victim, or both have been drinking.

Only a small minority of homicides appears to be the carefully planned acts of individuals with a single-minded intention to kill. Most gun killings are indistinguishable from nonfatal gun shootings; it is just a question of whether a vital organ is hit, the caliber of the bullet, and how much time passes before medical treatment arrives. One study found that 70 percent of all gun killings in Chicago were the result of attacks that resulted in only one wound to the victim, and most attacks with guns or knives that killed a victim looked quite similar to the gun and knife attacks that did not kill. In that study, for every homicide with a single bullet to the chest, there were two survivors of a bullet wound to the chest (Zimring 1968, 1972).

Domestic disputes are likely to be affected by the presence of a firearm (Reiss and Roth 1993). While many spousal homicides occur following a long history of violence in the home, spousal abusers are often impulsive and volatile (Hastings and Hamberger 1988). The availability and use of a firearm increases the likelihood that an attack will prove fatal (J. C. Campbell 1986; Saltzman et al. 1992).

Young people's easy access to firearms in the United States has been a particular problem. Many victims are extremely young. Our rate of firearm murder for children aged five to fourteen is seventeen times higher than the firearm murder rate of children in other high-income nations; our overall murder rate for five- to fourteen-year-olds is five times higher. Almost three-quarters of the children murdered in the developed world are Americans (Krug et al. 1998). Murder is the third-leading cause of death for children aged five to fourteen in the United States (CDC 1999b), following unintentional injuries and malignant neoplasms. In states where there are more guns, more women and children are murdered (Miller, Azrael, and Hemenway 2002a, 2002b), as are more citizens of all ages (Miller, Azrael, and Hemenway 2002c).

During the decade 1991–2000, on an average day in the United States, fifteen young people aged between fifteen and twenty-four were murdered with a gun. The numbers have fallen since the early 1990s; homicide, like

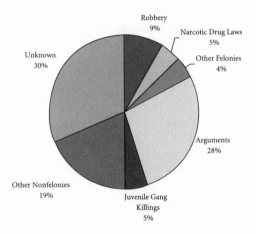

Fig. 3.1. Murder circumstances, 1997–2001. (From U.S. Department of Justice, FBI 2001, table 2.14.)

much crime, moves in somewhat unpredictable cycles (Philipson and Posner 1996; Blumstein and Rosenfeld 1998). Homicide is the second-leading cause of death for fifteen- to twenty-four-year-olds in the United States.

Youth have been disproportionately not only the victims but also the perpetrators of homicide. In the early 1990s, the rate of murder arrest was highest among eighteen- to twenty-year-olds, followed by seventeen-year-olds and sixteen-year-olds. Even fifteen-year-olds had a higher murder arrest rate than for any age over twenty-five. Adolescents were killing adolescents, and firearms were used in 80 percent of teenage homicides. Since the early 1990s, homicide perpetration and victimization rates have fallen, particularly among youth (U.S. Department of Justice 1994, 2003).

The distinctive feature of guns, as opposed to other weapons, is that they create a kind of judgment, or moment, that is often absolute and final. The use of guns in these settings does not allow one to change one's mind, to take it back; there is no opportunity to apologize. There was a time when fights among youth involved fists or occasionally knives. When brawls ended, there were opportunities for mediation, mending, and reconciliation. The kids doing the fighting sometimes would become friends. Now, when emotion overcomes a teenager's ability to make rational judgments, someone may die or become permanently disabled. The easy availability of guns has made it too easy for an impetuous youth to kill.

Kleck claims that "levels of general gun ownership appear to have no significant net effect on rates of homicide" (1997b, 383). That claim is contrary to the empirical evidence, which shows a strong link between the availability of firearms and homicide (Hepburn and Hemenway 2003).

Five types of empirical studies assess the association between gun availability and homicide: (1) cross-sectional studies of nations or U.S. regions, states, counties, and cities; (2) before-after studies of the effects of specific gun control laws; (3) case-control studies of the effects of gun purchase or household gun ownership; (4) time-series studies of the effect of individual gun purchases; and (5) time-series studies of the effects of aggregate levels of gun ownership or gun purchases. This fifth approach—areawide time-series analysis—can have serious methodological problems, and less confidence generally can be placed in the results. (See appendix A for a discussion of time-series analyses.)

As with the gun suicide literature, the small number of developed nations and U.S. regions and the lack of good data on gun ownership at the state and city levels reduce the likelihood of discovering a statistically significant relationship between gun availability and homicide. In addition, the percentage of households with guns may not be a good proxy for handgun availability, especially for inner-city teenagers. Nonetheless, most cross-sectional studies find a strong and significant relationship between gun availability and murder.

One international study examined fourteen developed countries for which gun ownership information was obtained from comparable telephone interviews. The rate of gun homicide and the overall homicide rate were significantly correlated with levels of gun ownership; there was no significant correlation between nongun homicide and gun ownership (Killias 1993).

Another international study examined twenty-six high-income nations with data from the early 1990s. Using various proxies for gun ownership, gun prevalence was strongly and significantly correlated with firearm homicide rates and with overall homicide rates (Hemenway and Miller 2000). (See appendix A for a discussion of international studies.) A related analysis of thirty-six high- and upper-middle-income countries also found a statistically significant association between firearm availability and homicide, even after statistically controlling for the possibility that high homicide rates may increase gun ownership for protection (Hoskin 1999).

Regional (Lester 1988; Miller, Azrael, and Hemenway 2002a, 2002b, 2002c), state (Brearley 1932; Seitz 1972; Lester 1990a; Birckmayer 1999; Miller, Azrael, and Hemenway 2002a, 2002b, 2002c; Hepburn et al. 2003), and county (Duggan 2001) cross-sectional analyses often find a significant relationship between gun ownership levels and homicide. One study (Lester 1990b) separated homicide into murders involving family and friends as victims and murders of strangers. Availability of firearms was significantly associated with the murder of family and friends at the state level but not with the murder of strangers, "perhaps because the presence of a firearm has more impact on impulsive assaultive behavior" (490).

The most recent state-level study finds a strong statistically significant association between gun availability and homicide rates between 1988 and 1997 for every age group. Using a validated measure of household gun ownership (Azrael, Cook, and Miller 2004), researchers found that high-gun states had three times the homicide rates of low-gun states. Results remained significant even after accounting for poverty, urbanization, alcohol consumption, unemployment, and violent crime (other than homicide) (Miller, Azrael, and Hemenway 2002a, 2002b, 2002c). The results were driven by the relationship between firearm availability and firearm homicide, although high-gun states also had somewhat higher levels of nongun homicide. (See appendix A for a discussion of the connection between gun prevalence and nongun homicide.) A compelling aspect of this series of studies is that the findings are robust to various measures of gun availability. For example, using data recently available for 2001 from surveys of household gun ownership for each state from the Behavioral Risk Factor Surveys produces similar findings.

Simple comparisons across cities also typically find significant correlations between gun ownership levels and homicides (Brill 1977; Kleck and Patterson 1993). A study of city homicide rates also tried to model a two-way causal relationship (homicide rates may affect gun prevalence as well as vice versa), but serious empirical mistakes make the results meaningless. (See appendix A for a discussion of reverse causation.)

Perhaps the strictest gun control regulation involving a major metropolitan area in the United States was the 1977 Washington, D.C., law that severely restricted the acquisition of firearms. A before-after analysis concluded that the law was effective—gun homicides fell by 25 percent, with little change in nongun homicides. No similar reduction in gun homicide occurred in the adjacent metropolitan areas of Maryland and Virginia (Loftin et al. 1991). This study is suggestive but not definitive, since other factors may have caused the reduction in gun homicides (Britt, Bordua, and Kleck 1996; McDowall, Wiersema, and Loftin 1996).

Case-control studies have examined the association between household gun ownership and homicide victimization. Results suggest that a gun in the home increases the likelihood of murder rather than providing protection against being murdered. One study used as cases approximately four hundred homicide victims from three metropolitan areas who were killed in their homes. Half died from gunshot wounds. About one-third were killed by an intimate, 12 percent by another relative, 31 percent by a friend or acquaintance, and 4 percent by a stranger. (The perpetrator was not determined for 17 percent.) Forty-four percent of the homicides occurred in the context of an altercation or quarrel, 11 percent in a romantic triangle or as part of a murder-suicide, 8 percent were drug related, and 22 percent occurred during the commission of another felony, such as robbery, rape, or burglary; no motive could be determined in 13 percent of the cases. In only 14 percent of the cases was there evidence of forced entry (Kellermann et al. 1993).

Controls were matched to cases by gender, race, age range, and neighborhood of residence. Handguns were kept in 36 percent of case households but only 23 percent of control households. After controlling for illicit drug use, fights, arrests, living alone, and whether the home was rented, the presence of a gun in the home remained strongly associated with an increased risk for homicide in the home (Kellermann et al. 1993).

The study did not present any evidence about whether a gun from the home was used in any of the homicides, relied on self-reports of household gun ownership, and was unable to include as confounders all potentially important risk factors for homicide. Nonetheless, the findings from stratified analyses are consistent with the notion that a gun in the home increases the risk of death. First, the link between gun ownership and homicide resulted entirely from a strong association between gun ownership and homicide by firearm; homicide by other means was not significantly linked to the presence or absence of a gun in the home. Second, gun ownership was most strongly associated with homicide at the hands of a family member or intimate acquaintance; guns were not significantly linked to an increased risk of homicide by other friends, unidentified intruders, or strangers. Finally, there was no evidence of a protective effect of keeping a gun in the home, even in the small subgroup of cases that involved forced entry.

A second case-control study examined whether the purchase of a handgun from a licensed dealer was associated with the risk of homicide occurring at any location (Cummings, Koepsell et al. 1997). More than one hundred cases and more than five hundred controls, matched on gender, age group, and zip code, were drawn from members of a large health maintenance organization in Washington state. For 22 percent of homicide victims but only 12 percent of controls, family members had purchased handguns. (Nine percent of victims and 5 percent of controls had purchased the handguns themselves.) The median interval between the first family handgun purchase and any homicide death was more than eleven years. The relative risk of death by homicide associated with a handgun purchase bore no statistically significant relationship to time since purchase. Indeed, no victim in this study was murdered with a gun within five years of any first handgun purchase, suggesting that in this population, deliberate legal purchase of a handgun to commit murder within a family was a rare event.

The study could not control for many differences (other than those characteristics the researchers matched between cases and controls) such as criminal history or substance abuse. Inclusion of such variables would probably lower the estimated risk of homicide associated with a handgun purchase. Conversely, the study examined only legal gun purchases from licensed dealers. If persons likely to be murdered or inclined to commit murder within their families are more likely to procure handguns exclusively from private or illegal sources, the study would underestimate the risks resulting from handgun ownership. The authors correctly conclude that "on average, the acquisition of a handgun appears to be associated with an increased risk of violent death" (Cummings, Koepsell et al. 1997, 978).

A third case-control study of homicide combined two national data sets for 1993/94. After controlling for family income, education, marital status, region, and other variables, a gun in the home was a risk factor for becoming a homicide victim. The risk was particularly high for women. A limitation of the study was that information on firearm presence was not available for over one-third of the homicide cases (Wiebe 2003b). Merrill (2002) uses similar data but found gun prevalence was associated with lower homicide rates. The differing results of these two analyses need to be reconciled.

Results from two offender-based case-control homicide studies find that gun ownership is a risk for homicide. One study of fifty Ohio offenders examined firearm homicides involving family members, relatives, and friends. Results indicate that offenders (cases) were far more likely to live in a household with a loaded firearm than were individuals (controls) who were similar to cases in terms of age, sex, and living in the same neighborhood (Rowland and Holtzhauer 1989).

Another case-control study compared prisoners convicted of homicide with an unmatched sample of national adults. Instead of a comparison of similar people (age, race, gender) from the same neighborhoods, the sample of cases is made up disproportionately of young, urban minorities, while older rural whites, with a hunting tradition, make up a disproportionate share of the controls who have guns. Although an attempt was made to control for some attributes, no variable held constant the neighborhood environment or even rural versus urban residence. Since rural areas have lower crime rates (in virtually all high-income countries, whether or not there are many guns available) but more guns (for hunting and shooting), the lack of neighborhood controls reduces the likelihood of finding any true relationship between gun ownership and homicide. Nonetheless, the authors still found that persons owning guns were 1.36 times more likely to commit homicides than persons without guns (Kleck and Hogan 1999). (See appendix A for a discussion of the importance of controlling for urbanization.)

Time-series analyses have also attempted to determine the association between gun availability and homicide. Studies trying to use the stock of firearms as the proxy for gun availability have been plagued with measurement problems. (See appendix A for a discussion of time-series studies.) Probably the most sophisticated study analyzed the relationship between handgun *sales* and homicide after accounting for beer sales, unemployment, migration, racial composition, and cohort size. Using data from California for twenty-two years, from 1972 to 1993, researchers found that the prior year's dealer sales of handguns were significantly linked to homicides of virtually every age group of black, Hispanic, and white males. There was no association with female homicides. The association of handgun sales with homicide was stronger for younger than for older males and was more closely related to firearm homicides than to all homicides. The associations were substantial. If causative, they suggest that almost five thousand fewer male Californians between the ages of fifteen and thirty-four would have died during this period if handgun sales had remained at 1972 levels (Sorenson and Berk 2001).

Overall, the literature on the link between gun availability and homicide is compelling. Most studies—whether cross-sectional or time-series, international or domestic—show that higher levels of gun prevalence are linked not only with higher levels of gun homicide but also with a higher overall homicide rate. These studies are perhaps more on point than the case-control studies, since other people's guns rather than one's own usually directly increase the risk of becoming a homicide victim. However the case-control studies suggest that a gun in the home increases the risk of becoming a victim of intimate-partner homicide (Hepburn and Hemenway 2003).

OTHER GUN-RELATED CRIMES

A gun in the home can also be used to terrify a spouse [or] intimidate a girlfriend.
—A. Kellermann and S. Heron

Focusing exclusively on incidents that result in injury or death would severely underestimate the extent of the gun violence problem in the United States. Guns are often used in crime with no bullets being fired and no one shot. Many such crimes, including cases of assault, rape, and robbery, are not reported to the police. To better estimate the actual rates of such crimes, the U.S. National Crime Victimization Survey (NCVS) has been created. This semi-annual survey asks a representative sample of the population whether they have been the victims of attempted or completed crimes.

International comparisons of victimization surveys suggest that U.S. citizens are neither clearly more violent nor more criminal than those of other developed nations but that guns are used far more often in the commission of crimes in the United States than elsewhere (R. Block 1993). The authors of one cross-national report on crime victimization conclude that American crime rates are comparable to other developed nations but that the United States is "unusual in the extent to which guns were mentioned in assaults and robberies" (Mayhew and van Dijk 1997, 67). Two longtime scholars of crime in the United States, F. E. Zimring and G. Hawkins, also conclude that "rates of crime are not greatly different in the United States from those of other developed countries. . . . Our extremely high rates of lethal violence are a separate phenomenon, a distinct social problem that is the real source of fear and anger in American life" (1997b, 3). As E. J. Dionne Jr. colorfully explains, "You're just as likely to get punched in the mouth in a bar in Sydney [Australia] as in a bar in Los Angeles. But you're 20 times as likely to be killed in Los Angeles" (1999).

On an average day in 2001, there were seventeen hundred robberies in the United States, including holdups, muggings, purse snatchings, and other violent confrontations motivated by theft. Guns were used in more than five hundred of these robberies (National Archive 2002). Higher levels of gun ownership appear to be associated with higher rates of robbery with guns but not with overall robbery levels (Cook 1979, 1987; Kleck 1997b). Victims of gun robbers are less likely to resist and less likely to be nonfatally injured than victims of robbers without guns (Conklin 1972; R. Block 1977; Skogan 1978; Cook 1987; Kleck 1997b; Wells 2000). Indeed, felons claim that a principal motive for having a gun is so they "don't have to hurt the victim" (Wright and Rossi 1986, 128).

Victims of gun robbers, however, are far more likely to be murdered (Cook 1987). Various studies have similar findings: robberies and assaults with guns are three to five times more likely to result in death than robberies and assaults with knives, six to ten times more likely to result in death than robberies or assaults with other weapons, and some forty times more likely to result in death than if no weapon were used (Zimring 1968; Cook 1991; Saltzman et al. 1992; Alba and Messner 1995). Unfortunately, compared to other high-income nations, in robberies in the United States the criminal is far more likely to have a gun.

While the law determines the seriousness of the crime by whether the victim lives or dies, neither the outcome nor the weapon used is a reliable indicator of the assailant's intent or state of mind (Cook and Moore 1999). There is no evidence to indicate that gun robbers have a greater intent to kill than other robbers. Many robberies are unplanned acts, committed by addicts in need of quick money for a fix. Some evidence does suggest that robbers who use the crudest weapons or none at all are often the most reckless, causing the most injuries and deaths and making the least profit (Gabor et al. 1987). Similarly, the seriousness of many nonfatal knifings indicates that many are attempted homicides. In general, there is a good deal of overlap in intent between fatal and nonfatal assaults and robberies (Zimring 1968). But one thing is clear: the probability that a victim will live or die depends in large part on the lethality of the weapon used. As researcher P. J. Cook put it,

> The relatively high death rate in gun robbery is the direct consequence of the fact that a loaded gun provides the assailant with the means to kill quickly at a distance and without much skill, strength, or danger of counterattack. A passing whim or even the accidental twitch of a trigger finger is sufficient. Thus a gun is intrinsically more dangerous than other types of weapons. (1987, 372)

Data on gun use in crime come from the NCVS, which is conducted by the U.S. Census Bureau. The NCVS provides detailed information from a sample of sixty thousand households on the incidence and circumstances of six specific attempted or completed crimes. However, much crime involving intimates is not reported to the NCVS, and it appears that many additional illegal gun uses—when guns are used to threaten, intimidate, or coerce—are also not reported on the NCVS.

In 1996 and 1999, the Harvard Injury Control Research Center sponsored the first two national nongovernmental surveys to ask detailed questions about both illegal gun use against and self-defense gun use by respondents. In the first survey, excluding police officers, security guards and military personnel, 3.1 percent of respondents reported hostile gun displays against them (after further excluding hostile gun displays by the police against respondents). By contrast, 0.7 percent of respondents reported self-defense gun uses in the past five years (Hemenway and Azrael 1997, 2000).

For many of those who reported experiencing hostile gun incidents, the guns were displayed during planned crimes. These crimes were primarily either assaults by strangers, which often occurred at work (e.g., restaurants, convenience stores), or assaults by acquaintances (e.g., ex-boyfriends). While police were notified in almost all the cases involving strangers, the police were not notified about some of the threats made by intimates, and these incidents may also not have been reported on the NCVS. For example, one young woman said, "My boyfriend was mad because I was seeing someone else. We broke up. Six months later he showed up at my house to talk. He showed me the gun to scare me into seeing him again" (Hemenway and Azrael 2000, 264).

For many respondents, the most recent threat with a gun had taken place during an argument that escalated into gun use. The majority of the cases involved family or acquaintances. Many of these incidents might not be reported as crimes on the NCVS. From the perspective of the other parties, some of these events might be called "self-defense gun use," even though they would not legally be considered thus. Examples of gun use during arguments include:

A young male said, "I was outside at a party—I was walking to my car. A guy was upset. He thought I was hitting on his girlfriend. He pulled out a gun. . . . He was pretty drunk. I laughed and then I drove away."

A middle-aged male was in the basement of his brother-in-law's house. The brother-in-law brandished a gun "to make a point and to be more aggressive during an argument about the safety of having a gun in the house."

A young male was in his car. A stranger "got upset because he thought I cut him off and began to throw objects at me. Then he pulled out the gun and waved it at me."

A woman in her thirties was walking with a female friend when a "guy across the street yelled something. My friend yelled back and he crossed the street and pulled out a gun from the front of his pants. He asked if she had said something. She said 'No,' and we left."

A number of respondents reported an unprovoked brandishing in which someone displayed a gun in a hostile manner against the respondent for no apparent reason. While such actions are crimes and are almost always committed by strangers, many may not be reported on the NCVS. Examples include:

A young female said, "I was driving with our family and stopped at an intersection. The individuals pulled alongside, pulled a gun out and pointed it at us, taunting us until the light changed."

A young male said, "I was on the curb in front of a friend's house. It was racially motivated. They shouted, 'Whitey go home.' They shot the gun at us and drove off."

A male in his forties was walking with his wife "down a sidewalk in a neighboring apartment complex. A teenager picked up a .22 and started pointing it at me, threatening to blow my head off. He was showing off."

An older male said, "This guy was next to me in his car. I just walked to my car from K-Mart, and he was mouthing off. He was cussing at me, threatening me. . . . He was messed up. I don't know if he was drunk or on drugs. Obscene, really talking. He saw I was leaving and he pulled out his gun and said, 'I'll just shoot you.' Then he drove off."

Eight respondents reported hostile gun displays when they were perceived to be criminals. Five of these gun displays were by the police; three were by civilians. These events would almost certainly be considered "self-defense gun use" if the other party had been surveyed. One example of a civilian thinking the respondent was a criminal is:

> The respondent was jogging in the woods. "Someone lived in a shack in the woods and thought I was getting too close to their house. They just displayed the gun and asked me to leave."

The survey results indicated not only that many hostile gun uses might not be included in the NCVS estimates but also that the number of respondents reporting that they were victims of gun threats greatly exceeded the number of respondents claiming to have used guns in self-defense. The second survey results were similar: 3.8 percent of respondents reported gun threats, compared to 1.2 percent who reported self-defense gun use in the past five years (Hemenway, Miller, and Azrael 2000).

At least five other surveys have asked about both offensive and defensive gun use; they, too, all find that the former is far more common than the latter (Gallup 2000; Hemenway and Azrael 2000). For example, a random survey of adolescents in California in 2001 asked if anyone had "brought out, showed, or used a gun to threaten" the respondent and if the respondent had ever "brought out, showed, or used a gun in self-defense." Eleven times more adolescents reported that they had been threatened with a gun than reported ever using a gun in self-defense (Hemenway and Miller 2003).

The NCVS also finds that criminal gun use is far more common than self-defense gun use, by a margin of about ten to one (National Archive 1998). No survey using similar questions for both types of events has ever found that self-defense gun use is more common than criminal gun use. A May 2000 national survey by the *Washington Post*/ABC News asked, "Excluding any time served in the military, have you EVER been threatened with a gun or shot at?" and 23 percent of respondents replied in the affirmative (Morin and Deane 2000). By contrast, a May 2000 national Gallup survey asked, "Not including military combat, have you ever used a gun to defend yourself either by firing it or threatening to fire it?" Seven percent of respondents said that they had done so.

It is thus quite surprising—and unfounded—that Kleck has repeatedly claimed that "the best available evidence indicates that guns are used defensively by crime victims four to five times more often than they are used by offenders to commit a crime" (1997a, 295). Kleck compares the results for offensive and defensive gun use from two different types of surveys—the NCVS for criminal gun use and private surveys for self-defense gun use. The NCVS has largely eliminated the large false-positive problem that plagues surveys looking for rare events. (See appendix A for a discussion of self-defense gun use.) Estimates of offensive and defensive gun use from the NCVS are more conservative than estimates from one-shot private surveys— typically an order of magnitude lower. Comparing the criminal gun use figures from private surveys with the self-defense gun use estimates from the NCVS (the reverse of what Kleck does) could lead to the conclusion that criminal gun use was fifty to four hundred times more likely than self-defense gun use. Neither comparison is legitimate.

It is generally accepted that the NCVS may underestimate certain crimes, particularly those involving intimate-partner violence, which respondents may prefer not to report. Surveys of batterers indicate that threats with a firearm are not uncommon in abusive relationships when there are guns in the household (E. F. Rothman 2003). As noted earlier, the NCVS may also miss many hostile gun displays during escalating arguments and many unprovoked gun brandishings. It may even miss many assaults in which the victims are shot (Cook 1985). All these are criminal gun uses and should be counted.

The NCVS probably also misses much so-called self-defense gun use during escalating arguments and other situations when the respondent would not initially report that a crime had been committed. However many of these gun uses are likely criminal acts (see chap. 4). If the story were told from the other combatant's perspective, it is likely that in many instances he or she would seem to have been the one who was assaulted and forced to act in self-defense. For example, in the Harvard Injury Control Research Center surveys, one man in his fifties reported a self-defense gun use in a reaction to an argument with a neighbor: "I was on my porch and this man threw a beer in my face so I got my gun." Another male reported a self-defense gun use against an acquaintance in his home: "I was watching a movie and he interrupted me. I yelled at him that I was going to shoot him and he ran to his car" (Hemenway, Miller, and Azrael 2000).

Criminal gun use is far too common in the United States. A public health approach to reducing gun use in assaults and robberies and in other forms of intimidation emphasizes prevention. Criminal justice plays an important role in deterring crime and separating violent offenders from society, but other measures are also crucial. Unfortunately, until recently,

> assaultive injuries have been subject to little prevention-oriented research. Typically, they have been regarded as a "crime problem" rather than as a health problem, and blame and punishment of the perpetrators have been emphasized, rather than measures to reduce the frequency and severity of such injuries. (Institute of Medicine 1985, 44)

Guns in criminal hands increase the risk of lethal violence. Many policies can reduce the ease with which known criminals have access to firearms. As I will argue, the most cost-effective interventions involve further restrictions of the secondary markets for guns—sales at gun shows, flea markets, and over the Internet.

One small step in reducing access to firearms is for police departments to destroy rather than sell used and confiscated firearms. More than 230 homicide-related gun traces between 1994 and 1998 ended at the doors of other law-enforcement agencies. For example, in August 1999, Buford Furrow used a Glock pistol sold by the Cosmopolis, Washington, police department to shoot children at a Jewish community center in Los Angeles (Olinger 1999b).

A 1998 resolution by the International Association of Chiefs of Police urged police departments to stop selling used and confiscated guns and to instead destroy them. This recommendation should be followed. Larry Todd, the chief of police in Los Gatos, California, who helped draft the resolution, stated, "It did not make sense for us to be reintroducing guns back into communities we were sworn to protect" (Shear and Jackman 1999).

SUMMARY

The United States has very high rates of death from guns—gun accidents, gun suicides, and gun homicides—compared to other high-income nations. Appendix B provides a list of well-known civilians shot in the United States. We have far more unintentional gun injuries per capita than any other high-income nation. Each day, some thirty Americans are accidentally shot with firearms; about two or three die. In states with more guns, there are more accidental gun deaths.

Suicides are a bigger problem for the United States. About fifty Americans die each day by their own hands. A gun in the home has been shown to be a risk factor for suicide, and areas in the United States with more guns have more suicides. Compared to other developed nations, our firearm suicide rate is high in all age groups, as is our overall suicide rate among children. However our adult suicide rate is comparable to that in other high-income countries.

The U.S. firearm and overall homicide rates are far higher than those of other developed nations for all age groups. Every other high-income country has fewer guns (especially handguns), stronger gun control regulations, and much lower homicide rates. Zimring and Hawkins have summarized the issue:

When discussing American lethal violence with any foreign criminologist, guns are always the first factor to be mentioned as an explanation of the distinctively high rates of death in the United States. What sets the foreign criminologists' comments apart from our American colleagues is not the unanimity with which they focus on guns, however, because this topic is inevitably mentioned by American criminologists as well. But our foreign colleagues are frequently unwilling to discuss any other feature of American society or government *except* gun ownership and use. In Europe or Japan, any mention of social, demographic, or economic factors as a cause of homicide is commonly regarded as an evasion of the most obvious reason why American violence is specially dangerous. . . . Firearms use is so prominently associated with the high death rate from violence that starting with any other topic would rightly be characterized as an intentional evasion. (Zimring and Hawkins 1997b, 106)

The United States might have a lethal violence problem even without guns. Our nongun homicide rate is higher than the total homicide rates of almost all other high-income nations. However, the evidence indicates that the current easy access to guns by all members of our society makes our proclivity toward lethal violence much worse. Historian R. Lane sums it up this way: "High American [homicide] rates, finally, owe much but not all to our gun culture" (1999, 191).

Within the United States, a wide array of empirical evidence indicates that more guns in a community lead to more homicide. Studies also indicate that a gun in the home increases the risk of murder for family members. Since a gun in the home tends to also increase the risk of suicide and unintentional firearm injury, many public health practitioners emphasize the dangers of bringing a gun into the home, particularly if children are present.

Many policies are readily available to reduce our gun injury problem. Gun accidents would be reduced if manufacturers made guns that were childproof and personalized. Unintentional injuries would also fall if new guns were equipped with a loaded-chamber indicator and a magazine safety. At the very least, mass-produced films and TV shows can help to educate the public by presenting more realistic depictions of the causes and consequences of gun accidents, suicides, and nonfatal firearm injuries.

Many groups can also play a more active role in reducing our gun suicide problem. Physicians and other medical providers can counsel their patients about the dangers of firearms in the home and suggest strategies to reduce suicide risk. Most family practitioners (Kirschner 2000) and psychologists (Brown 2002) apparently do not currently ask about guns in the homes of depressed patients, and a substantial minority of psychiatrists do not ask about guns even when a patient is suicidal (Gallagher et al. 2002); these practitioners should begin to routinely ask about gun ownership and access since guns are the most common agent of completed suicide in the United States.

Firearms are only a small part of the U.S. "crime problem" (guns are involved in some 4 percent of all serious crimes in the United States), but they are a large part of our violent death problem (guns are used in two-thirds of U.S. homicides and almost 60 percent of U.S. suicides).

Guns increase the lethality of violent crime. Robbers often use firearms so that they don't have to hurt the victim to steal the property, but when force is used, gun robberies are far more likely to end in murder than are robberies with other weapons or no weapons.

Many policies can reduce criminals' ability to obtain firearms, such as licensing of gun owners, registration of guns, and prohibitions on gun transfers without a criminal background check—policies common in many other industrialized nations. One small step directed toward reducing criminal access to firearms would be if police destroyed rather than resold confiscated weapons.

Guns are used not only to kill and to wound but also to intimidate and coerce. Criminal intimidation with firearms is far more common than self-defense gun use. Unlawful intimidation with firearms takes place not only during planned crimes but also escalating arguments, which generally occur between intimates, friends, and acquaintances.

Many of these criminal uses of guns against humans do not seem to be included in official statistics—crime reports, emergency room logs, death certificates, and so forth. When determining the benefits and costs of various measures to increase or reduce the availability of and access to guns, it is important to consider the effect not only on reported crime, suicide, and accidental injury but also on more hidden uses. The vast majority of these hidden uses appear to be against society's interests.

CHAPTER 4   SELF-DEFENSE
USE OF GUNS

There is little or no need for a gun for self-protection [for most Americans] because there's so little risk of crime. People don't believe it, but it's true. You just can't convince most Americans they're not at serious risk.

—Gary Kleck

The previous chapters highlighted some of the costs guns impose on society. But guns also provide some safety benefits. Guns may be used to thwart criminal acts, and awareness of their presence may deter individuals from attempting to commit crimes. But how common is self-defense gun use, and how much benefit do guns really provide for our society? This chapter describes the scientific evidence available on the role of firearms in deterring crime and thwarting criminals, discusses the frequency of self-defense gun use and whether such incidents are usually socially beneficial, and considers the evidence concerning whether armed resistance against attackers makes good sense.

THE MYTH AND REALITY OF DETERRENCE

Given the claims of the gun lobby, it is perhaps surprising that there is in fact little credible evidence that guns deter crime. Criminologist Gary Kleck (1988) claims that publicized police programs to train citizens in gun use in Orlando (to prevent rape) and in Kansas City (to prevent robbery) led to reductions in crime by changing prospective criminals' awareness of gun ownership among potential victims. However, a careful analysis of the data found no evidence that crime rates changed in either location after the training (McDowall, Lizotte, and Wiersema 1991). The deterrent effects of civilian gun ownership on burglary rates were also supposedly shown by the experiences of Morton Grove, Illinois (after it banned handguns), and Kennesaw, Georgia (after it required that firearms be kept in all homes) (Kleck 1988). Again, a careful analysis of the data did not show that guns reduced crime (McDowall, Wiersema, and Loftin 1989). Instead, in Morton Grove, the banning of handguns was followed by a large and statistically significant decrease in burglary reports (McDowall, Lizotte, and Wiersema 1991).

The fact that rural areas in the United States have more guns and less crime than urban areas has sometimes been claimed as evidence of the deterrent that firearms represent (e.g., Polsby and Kates 1998). The comparison, of course, is inappropriate. Cities in high-income countries generally experience more crime than rural areas, whatever the levels of gun ownership. A more valid comparison is between cities, between states, or between regions.

One study found a negative association between rates of gun ownership and crime rates (more guns, less crime) (Lott 1998a). However, in that study, gun ownership data came from election exit polls conducted in 1988 and 1996. These data on gun ownership levels are unreliable. According to the polling source, Voter News Service, the data cannot be used as the author uses them—to determine either state-level gun ownership levels or changes in gun ownership rates—for three reasons: (1) the survey sampled only actual voters, a minority of the adult population; (2) the gun ownership question changed between the two periods; and (3) the sample size was far too small for reliable estimates. In only fourteen states were there more than one hundred respondents to the 1996 poll, and for one such state, Illinois, the polls indicated, nonsensically, that personal gun ownership more than doubled between 1988 and 1996, from 17 to 36 percent of the adult population. Overall, the data from these exit polls indicate that gun ownership rates in the United States increased an incredible 50 percent during those eight years. Yet all other surveys of the general population show either no change or a decrease in the percentage of Americans who personally own firearms (Kleck 1997b). Analyses of guns and crime using the Voter News Service data are meaningless.

No other study finds that crime is lower in cities, states, or regions where there are more guns. Instead, the evidence indicates that where there are more guns, while there are no more robberies, there are more gun robberies and more robbery homicides (Cook 1987). Most studies find that where there are more guns, there are significantly more gun homicides and total homicides (Ohsfeldt and Morrisey 1992; Hepburn and Hemenway 2003).

A widely cited proponent of the supposed deterrent effect of guns has claimed that when gun prevalence is high, burglars seek out unoccupied dwellings to avoid being shot (Kleck 1988, 1997b). Yet the evidence comes not from a scientific study but from a flawed comparison using different victimization surveys in different time periods for four areas—the United States, Britain, the Netherlands, and Toronto. In the United States, compared to the other three areas, a higher percentage of burglaries are committed when no one is at home. Kleck's analysis does not take into account relevant factors that might explain the association (e.g., the percentage of time in which dwellings are occupied). The areas are compared to the United States but not to each other, and only four nations/cities are examined. One could just as well argue that since cigarette consumption is higher in Japan and Stockholm than in the United States, and the Japanese and Swedish live longer than Americans, cigarettes are good for longevity.

A more reliable study used data from the Uniform Crime Reports for all fifty U.S. states for 1977–98 and data from the U.S. National Crime Victimization Survey (NCVS) for 330,000 households for 1994–98. The findings from both analyses were that U.S. counties and states with more guns have higher rates of burglary and higher per capita rates of "hot burglary" (burglary when someone is at home) (Cook and Ludwig 2003). Homes with firearm collections are considered prime targets for burglars.

Surveys of burglars in the United States do indicate that most would prefer that no one is at home—and presumably that no one is armed—when they enter the premises (Rengert and Wasilchick 1985; Wright and Rossi 1986). There is little question that professional burglars, who are among the least violent of serious criminals, want merchandise and do not want to get arrested, bludgeoned, or shot. But there is currently no credible evidence that a high prevalence of gun ownership reduces burglary or any other crime or in any way reduces potential violent confrontations.

HOW COMMON IS SELF-DEFENSE GUN USE?

Much discussion about the protective benefits of guns has focused on the incidence of self-defense gun use. Proponents of such putative benefits often claim that 2.5 million Americans use guns in self-defense against criminal attackers each year (Kleck and Gertz 1995). This estimate is not plausible and has been nominated as the "most outrageous number mentioned in a policy discussion by an elected official" (Cook, Ludwig, and Hemenway 1997, 463).

The estimate comes from a national telephone survey in which respondents reported their own behavior. All attempts at external validation reveal it to be a huge overestimate (Hemenway 1997b). For example, in 34 percent of the cases in which respondents stated that they used guns for self-defense, they said they used guns to protect themselves during burglaries. If true, this would translate into guns being used in self-defense in approximately 845,000 burglaries each year. From sophisticated victimization surveys (the NCVS), however, we know that there were fewer than 6,000,000 burglaries in the year of the survey, and in only 1,300,000 of those cases was someone certainly at home. Since only 41 percent of U.S. households owned firearms, and since the victims in two-thirds of the occupied dwellings remained asleep, the 2.5 million figure requires us to believe that burglary victims used their guns in self-defense more than 100 percent of the time.

A more reasonable estimate of self-defense gun use during burglary comes from a retrospective analysis of Atlanta police department reports. Examining home invasion crimes during a four-month period, researchers identified 198 cases of unwanted entry into single-family dwellings when someone was at home (Kellermann et al. 1995). In only three cases (less than 2 percent) did a victim use a firearm in self-defense. If this figure were extrapolated nationally for the year the survey covers, it would suggest approximately twenty thousand gun uses against burglary.

If it were true, the estimate of 2.5 million self-defense gun uses per year would lead to many other absurd conclusions. There just aren't enough serious crimes for victims to use guns so many times. For example, the number of respondents who claim to have used a gun against rape and robbery attempts suggests that victims of these attempted crimes are more likely to use a gun against the offender than the attackers are to use a gun against the victim—even though the criminal chooses the time and place for the attack, most citizens do not own guns, and very few people carry guns. Similarly, the number of people who claim to use guns in self-defense and report the incident to police (64 percent in the Kleck survey) often exceeds the total number of such crimes reported to police, including all the crimes when the victim did not have a gun (Ludwig 2000).

Other results coming from this telephone survey are also grossly exaggerated. Respondents claim to have shot more than two hundred thousand criminals. Yet each year, only about one hundred thousand people total (typically victims of assaults, suicide attempts, or accidents) are treated in emergency departments for gunshot wounds (Annest et al. 1995). Kleck (1997b) makes the strange claim that most gunshot victims are criminals, and when criminals are shot they do not seek professional medical care. But surveys of jail detainees find that even among criminals, almost all go to hospital emergency rooms for treatment of their wounds. Of more than 380 surveyed criminals in jails in California, Ohio, Nevada, Georgia, Maryland, and Washington, D.C., who had been wounded in incidents, few of which were related to their incarceration, more than 90 percent went to the hospital for treatment (May et al. 2000a; May, Hemenway, and Hall 2002).

While the survey respondents claimed to be shooting more than 200,000 criminals, FBI's Uniform Crime Reports (UCR) for that year reported only 350 justifiable homicides by private citizens, and not all of these were with firearms (U.S. Department of Justice 1993). Per week, that would mean about 3,850 shootings of bad guys—but fewer than 7 died? Even if the UCR figure may be somewhat of an underestimate (discussed later in this chapter) the wounding/death rates just don't make sense.

Respondents from this telephone survey also report being victims of more than four times the number of robberies as is estimated by the NCVS, whose purpose is to determine rates of victimization. But none of these additional robberies seem to show up in police records or in hospital admissions of injured patients.

Survey respondents in the self-defense telephone survey also claim to have used their guns to save more than four hundred thousand people a year from death. Yet only twenty-seven thousand homicides occurred in the year of the survey. In other words, for every person actually murdered, gun owners claimed to be saving fifteen (usually themselves and their families) from certain death. One might then expect that non–gun owners, of whom few are saved by guns, would have much higher rates of homicide victimization than gun owners. Yet the evidence shows that non–gun owners are less likely to be murdered than are gun owners.

It is clear that the claim of 2.5 million annual self-defense gun uses is a vast overestimate. But what can account for it? The main causes are telescoping and the false-positive problem—a matter of misclassification that is well known to medical epidemiologists. (See appendix A for a discussion of self-defense gun use and the false-positive problem.) Fortunately, the NCVS, which includes information on self-defense, drastically reduces these problems.

Housing units in the NCVS remain in the sample for three years, and residents are interviewed every six months. To eliminate telescoping—the reporting of events that occurred outside the time frame in question—incidents reported in the first interview are excluded. Residents are asked in subsequent interviews only about events that occurred since the most recent interview. In surveys of criminal victimization, telescoping can increase estimates "by between 40% and 50% depending on the type of crime; the inflation rate is greatest for violent crimes" (Skogan 1990, 262; see also Cantor 1989).

More important, the NCVS properly restricts claims of self-defense gun use to those who report a threatened, attempted, or completed victimization; it cannot be a genuine self-defense gun use unless there is an actual threat. Limiting the defensive gun use issue to this group eliminates most of the false-positive problem. The resulting estimate for annual defensive gun uses is between 55,000 and 120,000 per year, less than one-twentieth of the 2.5 million figure (Cook 1991; McDowall and Wiersema 1994; National Archive 1998).

The NCVS estimate has some limitations. It does not ask about all crimes (e.g., trespassing or vandalism), but only about six serious ones—rape and sexual assault, robbery, assault, burglary, nonbusiness larceny, and motor vehicle theft. However, no one claims that instances of self-defense gun use for the minor crimes that are omitted would dramatically swell the total. We also might expect the NCVS to give an underestimate of self-defense gun use since it prompts respondents not by asking directly whether they used a gun in self-defense but only by asking, "What did you do?" and "Anything else?" However, there is little reason to expect that respondents might forget or might be unwilling to report using a gun to protect themselves against a crime that occurred within the past six months. (See appendix A on self-defense gun use.)

Whatever its limitations, it seems clear that the NCVS estimates of self-defense gun use are more valid than the private telephone survey estimates of millions of self-defense gun uses each year.

IS MORE BETTER?

A presumption exists that the higher the number of reported self-defense gun uses, the greater the benefit of guns, both to the user and to society generally. This assumption may be incorrect.

An increased likelihood of self-defense gun use may change the behavior of criminals in a perverse direction. Rather than being deterred from committing crimes, criminals may instead increasingly arm themselves in the belief that the defender might be armed (Wright and Rossi 1986; Green 1987). Most delinquents and criminals claim that they are carrying and using guns primarily for self-protection (Wright and Rossi 1986; Hemenway et al. 1996). In a large survey of felons, half said a very important reason why they carried a gun was the chance that the victim might be armed (Wright and Rossi 1986). An arms race explains the sharp rise in homicide in many underclass neighborhoods in the late 1980s and early 1990s. Escalating murder rates increased the demand for guns for protection, which led to increases in murders, which led to further need for guns, turning these inner-city areas into "killing fields" (Wright, Sheley, and Smith 1992).

Having a gun for self-defense may also change the behavior of the gun owner in a perverse direction. For example, an individual who has a gun may become overconfident and put himself in dangerous situations he would have otherwise avoided. Even more important, he may use the gun inappropriately.

Police officers, who receive large amounts of training, are still often inadequately prepared to handle ambiguous but potentially dangerous situations. Intense stress, confusion, and fear are inherent in most possible shooting situations. Heart rates skyrocket, and it is difficult to think clearly and to act deliberately (Diaz 2001a). Not surprisingly, even police make serious mistakes. Individuals without training are likely to do much worse.

Attempts by civilians to use guns in self-defense sometimes end in catastrophe.

- A sixteen-year-old Japanese exchange student, Yoshihiro Hattori, in a suburb of Baton Rouge, Louisiana, was with an American friend on the way to a Halloween party. They missed the correct house by a few doors and rang the wrong doorbell. The frightened woman who answered the door called for her husband to get a gun. The boys left the property, but Hattori returned, probably because he mistook the homeowner's command of "Freeze" for "Please." The homeowner shot Hattori in the neck, killing him (Blakeman 2000).
- A fourteen-year-old girl jumped out of a closet and shouted "Boo" when her parents came home in the middle of the night. Taking her for an intruder, her father shot and killed her. Her last words were, "I love you, Daddy" (*Boston Globe* 1994).
- A twenty-year-old mother heard crunching noises on the gravel outside her home. Remembering reports of a recent burglary, she ran to

a bedroom and grabbed a small-caliber handgun. As she looked out the window for an intruder, the gun went off, striking her eight-month-old son in the head. The boy died seven hours later. The shooter's mother, stepfather, and thirteen-year-old sister returned home seconds after the shooting occurred (Moxley 2000).

- An eleven-year-old boy was trying to get three other boys, aged nine to eleven, to leave his trailer. He got his shotgun from his mother's room. He began arguing with his fifteen-year-old sister, and the gun went off, killing her. Neighbors said the boys had previously beaten up the eleven-year-old shooter (Vance 1999).
- A sixty-nine-year-old man critically wounded his seventy-two-year-old brother, thinking he was an intruder. The brothers lived together. The victim was shot by a .357-caliber revolver as he opened the front door (Craig 2000).
- A twenty-one-year-old woman wanted to surprise her new fiancé. With her eleven-year-old sister, she hid in his basement closet. When they jumped out, he killed her with a .40-caliber Glock handgun that he kept for protection (J. Anderson 2002).

Gun training in self-defense itself is not free of potential tragedy.

- A state trooper was shot and killed in a self-defense exercise by a fellow officer who forgot his gun was loaded (*Chicago Tribune* 1999).
- A co-owner of a music store was accidentally shot to death by his partner while the two men staged a mock robbery to rehearse how they would handle such an incident (*Boston Globe* 1999f).

Many reported self-defense incidents do not seem to be in society's interest. Our knowledge of these events comes primarily from surveys in which respondents report their side of a hostile interaction that usually occurred many months or years in the past. Still, many incidents appear to occur during escalating arguments; an objective observer indeed might classify them as criminal gun uses.

Since the early 1990s, at least six private surveys have asked adults whether they had ever used a gun in self-defense and followed up with detailed questions for those who answered in the affirmative. The first survey, by Kleck and Gertz (1995), produced the notorious 2.5 million estimate of self-defense gun use. Cook and Ludwig (1998) and McDowall, Loftin, and Presser (2000) analyzed two additional surveys. And the Harvard Injury Control Research Center sponsored three national telephone surveys (Hemenway and Azrael 1997, 2000; Hemenway, Miller, and Azrael 2000). The Harvard surveys seem to be the only ones to ask open-ended questions about the event. Some conclusions from the Harvard surveys follow.

First, many more people report a self-defense gun use against an animal than against a human (those surveys that find a lower rate often ask about animals only if the respondent first answered in the affirmative to "any self-defense gun use"). The main animals defended against were, in descending order, snakes, dogs, bears, raccoons, and skunks.

Second, police reported more total self-defense gun uses than did all civilians combined. This result is different from the NCVS, since, in those surveys, law enforcement officers can report using a gun in self-defense only if they personally were the victims of an attempted crime. Since police often use their weapons against criminals who have committed crimes against other people, the NCVS may miss some of the on-the-job police gun use that is reported on private surveys.

Third, excluding police, a handful of civilians report most of the self-defense incidents. For example, in a 1994 Harvard survey of eight hundred gun owners, five respondents reported 70 percent of the total self-defense gun incidents in the past five years; in a 1996 Harvard survey of nineteen hundred individuals, three respondents claimed 74 percent of the total incidents reported; and in the 1999 Harvard survey of more than twenty-five hundred adults, one respondent reported fifty self-defense gun uses (54 percent of the total incidents reported). One might ask, who are these people who continually use guns, and are all these events really self-defense?

Finally, and most importantly, many of the self-defense uses that were reported appear both illegal and undesirable. Five criminal court judges from across the United States read the thirty-five descriptions of the reported self-defense uses from the 1996 and 1999 surveys. Even assuming the gun ownership and carrying were legal and the description of the event was accurate, in more than half the cases, the majority of judges rated the self-defense gun use as probably illegal (Hemenway, Miller, and Azrael 2000). Three criminology students read a summary of the respondents' accounts from the 1996 survey and rated only 25 percent as socially desirable (Hemenway and Azrael 2000).

McDowall, Loftin, and Presser (2000) used a split-survey technique: for half of respondents, they used the NCVS approach, asking first about attempted crimes against the respondents and then about self-defense gun use; for the other half they used the Kleck approach, asking first about self-defense. The researchers found that the second group reported many more gun uses. After analyzing the follow-up questions, they concluded that many of these incidents "relied heavily on respondent judgments about the motives of possible offenders, and motives may be murky if the respondents acted quickly. . . . The gun use may follow mistaken perceptions of innocuous actions by the supposed criminal. These cases of armed resistance would then legally amount to aggravated assaults" (14–15).

Cook and Ludwig also found in their survey that many of the incidents described by respondents as self-defense gun uses might well be illegal and were certainly of questionable social value. The authors concluded,

> Most commentators have assumed that the [defensive gun uses] reported by survey respondents are actions that would be endorsed by an impartial observer who knew all the facts. Yet the sketchy and unverified accounts available from surveys leave considerable uncertainty about what actually happened, whether the respondent was the victim or the perpetrator, and whether the respondent's actions were otherwise legal, reasonable, and in the public interest. (1996, 58)

Information is often available on self-defense gun uses that result in death. In 2001, the UCR reported 585 justifiable homicides, 63 percent by the police. Of the 215 civilian justifiable homicides, 176 were with firearms (U.S. Department of Justice, FBI 2003). The UCR's annual justifiable homicide figure may be an underestimate since some jurisdictions also have an "excusable" homicide category, and many homicides ultimately ruled noncriminal by prosecutors or judges are reported as criminal since that is how they were treated in the initial police investigation (Kleck 1991). However, in many instances when grand juries decline to indict, the shooting remains questionable. Examples from Texas include:

- Tommy Dean Morris, fifty-four, a twenty-one-year veteran of the repossession business, was shot dead when he tried to repossess a pickup truck. The owner, who was behind on his payments, shot Morris twice with a rifle and claimed to have thought that Morris was stealing the truck (Locy 1994).
- Andrew DeVries of Scotland was fatally shot by a Houston home-owner who thought DeVries, who was knocking on the door, was try-

ing to break into the house. DeVries was intoxicated, lost, and trying to find his way back to his hotel (Locy 1994).

- Jason Williams, seventeen, was shot when a man found Williams in bed with his fourteen-year-old daughter. The father claimed he thought Williams was an intruder in his home (Locy 1994).
- Delivery driver Kenny Tavai, thirty-three, was fatally shot by Gordon Hale, forty-two, during an argument after Tavai's side mirror grazed Hale's pickup. Witnesses said Hale fired after Tavai left his car and punched Hale. Hale was the first Texan to use his legally concealed handgun in a fatal shooting (*Boston Globe* 1996).

A 1994 ABC News report on guns and self-defense also described shootings in self-defense. In one case, in Colorado Springs, Colorado, fifty-five-year-old Vern Smalley told police that seventeen-year-old Carmine Tagliere was tailgating Smalley's car. Smalley admits that the two exchanged obscene gestures. When Tagliere tried to pass Smalley on a highway on-ramp, Smalley cut him off. Smalley abruptly motioned for Tagliere to pull over, claiming to have intended to scold the youngster for his driving. Tagliere got out and angrily approached the car. Smalley reached into his glove compartment and placed a gun in his lap. Smalley says that Tagliere came up to the car and punched him in the face. Tagliere turned and started to walk away from the vehicle. Witnesses say that Smalley said something and the young man returned to the window. Smalley shot Tagliere in the neck, killing him. The jury found Smalley not guilty of murder in the second degree. Diane Sawyer summed up the various cases on the show: "By and large, victims who claim they pulled a gun in self-defense seem to get the benefit of the doubt from juries" (ABC News 1994).

Few statistics are available on nonfatal self-defense shootings. However, some illuminating results come from surveys of criminals who have been shot. For example, in one study of detainees being held for crimes in Washington, D.C., 24 percent had previously been shot. Of the shootings, 4 percent were by police, and none were by civilian victims of crime. These criminals were not shot while they were committing crimes but instead were shot while they were being victimized—such as during robberies and assaults, during arguments, or when they were caught in cross fire (May et al. 2000b). If criminals are not being shot by decent, law-abiding citizens, who are these self-defense gun users shooting?

There is no question that citizens sometimes justifiably shoot criminals.

For example, in Jacksonville, Florida, in 1997, a seventeen-year-old with a shotgun tried to rob the cashier at a restaurant full of senior citizens. The teen ordered the thirty patrons to hit the floor and told the waitress to open the cash register. Two elderly, armed patrons (one eighty-one years old) opened fire on the robber. One of the bullets hit the teen in the stomach. He fled and was subsequently arrested (*Boston Globe* 1997a). Yet even in this type of case, when there is no ambiguity about the criminal or the self-defense gun use, one wonders whether, on average, having seniors shooting in restaurants increases or decreases the chance of injury to other patrons.

Some self-defense gun uses certainly are in the public interest. However, from society's point of view, a problem exists analogous to the false-positive problem that plagues estimates of rare events. The possibility of using a gun in a socially useful manner—against a criminal during the commission of a crime—will occur, for the average person, perhaps once in a lifetime (or less often). It is an extremely rare event. By contrast, at any other moment, the use of a gun against another human is socially undesirable. Regular citizens, who are sometimes tired, angry, drunk, or afraid and who are not trained in dispute resolution, have lots of opportunities for inappropriate gun use. People engage in innumerable annoying and somewhat hostile interactions with each other in the course of a lifetime. It is not surprising that, from an objective public health perspective, false-positive "self-defense" gun uses by people who believe they are "decent, law-abiding citizens" may outnumber their legitimate and socially beneficial uses of guns (Hemenway, Miller, and Azrael 2000).

HOW EFFECTIVE IS SELF-DEFENSE GUN USE?

With respect to self-defense gun use, *effectiveness* can have two meanings: preventing the crime and catching the criminal. Some of the proponents of self-defense gun use tend to focus on the latter meaning. Tom Diaz, a writer formerly immersed in the gun culture, says gun owners often fantasize about using their guns against intruders. They fantasize about the kill. "It was almost as if they wanted someone to break in because they wanted to shoot someone. I think that's very scary, and dangerous. But that's the way people think about guns. I know because I was around it, and I talked to those people all the time" (Frey 1999).

A study of Good Samaritans—specifically, private citizens coming to the aid of victims during crimes—found that the Good Samaritans were often gun owners and gun carriers. The prime motive for the intervention was often anger against the criminal rather than concern for the victim. The authors concluded that the Samaritans have a low boiling point and seem to see their intervention as a contest between themselves and the criminal, while the victim is the occasion rather than the reason for action. As an example, the authors provided a story from the *Los Angeles Times.*

> A motorist saw a truck strike a pedestrian and then drive away. The motorist gave chase and forced the hit-and-run driver to the side of the road. He then took out a shotgun he had in his car and held the truck driver at gunpoint until the police arrived. Meanwhile, the woman who had been hit by the truck was left lying in the road, and died an hour later in the hospital. (Huston, Geis, and Wright 1976, 64)

The second issue is whether guns are useful in trying to stop crimes. The issue is controversial. Even given a completely unambiguous interaction—when the other party is definitely a robber or assailant—whether one should resist the criminal at all is much debated. More difficult is the question of whether it makes sense to try to use a firearm to resist. Kleck claims that NCVS data show that guns help prevent robberies from being completed and reduce the chance of injury to the victim. For example, in the NCVS, while 25 percent of robbery victims who did nothing were injured, only 17 percent of those who defended themselves with a gun received a physical injury (Kleck 1997b). More pertinent NCVS data provide information on whether victims were injured after (and not before) they tried to act in self-defense. Such data indicate that using a gun may not be much better at preventing injury than various other self-defense measures. For example, victims appear no more likely to be injured once they threaten the criminal with any weapon, or call the police (table 4.1). In addition, other data suggest that while resisting with a gun might reduce the chance of being injured, it increases the likelihood of being killed (Zimring and Zuehl 1986).

The most careful study of the relationship between victim resistance and injury and death in robberies finds that the existing data do not sufficiently take into account the differences in circumstances or type of robberies and thus do not support any conclusions about the victim's safest course of action when confronted by a robber. Author P. J. Cook concludes,

> I am convinced that victims should comply with an armed robber's demands in most cases and that it is a particularly dangerous and fool-

hardy act to forcefully resist a robber with a gun. This judgment is based on what I like to think of as common sense. The data indicate that most victims act as if they agree with this judgment. I further believe that there are exceptions to the "no forceful resistance" rule, cases in which the robber intends to inflict serious injury on the victim. The upshot is that some victims save their lives by resisting and some lose their lives by resisting. Currently available data are not helpful in suggesting how to increase the former or to reduce the latter. (Cook 1986, 416)

Results from the NCVS and the Harvard Injury Control Research Center surveys indicate that self-defense with weapons other than guns is far more common than self-defense gun use. Indeed, in the Harvard surveys, there were more incidents of successful self-defense with a baseball bat than with a firearm. A principal conclusion from these surveys is that individuals without guns are not necessarily unarmed (Hemenway and Azrael 1997; Azrael and Hemenway 2000; Hemenway, Miller, and Azrael 2000). Self-defense is not solely or even primarily for those with guns readily at their disposal.

SUMMARY

Self-defense gun use is a somewhat nebulous concept. Criminals, for example, often claim that they carry guns for protection and use them during crimes in self-defense because they felt threatened by the victim. Most of the

TABLE 4.1. Victims Physically Injured After Self-Defense, 1992–98 (in percentages)

Selected Types of Victim Action	Robbery	Assault	Burglary
Threaten or Attack with Gun	8	4	2
Threaten with Other Weapon	0	3	0
Run/Drive Away/Tried to	5	5	29
Call Police, Guard	3	5	3
All Incidents with Self-Defense	7	8	4

Source: Data from National Crime Victimization Surveys, 1992–98; Kleck and Kates 2001 (289).

self-defense gun uses reported on private surveys appear to be both illegal and against the public's health and welfare. Of course, there are undoubtedly many instances of successful and socially beneficial self-defense gun uses. Each month, the *American Rifleman*, the magazine of the National Rifle Association, features about a dozen accounts of armed citizens defending themselves based on newspaper clippings submitted by NRA members. Yet even these stories may not always be what they purport to be (Magnuson 1989).

Surprisingly, although protection and self-defense are the main justifications for a heavily armed citizenry, there is little evidence of any net public health benefit from guns. No credible evidence exists for a general deterrent effect of firearms. Gun use in self-defense is rare, and it appears that using a gun in self-defense is no more likely to reduce the chance of being injured during a crime than various other forms of protective action. No evidence seems to exist that gun use in self-defense reduces the risk of death; case-control studies of firearms in the home fail to find any lifesaving benefit, even when exclusively considering cases involving forced entry (Kellermann et al. 1993).

Whatever one thinks about the benefits of self-defense gun use, reasonable gun policies—such as requiring manufacturers to meet minimum safety standards or requiring background checks on sales at gun shows—would have little effect on the ability of responsible adults in the United States to defend themselves with guns.

CHAPTER 5   LOCATION

Dear Miss Manners: When my little Johnny wishes to play at Jimmy's house, how do I ask Jimmy's parents if they keep firearms, and if so, whether they store them in a locked cabinet?

Dear Gentle Reader: When one child visits another, the visitor's parent uses an apologetic tone—as if to admit that her fastidiousness is slightly comic—when she explains rules that may conflict with the standards of the household visited: "I'm afraid we feel Johnny is too young to play in houses where there are firearms. If that is a problem, perhaps you would send Jimmy to play with him here instead" (Never mind the fact that Johnny may be 40).

—Miss Manners

Gun use can occur in various locations, including at home, at school, and on the street and in other public venues. This chapter examines guns in these three settings, starting with the home. The first section describes empirical evidence on the actual and psychological risks and benefits of having a gun in the home, the way Americans store their guns at home, and the effects of firearms training on gun storage and use. The second section discusses the prevalence and consequences of guns in schools, including colleges. The final section describes public opinion about carrying guns in public and the evidence concerning the effects of state gun-carrying laws.

GUNS IN THE HOME

While firearms have a variety of purposes, the principal reason most Americans claim for having a handgun is protection. Yet the evidence indicates that, in most households, a gun makes the home less safe.

Having a gun in the home has many risks and benefits. Early studies focused on one of the most palpable and easily measured uses of a gun at home—to kill. Researchers found that a gun in the home was much more likely to kill innocent victims than criminals. For example, a study using medical examiner records from Cuyahoga County (Cleveland), Ohio, for 1958–73 found 115 fatal gun accidents occurring at home, compared to killings by residents of 23 burglars, robbers, or intruders who were not relatives or acquaintances, a five-to-one ratio (Rushforth et al. 1975).

A study in King County, Washington, which includes Seattle, examined a more complete record of gun deaths occurring at home, including family suicides and murders, in the period 1978–83. Only 2 of the 398 gun deaths at home involved intruders who were shot during an attempted entry, and only 9 were "self-protection" homicides. For every self-defense homicide involving a firearm kept in the home, there were 1.3 accidental deaths, 4.6 criminal homicides, and 37 firearm suicides (Kellermann and Reay 1986).

In an even more complete study of gunshot injuries in the home, researchers examined nonfatal injuries as well as deaths. A study of firearm injuries in three cities (Memphis, Tennessee; Seattle, Washington; and Galveston, Texas) in 1992–94 found 626 fatal and nonfatal shootings occurring at residences. Only 13 injuries were considered legally justifiable or acts of self-defense. Three of these self-defense shootings were by law enforcement officers acting in the line of duty; 3 women shot former boyfriends; 1 man shot his brother; and 6 citizens shot strangers, nonintimate acquaintances, or unidentified assailants. Examining only cases in which the gun involved was known to be kept in the home, guns in the home were four times more likely to be involved in accidents, seven times more likely to be used in criminal assaults or homicides, and eleven times more likely to be used in attempted or completed suicides than to be used to injure or kill in self-defense (Kellermann et al. 1998).

A similar study of all gunshot injuries in Galveston, Texas, over a three-year period found only two incidents that were related to residential burglary or robbery. In one, the homeowner was shot and killed by a burglar; in the other, the homeowner shot the burglar. During the same interval, guns in the home were involved in the death and injury of more than one hundred residents, family members, friends, or acquaintances (Lee et al. 1991).

It is more difficult to measure other risks and benefits of having a gun in the home, including the use of guns to threaten and intimidate family, friends, and acquaintances. Guns in the home, particularly gun collections, may increase the likelihood of burglary by criminals enticed by these valuables (Cook and Ludwig 2003). And an intruder may gain access to a gun in the home and use it against the resident (Kellermann et al. 1995).

Guns in the home may also provide benefits to the owner and to the community. Guns may deter intruders who fear confronting homeowners armed with firearms; high gun prevalence in the community may deter intruders from all homes, since they may not know who has firearms. Guns may be used to thwart attempts at crime. And guns may provide psychological benefits if they make household members feel more secure. However, while the evidence on these issues is scattered and only suggestive, it indicates that overall, guns in the home increase the danger for the family and for the community.

In one study, guns were used far more often in the home to intimidate and frighten intimates than to protect against intruders. Other weapons (e.g., baseball bats, clubs, knives) were used far more often for protection than were firearms (Azrael and Hemenway 2000). A household without a firearm is not an unarmed household or one incapable of defending itself.

In another study, researchers reviewed Atlanta police records to identify every reported case of unauthorized entry into an occupied, single-family dwelling. Of the 197 cases found, only 3 victims (1.5 percent) successfully used guns to defend themselves (2 only brandished the gun, and the other fired but missed the intruder), while in 6 of the cases (3 percent), the victim lost his or her firearm to the intruder (Kellermann et al. 1995). It would be useful to have prospective studies of this sort, where a priority would be to ask specifically about self-defense gun use.

Guns in the home increase the risk of unintentional firearm injury, suicide, and homicide. For example, a recent case-control study found that a gun in the home is a large risk factor for accidental firearm fatality (Wiebe 2003a). All nine case-control studies of guns and suicide in the United States found that a gun in the home is a significant and substantial risk factor for suicide. Not surprisingly, states with more guns have higher suicide rates (Miller and Hemenway 1999; Miller, Azrael, and Hemenway 2002a, 2002b, 2002d). Two case-control studies found that a gun in the home doubled the relative risk for homicide (Kellermann et al. 1993; Cummings, Koepsell et al. 1997). Kellermann and coauthors (1993) found that almost all of the higher risk for homicide resulted from a greater risk of homicide by a family member or close acquaintance; no protective lifesaving benefit was found for gun ownership, even in the homicide cases involving forced entry.

Theoretically, guns in the home can potentially deter and thwart burglaries and home invasions. However, no study has found such an effect. Instead, states and counties with more guns have more burglaries and more burglaries when someone is at home (Cook and Ludwig 2003). Guns are highly desirable items for burglars; it is estimated that almost half a million guns are stolen each year (Cook and Ludwig 1996), and many of them are subsequently used in crime.

A gun in the home can have psychological benefits for members of that household. For example, in one telephone survey of individuals who stated that protection was the main reason they owned a gun, 89 percent answered "yes" when asked "Do you feel safer because you have a gun at home?" (Kleck 1991). Such a finding is not surprising. If the guns made them feel less safe, owners could simply get rid of them.

But gun ownership can also have a psychological impact on other people, and here the evidence is less positive. Theoretically, a gun in household A could make neighbors feel more safe (e.g., because they believe household A's gun will help deter crime in the neighborhood) or less safe (e.g., because they believe the gun will increase the likelihood of accidents, might be used against others during an argument, or might be stolen and used by criminals).

To try to address this issue, a 1994 national survey of adults asked, "If more people in your community were to acquire guns, would that make you feel more safe, less safe, or the same?" The large majority of respondents—more than 85 percent of non–gun owners and a plurality of gun owners—said "less safe." Women in particular were likely to feel less safe (Hemenway, Solnick, and Azrael 1995a). A 1999 national random-digit-dial survey obtained similar results: 50 percent would feel less safe, and 14 percent more safe. By a ratio of seven to one, women would feel less (60 percent) rather than more safe (8 percent). Nonwhites were also especially likely to feel less safe (61 percent) rather than more safe (11 percent) (Miller, Azrael, and Hemenway 2000).

Certain individuals are at high risk for gun mishaps in the home. For example, elderly Americans with Alzheimer's disease or other forms of dementia are often a danger to others as well as to themselves. Assault by demented persons is a common reason for their psychiatric hospitalization. Yet psychiatric patients commonly have access to loaded firearms. One study of dementia patients at a southern hospital found that 60 percent lived in households with firearms and that fewer than 20 percent of these families knew for sure that the guns were unloaded (Spangenberg et al. 1999).

The danger of having a gun in the home is especially serious for children and adolescents. In one study of youth under the age of twenty in a metropolitan area, 76 percent of firearm suicide attempts and more than 50 percent of accidental firearm injuries occurred in the victims' homes. An additional 8 percent of firearm suicide attempts and almost one-third of firearm accidents occurred at the homes of friends or relatives. More than 90 percent of the unintentional shootings occurred in the absence of adult supervision (Grossman, Reay, and Baker 1999).

A goal of the Healthy People 2000 was to reduce the percentage of people living in homes with improperly stored firearms (U.S. Department of Health and Human Services 1990). If a gun is to be kept in the home, experts agree that it should generally be stored unloaded and locked up, with the ammunition stored separately—whether or not there are children in the household (Police Executive Research Forum 1990; American Academy of Pediatrics 1994; International Hunter Education Association 1998; Glock 2002; Remington 2002; Sporting Arms and Ammunition Manufacturers' Institute 2002). A few experts make a partial exception for guns owned for self-protection. An undated National Shooting Sports Foundation brochure, *Firearm Safety in the Home,* says, "Unload all firearms before taking them into the home. . . . Handguns should be stored in a locked cabinet or drawer. Locked storage is particularly important if there are children in the home." The same organization's *Handgun Guide* states, "Bring only unloaded handguns into the home and then lock them up out of reach of children. . . . Lock your ammunition in a safe place away from the firearm." However, this publication adds, "If self-protection is an overriding consideration, you may keep the handgun readily available but *unloaded* and the cartridges separate from it." In what appears to be their latest brochure, *Firearm Responsibility in the Home,* a loaded gun is permitted for protection, but "you must exercise full control and supervision over a loaded firearm at all times. This means the firearm must be unloaded and placed in secure storage whenever you leave your home. Secure ammunition separately." The National Rifle Association (NRA) training curriculum seems to go the farthest in relaxing the storage rules. A gun kept in the home for protection, according to the NRA, is "always in use" and may be stored loaded, although in a secure place, inaccessible to unauthorized users and in accordance with local laws (NRA 1990).

The evidence shows that many gun owners report following the most stringent guidelines, but a sizable minority do not. Two national telephone surveys have found that 21 percent of gun owners store a firearm both loaded and unlocked in the home and that, of gun owners with children under eighteen at home, as many as 14 percent store at least one gun loaded and unlocked (Hemenway, Solnick, and Azrael 1995b; Stennies et al. 1999). Similarly, a large study of parents with children found that 12 percent of handgun owners stored a gun both loaded and unlocked (Senturia, Christoffel, and Donovan 1996).

Gun safety training is often suggested as a way to increase responsible use and storage of firearms (Koop and Lundberg 1992; Zwerling, McMillan, and Cook 1993), and the majority of gun owners favor "requiring people to take safety classes in order to qualify to own a gun" (Teret et al. 1998). However, a national telephone survey found that gun owners who had received formal training—training that almost always covered gun storage practices—were more likely to store their guns in the least safe way (loaded and unlocked), even after controlling for more than a dozen factors, including whether the gun was kept for protection (Hemenway, Solnick, and Azrael 1995b). A more recent national survey also found that gun training was associated with inappropriate storage practices (Harvard Injury Control Research Center 2001). Similarly, a survey in rural Iowa found that having taken a gun safety course was associated with more than double the likelihood of storing a gun loaded and unlocked. In addition, households with someone with a lifetime prevalence of alcohol abuse or dependence were twice as likely as other households to report having loaded, unlocked firearms (Nordstrom et al. 2001).

Other surveys also find no evidence of any beneficial effect of gun training on storage practices (Weil and Hemenway 1992; Goldberg et al. 1995; Cook and Ludwig 1996), except possibly for training provided by the National Safety Council (Cook and Ludwig 1996). Mandatory training, at least the kind that has generally been provided, may not be the most effective way of improving storage practices and reducing gun accidents.

Another popular panacea often put forth by gun advocates are programs that educate children about the dangers of guns, such as the NRA's Eddie Eagle. Although the NRA continuously touts Eddie Eagle, no evaluation study shows that it or any similar program reduces inappropriate gun use. A randomized control study of children four to seven years old found that those who had participated in weeklong firearm safety programs were no less likely to play with guns (about 50 percent of the children) than those who had not (Hardy 2002). An earlier study had a police officer instruct a class of children four to seven years of age, "Don't touch guns—they're dangerous. If you see a gun, leave the area. Go tell an adult." The children learned the lesson—they could tell you what they would do if they saw a gun. But when they were left alone with real guns, they picked them up and shot at everything in sight. The results were shown dramatically on ABC's *20/20* on May 21, 1999.

Other television programs have run similar hidden-camera experiments with children, with similar findings that stunned the parents (MSNBC, "Topeka, Kansas" 1999). The psychologist who directed the ABC study asked, "Would your child pick up a gun? Would he shoot a friend? Shoot himself? Mine would, and so would dozens of other children at his day-care center. . . . We childproof medicine bottles and swimming pools. But we put loaded handguns in bedroom drawers" (Hardy 1999).

A study of eight- to twelve-year-old boys reported similar findings. Separated into small groups and placed in a room for fifteen minutes with a handgun hidden in a drawer, more than two-thirds discovered the handgun, more than half of the groups handled it, and in more than one-third of the groups someone pulled the trigger. More than 90 percent of the boys who handled the gun or pulled the trigger reported that they had previously received some sort of safety instruction (Jackman et al. 2001).

Another study of children four to six years of age in day-care centers further illustrates why it is so important for parents who own guns to store them properly. All of the children whose parents owned a gun were aware of that fact, including 24 percent whose parents claimed the children were unaware. And almost 20 percent of the children with guns in their houses reported that they had played with the guns without their parents' permission or knowledge (Hardy et al. 1996).

One of the strongest arguments against child gun-safety programs like NRA's Eddie Eagle is that rather than encouraging parents to acknowledge the inherent dangers guns in the home pose for children, these programs place the onus of responsibility on the children themselves. Yet as one team of pediatricians concluded,

> There is no evidence that safety lessons are retained by children at the critical times when they confront a loaded weapon. Indeed, the combination of the high stakes involved, death or disability, and the propensity of children to forget rules while playing or upset makes [safety education] a dubious approach at best. (Dolins and Christoffel 1994, 646)

Frighteningly, many gun-owning parents do not have a good understanding of child development and have unrealistic views concerning their child's safety around guns. In a study of suburban Atlanta-area parents with children aged four to twelve years old, 87 percent believed that their children would not touch a real gun if given the opportunity. Fourteen percent said they would trust their four- to seven-year-old with a loaded gun. Fewer than half of the parents stored all their guns unloaded and locked up (Farah, Simon, and Kellermann 1999). In a randomized telephone survey of urban and rural parents in northeast Ohio who had children aged five to fifteen in their homes, 87 percent believed that their children would not touch guns they found (Connor and Wesolowski 2003). Given the prevalence of guns in the United States, our gun storage practices, and our parental misunderstanding of children's capabilities, is it any wonder that our unintentional death rate from guns for five- to fourteen-year-olds is seventeen times higher than that of the other high-income nations?

Methods exist to improve gun storage and handling practices. These include community, city, and statewide prevention programs (Becker, Olson, and Vick 1993; Horn et al. 2003), such as the community handgun safety campaign in Charlotte, North Carolina, that led to a significant increase in the number of firearms locked up (though no change in other gun-related behaviors, including whether the gun was stored loaded) (Vogel and Dean 1986).

More generally, candid advice and counseling from physicians, particularly pediatricians and family physicians, might have an impact on gun storage and gun handling practices. Most pediatricians and family practitioners believe that physicians have a responsibility to counsel families about firearms, though most doctors rarely give such advice (Grossman, Mang, and Rivara 1995). The large majority of patients with children would find physicians' advice and information on safe storage practices helpful and would consider or follow a provider's advice not to have a gun in the home (Haught, Grossman, and Connell 1995). A recent study of a brief office counseling by family physicians found a significant reported change in safe storage habits two to three months after intervention (Albright and Burge 2003).

Getting patients to remove guns from the home, even for high-risk families, appears to be a more daunting task. In a study of adolescents with major depression, clinicians urged the removal of firearms from the home. By the end of the intervention, 27 percent of the families with firearms had removed them from the home; unfortunately, however, 17 percent of families without firearms had acquired them (Brent et al. 2000). A study of psychiatric patients who had threatened to harm themselves or others with firearms or had access to firearms showed more success. Treatment and discharge planning focused on removing firearms from the home was fully successful at discharge, though some discharged patients were able to gain access to firearms within twenty-four hours (Sherman et al. 2001).

Rather than trying to teach all children about gun safety (which may just increase their curiosity and interest in guns), many pediatricians and public health and child advocates believe we should target parents, teaching them how to prevent firearm injuries. A Massachusetts nonprofit group, Common Sense about Kids and Guns, uses public service ads to try to make unloading, locking, and storing guns properly as automatic as buckling a safety belt (Robinson 1999).

Another approach, also focusing on adults, is a hospital-based speakers' bureau to help educate parents in the community. In Kansas City, nurses were trained to use the American Academy of Pediatrics–developed speaker's kit that emphasizes developmental risk factors for children and the importance of safe gun storage. On a prepresentation survey, only 10 percent of participants asked the parents of their children's friends if they had guns in their homes. On a postpresentation survey, 75 percent indicated that they would be likely or very likely to ask that question (Dowd et al. 1999). The national ASK campaign, in collaboration with the American Academy of Pediatrics, encourages parents to "Ask your neighbor if they have a gun before sending your kids over to play" (PAX 2002). Changing such social norms is an important part of the public health approach to reducing firearm injuries.

Retailers could provide better point-of-sale education on safe firearm storage. Few firearms salespeople currently seem to provide relevant information. In visits to nearly one hundred dealers in two metropolitan areas, researchers asked for suggestions about keeping their four-year-old children safe with a gun in the home. They discovered that only 8 percent of dealers had any safe storage educational materials on site, and only 9 percent offered advice that included keeping guns locked and unloaded with the ammunition stored separately (Sanguino et al. 2002).

Liability laws also might alter gun storage behavior. In an attempt to reduce firearm accidents involving children, a number of states have added to existing tort liability by passing statutes holding adults criminally liable for a child's death resulting from the negligent storage of a gun. Most statutes declare that use of a locked box, container, or a trigger lock constitute legal storage. One study of state fatalities estimated that these laws may have reduced accidental shooting deaths among children under age fifteen by at least 6 percent and perhaps much more (Cummings, Grossman, Rivara, and Koepsell 1997); however, the results occurred because of a large reduction in only one state (Webster and Starnes 2000). Another study found that these laws had no effect on accidental shooting deaths among children (Lott and Whitley 2001).

While many policies could reduce gun injuries at home, changing attitudes and behavior is never easy. In the *New England Journal of Medicine*, editor Jerome Kassirer related the story of a letter he received from a surgeon on the West Coast, who said,

> Guns are single answers for situations they [members of the NRA] fear they will face. If anyone asks you, send them to me. I once had to go from the operating room to tell a young couple that their little boy was dead—shot while playing with his father's handgun. The mother collapsed into tears. The father, who told me he was an NRA member, did not cry, but became visibly angry, saying, "I taught the dumb kid how to use it right." (1993, 1119)

As Kassirer pointed out, "That kind of passion dies hard" (1993, 1119). But that is no reason not to try to reduce the risk—to gun owners, their families, and others—that guns in the home can present.

GUNS IN SCHOOLS

In prison in the 1990s when someone was losing control, inmates would often say, "Now don't go postal on me." Beginning in 1999, they began saying, "Now don't go high school on me."

—A. Browne

Schools are among the safest places in America in terms of homicide—less than 1 percent of all homicides among school-aged children occur in or around school grounds or on the way to and from school (Kachur et al. 1996). The number of students murdered while at school has remained fairly constant for the past decade, staying between thirty and thirty-five each year (Small and Tetrick 2001). Yet our schools are far less safe than those of other high-income countries, just as our streets and homes are far less safe. The easy access to firearms allows such lethal violence.

In the past few years, the violent and suicidal fantasies of a small number of adolescents have been played out for real in our nation's classrooms. The shootings have had terrible consequences—for the shooters, the victims, the witnesses, the local community, and our broader society. It is a sad sign of the times that the National Education Association, the leading teaching union in the United States, now offers its 2.6 million members a special insurance deal for an "unlawful homicide" benefit worth $150,000 to the families of those killed at work (D. Campbell 2001). It is also a sad sign that many high schools in the United States now believe it necessary to run "code red" drills or lockdowns, the modern version of the 1950s nuclear war drill. Students are trained to lock the classroom door and make the room look empty so potential killers will move on to easier targets (Ruane 2001).

Although the frequency of school shootings has not changed, the type of killing has, as has the amount of media attention and the public perception of a substantial problem. Most of the killings in the earlier 1990s were in urban schools, and many were gang-related or single-victim stabbings or fights over girlfriends. These incidents prompted a federal law banning guns from schools, security measures such as metal detectors, and efforts to control the gang influence. In the late 1990s, however, the major events occurred in white rural or suburban areas, with little gang involvement. These more recent killings involved multiple victims. Indeed, the proportion of all school-associated student homicides that involved multiple victims rose from 0 percent in 1992 to 42 percent in 1999 (M. Anderson et al. 2001). Ten of the most notorious incidents occurred in the late 1990s.

1. *Moses Lake, Washington, February 2, 1996.* A fourteen-year-old honor student opens fire in his junior high algebra class, killing the teacher and two students and wounding another. The perpetrator, who learned how to shoot firearms from his father, is armed with three family firearms, including a .25-caliber semiautomatic pistol; the guns were taken from an unlocked cabinet and the family car. The shooting ends when he is tackled by a teacher.

2. *Bethel, Alaska, February 19, 1997.* A sixteen-year-old kills a student and the school principal and wounds two other students. The perpetrator uses a twelve-gauge shotgun kept unlocked at the foot of the stairs in his foster home. A friend had dissuaded him from killing himself, convincing him instead to murder. The killer exchanges shots with the police before surrendering.

3. *Pearl, Mississippi, October 1, 1997.* A sixteen-year-old stabs his

mother to death, then kills two students and wounds seven others at his high school with his .30-.30 deer rifle. The youth leaves the school and is driving away in his mother's car when he is stopped by the assistant principal, who has grabbed a .45-caliber pistol from his pickup truck.

4. *West Paducah, Kentucky, December 1, 1997.* A fourteen-year-old kills three students and wounds five others at a prayer group meeting in a high school hallway. The perpetrator uses a .22-caliber Ruger automatic pistol stolen from a neighbor's garage. Although a round remains in the chamber and he has brought along four other firearms, he drops the pistol when approached by the principal and another student and is led to the principal's office without a struggle.

5. *Jonesboro, Arkansas, March 24, 1998.* From the woods, an eleven-year-old and a thirteen-year-old shoot and kill four girls and a teacher and wound another ten students after setting off a fire alarm at a middle school. The perpetrators, who were trained with guns (one took along his hunter education card), took a cache of firearms from one boy's grandfather's unlocked closet, including a .44 Magnum semiautomatic hunting rifle with a telescopic sight and an M-1 carbine Remington .30-.06 hunting rifle. Police capture the shooters running through the woods.

6. *Edinboro, Pennsylvania, April 24, 1998.* A fourteen-year-old uses a .25-caliber handgun registered to his father to shoot a science teacher to death in front of students at a middle school graduation dance being held at a restaurant. The youth walks out of the dance and is coaxed into giving up his weapon by the restaurant owner, who has grabbed his shotgun.

7. *Springfield, Oregon, May 21, 1998.* A fifteen-year-old opens fire in a high school cafeteria, killing two students and wounding eighteen. His parents are later found dead in his home. Taking his own guns, locked away by his father, the perpetrator shoots fifty rounds from a .22 semiautomatic Ruger rifle. While reaching for his Glock handgun, he is wrestled to the ground by other students.

8. *Littleton, Colorado, April 20, 1999.* Two heavily armed seniors storm a suburban Denver high school, and, in a shooting rampage on a scale unprecedented in an American school, kill thirteen people and wound another twenty-eight. They primarily use a TEC-DC9

semiautomatic handgun and 9mm 4-point carbine rifle purchased by a girlfriend at a gun show. Early on in their rampage, the shooters trade shots with an armed school guard. Hours before a SWAT team enters the building, the perpetrators shoot and kill themselves.

9. *Conyers, Georgia, May 20, 1999.* A fifteen-year-old wounds six students twenty minutes before classes start. The perpetrator, a trained marksman who often went hunting, breaks into his stepfather's locked gun cabinet and takes a rifle and pistol. He shoots below the knees with the rifle, seeking to wound rather than to kill. Then he falls to his knees and sticks a .22-caliber pistol in his mouth. The assistant principal approaches and asks for the gun. The boy gives the man the gun and starts crying, "Oh my God, I'm so scared, I'm so scared." The mostly white, suburban school had video surveillance cameras and an armed sheriff's deputy on duty.

10. *Fort Gibson, Oklahoma, December 7, 1999.* A thirteen-year-old wounds four classmates outside a middle school building in this small rural town before classes start. The perpetrator, described as a popular, churchgoing, honor roll student, uses a 9mm semiautomatic pistol his father had purchased a few years previously at Wal-Mart. The youth fires at least fifteen times; he drops the gun when a science teacher approaches and pins the boy against a wall.

What is most striking about these ten incidents is the young age of many of the shooters and that these were multiple shootings, with many of the victims killed almost at random. The shootings had many similarities, and some may have been copycat assaults (Egan 1998; Lawrie and Kuesters 1999).

All the shooters were male. In most cases, the perpetrators were children who felt inferior or picked on, with grudges against other students or teachers. The shooters were typically immersed in violent pop culture, from movies to rap music to video games. Many of the shooters were suicidal (M. Anderson et al. 2001). And most were of above-average intelligence. Their killings may be viewed as a way to end their lives in a blaze of terror. Part of the tragedy of all these killings is the tragedy to the shooters and their families. Most could have led normal and productive lives had they gotten through the difficulties of adolescence. In hindsight, the shooters gave many warning signals, from detailed school essays to verbal and physical threats and assaults. And, finally, and perhaps most significantly, all the killings involved firearms, which were readily available to these young people. The specific firearm used—its capability for rapid-fire and bullet caliber—seems to have influenced the number of victims who were shot and killed.

In two cases (Edinboro and Pearl) civilian guns may have helped capture the perpetrator, but they did not seem to limit the number of people injured. Heroic civilian action without guns limited the number of victims in some cases (Springfield, West Paducah, and Moses Lake) and may have prevented a suicide (Conyers).

Each year brings new tragedies. In February 2000, in Flint, Michigan, a six-year-old boy shot a schoolmate named Kayla to death in their first grade classroom. The boy waved his weapon at several classmates before leveling it at Kayla, saying, "I don't like you," and pulling the trigger. He put the gun in his desk and ran into the hallway, where he was caught by school officials. The gun was a .32-caliber Davis automatic pistol, described in dealer literature as "our original pocket pistol" (Goldberg 2000; Naughton and Thomas 2000).

In March 2001, at a high school in Santee, California, a San Diego suburb, a fifteen-year-old fired about thirty rounds from his father's .22-caliber Arminius revolver, killing two students and wounding thirteen others. The shooter reloaded four times, ducking inside the boys' bathroom to reload. Armed officers burst into the rest room and pointed their guns at the perpetrator, preventing further shootings (Dillon 2001; Fox 2001).

The shootings never seem to stop. For example, a quick web search for September 26, 2003, found three news reports concerning school shootings. In Cold Spring, Minnesota, a fifteen-year-old high school freshman killed one student and wounded another; the shooter then pointed the gun at a gym coach but put it down when the coach yelled "No" (*Minneapolis-St. Paul Star Tribune* 2003). In Los Angeles, students and teachers praised the surrender of two reputed gang members sought for a drive-by shooting at a crowded bus stop outside Taft high school in which three students were shot in the chest (*Mercury News* 2003). And in Lawndale, North Carolina, a thirteen-year-old middle school student brought a 9mm semi-automatic gun to school and fired two shots into the ceiling. Fortunately no one was injured, though students and parents were nervous and scared, and the shooter was taken into custody by a school resource officer (News 14 Carolina 2003).

In the wake of any gun tragedy, the response of one extreme faction in the American gun debate is to call for a ban on all guns; the response of the other extreme is to advocate the arming of citizens. The *Wall Street Journal,* for example, ran op-ed pieces claiming that the way to reduce school lethal violence is to arm teachers and train them in self-defense (Lott 1998b; Ayoob

1999). Fortunately, this is not the way we handled the cowboy problem of the 1880s or the airline hijacking problem of the 1970s. Nor is it the way any other country has responded to school shootings.

With a few terrible exceptions (e.g., Dunblane, Scotland), school violence in other developed countries throughout the 1990s was typically less deadly than in the United States, for guns were less available. For example, in Wolverhampton, England, in 1996, a crazed thirty-five-year-old attacked pupils picnicking at St. Luke's Infants' School, where students were aged four to seven. Police arrested the man after a search of the area, and three adults and four students were taken to the hospital. None of the wounds were fatal—the man was wielding a machete (BBC 1996).

Surveys sponsored by the World Health Organization find that the United States is an average high-income country in terms of school bullying (*Louisville Courier-Journal* 2001), but we are an exception in terms of lethal school violence. Unfortunately, in the past few years, copycat school shootings were seen throughout the industrialized world, though still far below the rate of the U.S. school shootings.

In the United States, more than six thousand students were expelled from schools in 1996–97 for bringing guns to school (U.S. Department of Education 1998). In surveys, about 3 percent of high school respondents claim to have carried guns to school. For example, a survey of high school seniors found that 3 percent reported carrying guns to school in the past month (National Center for Education Statistics 1999). A 1995 nationally representative school-based sample of adolescents in grades seven to twelve found that access to a gun at home was associated with carrying a gun to school (Swahn and Hammig 2000).

In a survey of more than two thousand middle school students in North Carolina in 1995, 3 percent reported carrying a gun to school. Gun carrying was associated with cigarette, alcohol, and illegal drug use (DuRant et al. 1999). In a survey of more than twelve hundred seventh and tenth graders in inner-city schools in Boston and Milwaukee in the mid-1990s, 3 percent reported bringing guns to school in the past month (Bergstein et al. 1996). Our analysis of this data indicates that those carrying a gun to school were more likely to smoke, to have poor grades, and to live in households with firearms. In a 1993 national survey of sixth- to twelfth-graders, about 4 percent said that they had taken guns to school in the previous year. Because of the false-positive problem for rare events described in appendix 1, an extrapolation of these figures will probably lead to an overestimate. Nonetheless, it suggests that while school officials have been cracking down on gun carrying, they are probably not catching most carriers.

A recent National Academy of Sciences report on school shootings concludes that it is virtually impossible to identify the likely offenders of rampage school shootings in advance and emphasizes the fact that all these young people had easy access to firearms. A key policy recommendation of that research team is to find more effective means of realizing "the nation's long established policy goal of keeping firearms out of the hands of unsupervised children and out of our schools" (Moore et al. 2002, ES-6). A Centers for Disease Control study of school shootings between 1992 and 1999 found that the majority of the firearms came from the perpetrators' homes or from friends and relatives. That report emphasized the need for safe firearm storage (CDC 2003a).

The danger to adolescents in the United States from firearm availability and use is illustrated by the life of Richard Peek Jr., who was wounded in the 1998 school cafeteria shooting in Springfield, Oregon, and whose parents filed a $250,000 lawsuit against the student shooter and his parents. In October 1999, a little over a year after those shootings, Richard was hunting deer with his seventeen-year-old brother and was shot in the head and killed when his brother's rifle accidentally discharged (*Boston Globe* 1999g). Guns are dangerous consumer products; it is not only during intentional attacks that firearms can turn deadly.

It is also not only in junior and senior high schools in the United States where guns have been used to kill or maim: college campuses are not immune to the danger. Spectacular news coverage of shootings at colleges offers a sharp contrast to the idyllic images of sanctuaries far removed from the violence that characterizes life outside the walls of higher learning. For example, in 1991, at the University of Iowa campus in Iowa City, a disgruntled doctoral student killed three professors, a student he saw as a rival, and an administrator and paralyzed a staff member—using a legally purchased handgun (Cotton 1992). In 1995, a student at the University of California at Davis accidentally shot himself twice in the hand and another student four times in the chest while converting a semiautomatic firearm to an automatic weapon (*New York Times*, Jan. 24, 1995). In 1998, at North Carolina State University, a twenty-one-year-old student fired several shots from his handgun at a party across the street from his town house. One of the bullets grazed a North Carolina State wrestler, and a half dozen people from the party went to the town house and assaulted the shooter. The shooter's gun somehow went off, and he was killed. Alcohol was a contributing factor in the entire episode (Fitzsimon 1998).

In the mid-1990s, some writers claimed that guns at college were becoming a public health problem. For example, one article reported, "Guns—for years a scourge of the nation's high schools—are a growing menace on college campuses" (Lederman 1994, 33). Another piece contended, "Each year, campus violence with injuries increasingly involves firearms. . . . The prevalence of alcohol and firearms on and around college campuses has had deadly effects" (Nichols 1995, 2). Responding to such reports, the Association for Student Judicial Affairs unanimously adopted a 1994 resolution urging colleges to support tough rules and laws to keep guns off campuses (Lederman 1994). More than 90 percent of American adults want to outlaw gun carrying on college campuses (Hemenway, Azrael, and Miller 2001).

Two recent surveys provide some information about the availability of guns at colleges. In a 1997 national random survey of students at 130 four-year colleges, 3.5 percent of students (6 percent of male students) reported having a working firearm at college. Students with guns were more likely to attend public rather than private colleges, to attend school in the South or West, to belong to fraternities or sororities, to live off campus, and to have various alcohol problems. After accounting for age, gender, race, and other factors, individuals with guns were found significantly more likely to engage in reckless behavior involving alcohol, including driving while intoxicated, damaging property, and sustaining an alcohol-related injury (Miller, Hemenway, and Wechsler 1999).

A 2001 national random survey found that 4 percent of students reported having guns at college. Those with guns were much more likely to smoke, binge drink and drive, and, when under the influence of alcohol, to vandalize property and get into trouble with police. In regions with high levels of firearm ownership, there were many more guns on college campuses, and students reported being the victims of many more threats with guns (Miller, Hemenway, and Wechsler 2002).

Many colleges and universities forbid gun possession on campus, but this policy may not be well enforced. In 1996, the University of Northern Arizona's student newspaper reported that although guns were not allowed on campus, some students kept them in their dorm rooms. At that school, the police department maintains a locker in the station house where students are encouraged to store their firearms. A spokesman for the campus police said the locker contains forty to fifty guns at any one time (Join Together Online 1999).

In Iowa, some town-gown cooperation exists regarding handguns. Iowa state law requires each handgun-purchase applicant to file a petition with the local police chief, who conducts a background check. The sheriff contacts the University of Iowa whenever a student applies for a handgun permit so that university officials can inform the sheriff if they know of any problem with granting the petition (Join Together Online 1999).

GUNS IN PUBLIC

We have law-abiding citizens who have to leave their weapons in their car when they take their family out for a nice dinner. . . . This is just a major inconvenience.
—Virginia State Senator Stephen H. Martin

Most homicides, robberies, and stranger victimizations occur outside the home. When guns are involved, as they are for most homicides and many robberies, the gun is usually being carried illegally.

Illegal gun carrying became common among inner-city youth in the early 1990s. Studies conducted at that time consistently found that approximately one-quarter of teenage boys in the inner city had carried handguns at some time and that the principal reason for carrying was protection against other teenage boys (Blumstein and Cork 1996; Hemenway et al. 1996).

In the past few years, a variety of national surveys have examined gun carrying among adults (Cook and Ludwig 1996; Hemenway and Azrael 1997; Kleck 1997b; T. W. Smith 2001). Data are now available on the percentage of people reporting that they carried guns within the past year or the past month; whether the firearm was a handgun or long gun; whether the gun was carried in a vehicle or on the person; whether the gun was carried for work; whether the gun was carried primarily for protection or for some other reason; and whether the gun was carried for protection against people or against animals.

T. W. Smith (2001) estimates that more than 8 percent of adults carried a gun for protection at least once in the preceding year. Cook and Ludwig (1996) estimate that 7.5 percent of the adult population carried a gun for protection in the preceding year. After eliminating those carrying only for work, the Cook and Ludwig figure becomes 5.4 percent of adults. Of these, about half (2.6 percent) carried a gun on their person rather than only in their vehicle.

Two Harvard Injury Control Research Center national surveys asked about gun carrying in the preceding month and obtained roughly comparable results. For example, on the 1996 survey, after excluding police, security guards, and military personnel, about 3 percent of adults reported carrying guns on their persons during the previous month. Of these, a little more than half claimed that they carried a gun to protect themselves from people; the rest cited protection against animals, recreation, or some other reason.

Compared to the rest of the adult population, those carrying guns on their persons were more likely to be male, to live in rural communities, to lack confidence in the police, to smoke, and to binge drink (Hemenway and Azrael 1997). A 1994 survey also found that, like gun owners generally (Cook and Ludwig 1996), those who carry for protection are more likely than the rest of the adult population to have been arrested for a nontraffic offense (12 percent of those arrested carry a gun, compared to 8 percent of those never arrested) (T. W. Smith 2001).

The gun carrying–arrest association is disturbing. So too is the gun-alcohol connection, which turns up in many studies. A study of adults in Oregon found that gun carriers were more likely than non–gun carriers to be current alcohol users and to have consumed five or more drinks on one or more occasions in the past month; they were also less likely to use seat belts (Nelson et al. 1996). Following the passage of a Kentucky concealed-gun-carrying law, a telephone survey in one county there found that, compared to other citizens, heavy drinkers were more likely to want concealed-gun licenses (Schwaner et al. 1999). Adolescent gun carriers in Boston and Milwaukee have also been found to be more likely than other teens both to smoke and to binge drink (Hemenway et al. 1996).

National surveys find that gun carrying in a vehicle is more common than gun carrying on the person. The surveys also find that adults who carry guns, whether on their persons or in their vehicles, tend to have higher-than-average incomes.

A 1999 survey in Arizona found that 11 percent of motorists always or sometimes carried guns in their cars. Those carrying were significantly more likely than other respondents to have closely followed other cars and to have made rude gestures at other drivers during the past year. Data were not available on whether motorists with guns typically drove more or less often than other respondents (Miller et al. 2002).

A 1999 death in Alabama illustrates the dangers of having a gun in the car. Two women, aged thirty-four and forty, were driving home from work when one cut the other off on a congested highway. Their rage escalated as traffic crawled for miles and the women flashed their headlights and hit their brakes.

Both vehicles left the interstate, heading for home. At the first traffic light, one woman left her car and approached the other, perhaps to put an end to the confrontation. The woman in the car shot the approaching woman in the face, killing her. The shooter wept, repeating, "Oh my God, I shot her, Oh my God, I can't believe I shot her, Oh my God, I can't believe she's dying" (Sipress 1999). Events like this occur far more frequently in the United States than in any other high-income country.

Public opinion polls consistently show that the large majority of Americans do not favor civilian gun carrying. For example, a 1991 CBS News/*New York Times* national telephone poll asked, "Do you think that when ordinary people carry weapons like guns or knives or mace they make the streets safer, or do you think carrying weapons creates more problems than it solves?" Sixty-nine percent answered "more problems," 15 percent said "safer," and 16 percent either said "don't know" or did not answer.

A 1996 national telephone survey conducted by the National Opinion Research Center asked, "Do laws allowing any adult to carry a concealed gun in public provided that they pass a criminal background check and gun safety course make you feel more safe or less safe?" Fifty-six percent of respondents replied "less safe," compared to 36 percent who said "more safe" (Hemenway, Azrael, and Miller 2001).

The 1996 Harvard Injury Control Research Center national survey asked, "Some states have recently changed their laws concerning gun carrying. . . . If more people in your community begin to carry guns, will that make you feel more safe, the same, or less safe?" Sixty-two percent said "less safe," and 12 percent said "more safe." A majority said they would feel less safe rather than more safe, independent of their age, race, gender, income, or region or whether they lived in a city, suburb, or rural area. The groups significantly more likely than others to believe that they would feel less safe were non-whites, women, urban dwellers, individuals with children, and people who do not own guns (Hemenway and Azrael 1997; Hemenway, Azrael, and Miller 2001). A 2001 national poll by the National Opinion Research Center asked an almost identical question and obtained nearly the same results: 64 percent said they would feel less safe, and only 9 percent said they would feel more safe if more people in their community began carrying guns (T. W. Smith 2001).

In 1999, Missouri held the first state referendum on a permissive gun-carrying proposal. (Missouri had initially banned the carrying of concealed weapons in 1875, when Jesse James was still at large.) Professional sports teams in Missouri, fearing for the safety of players, fans, and referees, strongly opposed the relaxation of the state's gun-carrying laws. The chiefs of the baseball and football players' unions were similarly opposed. Don Fehr, executive director of the baseball players' association, declared that the proposition was "one of the most dangerous ideas we have had to confront" (*Hannibal Courrier-Post*, March 25, 1999).

Although the gun lobby spent some $3.8 million on the campaign, an amount far greater than its opponents, the measure went down to defeat, as suburban white voters and black city voters more than offset the support of rural Missourians. Preelection polling had shown that women were far more opposed to the permissive gun-carrying proposal than men (Edsall 1999). Nonetheless, in 2003, state lawmakers, overriding the governor's veto, voted to make Missouri a permissive gun-carrying state (*Kansas City Star* 2003).

At one extreme in the contentious American gun debate are those who would ban all gun carrying. At the other extreme are those who would allow gun carrying anywhere for virtually anyone who is not an already convicted felon. The latter view is reminiscent of Archie Bunker's solution to the airline hijacking problem of the 1970s: "If everyone was allowed to carry guns, them hijackers wouldn't have no superiority. All you gotta do is arm all the passengers. Then no hijacker would risk pullin' a rod" (Landes 1978, 1).

In most places, more guns typically mean more danger. The airlines took the disarmament route, checking everyone to prevent guns being taken onboard planes, and until the terrorist suicide attacks of September 11, 2001, hijacking problems had largely disappeared. However, since those attacks, pilots have received permission to carry firearms on their planes if they desire. No evidence yet exists on the effect of this new policy. By contrast, inside prisons, which are filled with the most violent members of society, guards on the prison floor do not carry guns, as it is widely agreed to increase the danger for everyone.

In 1999, a Harvard Injury Control Research Center national survey asked, "Do you think regular citizens should be allowed to bring their guns into (a) restaurants, (b) bars, (c) college campuses, (d) hospitals, (e) sports stadiums, and (f) government buildings?" The overwhelming majority of Americans— generally more than 90 percent of respondents—said "no" to each location (Hemenway, Azrael, and Miller 2001a). A 2001 national poll by the National Opinion Research Center obtained similar results (T. W. Smith 2001).

Yet state gun-carrying laws are typically quite permissive; for example, in 2000, twenty-two states allowed gun owners to carry concealed weapons into places of worship (Black and Bush 2000). Yet even the Mormon church, based in Utah, where most households own guns, says that even legally concealed firearms do not belong in houses of worship (Harrie 1999).

Four generic types of state gun-carrying laws currently exist: (a) carry prohibited; (b) "may issue" (police have some discretion over who receives a permit); (c) "shall issue" (police must provide a permit to anyone who is not expressly prohibited by statute); and (d) no carry restrictions. Currently, seven states effectively prohibit concealed carry, eight states let police authorities use discretion in granting permits, thirty-four states require licensing authorities to issue permits to any applicant who meets the specific criteria, and one state (Vermont) does not regulate concealed carry. Although popular opinion prefers more stringent gun-carrying laws, the trend is toward the more permissive. Between 1985 and 1991, thirteen states moved from may-issue to shall-issue status; between 1994 and 1996, another fifteen states became shall-issue; and between 2000 and 2003 another five states became shall-issue. These changes have created something of a natural experiment, and many studies have tried to evaluate the effects of these changes to more permissive concealed carrying laws.

The first study examined the effects on homicide in the large urban areas of Florida, Mississippi, and Oregon before and after the change in the law. Results showed that firearm homicides increased after the law became more permissive, with little change, on average, in nongun homicides (McDowall, Loftin, and Wiersema 1995).

Since then, many large statistical (econometric) studies have used data from all states to examine the effects on crime of more permissive gun-carrying laws. The most sophisticated studies try to take into account that the effect of the law may differ among states, that crime moves cyclically, and that crime rates may influence the passage of gun-carrying legislation.

One such study that included state-specific nonlinear trends found that permissive gun-carrying laws appeared to increase the number of assaults but had no significant effect on homicides, rapes, or robberies (Black and Nagin 1998). Another sophisticated study exploited the minimum age requirements for concealed-carry permits to control for omitted variables. Using adolescent crime rates as controls, the analysis found that shall-issue laws resulted, if anything, in an increase in adult homicides (Ludwig 1998).

Still another study attempted to account for the fact that the effect of the law depends on economic and demographic characteristics. It found that permissive gun-carrying laws appeared to increase robbery and usually increased aggravated assault and perhaps even rape but reduced homicide (Dezhbakhsh and Rubin 1998). Conversely, other statistical studies found evidence that permissive gun laws reduced violent crime (Olson and Maltz 2001; Plassmann and Tideman 2001). These studies looked at data only through 1992 and one of the authors (Maltz) subsequently realized that the county-level data used in these analyses had so many errors (e.g., missing values) that the results lacked any degree of reliability (Maltz and Targonski 2002, 2003).

Because so many state gun-carrying laws have been recently enacted, it is important to analyze recent state data. A study using data through 1997 (Donohue 2003) disaggregated the results by state and found that murder rates increased significantly in nine states and decreased in four states following the passage of permissive gun-carrying laws. Another recent study using more current data compared the change in homicide rates for each state enacting shall-issue laws with the other forty-nine states and with states without such laws; again, most states that changed to permissive gun laws saw a relative increase in their homicide rates after the laws were enacted. Overall, gun-carrying laws had no statistically significant effect on homicide (Hepburn et al. 2003).

One study by John Lott (1998a) has frequently been cited in the national gun debate. The initial results seemed to show that permissive gun-carrying laws significantly reduced murder, rape, and aggravated assault but not robbery and increased larceny, auto theft, and property crimes generally (Lott and Mustard 1997).

In at least eight published articles, more than a dozen academics have found enough serious flaws in Lott's model to discount his findings (Alschuler 1997; Webster, Vernick, and Ludwig 1997; Zimring and Hawkins 1997a; Black and Nagin 1998; Dezhbakhsh and Rubin 1998; Ludwig 1998; Duggan 2001; Ayres and Donohue 2003a, 2003b). These studies found, among many other problems, that Lott did not sufficiently account for the cyclical nature of crime or the differing nonlinear effects of the laws on various localities. The general consensus among those who have seriously analyzed the results is that any "inference that is based on the Lott and Mustard models is inappropriate, and their results cannot be used responsibly to formulate public policy" (Black and Nagin 1998, 219). The results of extending Lott's model through 1999, once his data coding errors are eliminated, show no significant effect of concealed carry laws on crime, except to increase property crime (Ayres and Donohue 2003a). Results from a more appropriate model suggest that permissive gun carrying laws increase violent crime in most states (Ayres and Donohue 2003b). Lott's conclusion (2003) that concealed-carry laws have reduced multiple-victim public shootings also appears to be incorrect (Duwe, Kovandzic, and Moody 2002). (See appendix A on gun carrying.)

Overall, the results of the econometric analyses of concealed-carry laws have been inconsistent. The evidence from the most credible analyses and those with the most recent data (e.g., Duggan 2001; Ayres and Donohue 2003; Hepburn et al. 2003) suggest that permissive gun-carrying laws may not have had large effects but that, if anything, they may have led to increased levels of violent crime: "The best evidence suggests overall small *increases* in crime associated with adoption of concealed-carry laws" (Ayres and Donohue 2003a, 1397).

The studies discussed here investigate the association between types of gun-carrying laws and crime rates. None examine actual gun carrying. A recent study investigated the effects of changes in concealed carry permits on crime in Florida counties, 1980 to 2000. Florida was an important state to examine because many beneficial effects of permissive carrying laws in Lott's model disappear if Florida is excluded from the analysis. The study found little evidence that changes in gun carrying permits had any effect on violent crime in Florida (Kovandzic and Marvell 2003).

Three pieces of the evidence about actual gun carrying suggest that the effects of the passage of the shall-issue laws should be fairly modest. First, not many people are obtaining permits. In Florida, for example, seven years after the state passed a permissive law, well under 2 percent of adults had obtained permits. A review of sixteen other concealed-carry states also found that in most, fewer than 2 percent of adults had obtained permits (Hill 1997).

In addition, many permitted carriers seem to have simply moved from illegal to legal status: in North Carolina, 85 percent of those who carry permitted guns in their cars did so before they had obtained permits, as did 34 percent of those permitted carriers who carry guns on their persons (Robuck-Mangum 1997). In a recent national survey, only 31 percent of self-reported concealed-gun carriers said they had permits to carry concealed weapons; among those who said they had permits, 73 percent said there was no change in gun carrying after they obtained the permit, 14 percent reported an increase in carrying, and 9 percent reported a decrease (T. W. Smith 2001).

Finally, most of the people who are obtaining permits are at low risk for victimization. In Dallas, less than 1 percent of the population had obtained a permit, and most lived in zip codes with very low levels of crime (Hood and Neeley 2000). In North Carolina and Texas, about 75 percent of those obtaining permits were over the age of forty, almost all were white, and more than half lived in rural areas. By contrast, those at highest risk to be victims of violent crime are the young, the poor, urban dwellers, and members of ethnic minorities (Hill 1997).

Nonetheless, evidence suggests that permitted carriers may give cause for concern. First, many were formerly carrying guns without permits, thereby willingly breaking the law. Second, information on the behavior of the specific people who obtain permits indicates that many are not particularly law-abiding.

In Texas, from 1996 to 1998, more than two thousand concealed-handgun-license holders were arrested for crimes. While license holders represent 1.4 percent of the state's population, they account for only 1.1 percent of those accused of crimes. But the rate of weapon-related offenses was higher among this group than among the general adult population (Violence Policy Center 1998).

In Florida, an MSNBC investigation reported,

During the past 11 years, the Secretary of State's Office has issued more than 535,000 licenses and revoked very few. Only about 1,100 permit holders have seen their licenses taken away after committing crimes or otherwise disqualifying themselves. That's an extremely small number of revoked licenses—that is, until you take a closer look. (MSNBC, "Special Report" 1999)

This investigation revealed that in one Florida county, many people who had licenses to carry were not the type of individuals who most of us would want legally packing heat. For example, Wayne W. was driving his pickup truck when he crossed paths with another motorist. Tempers flared, road rage escalated. Wayne rammed the stranger's vehicle with his pickup and got out with a loaded gun in his hand. Wayne ended up shooting his own finger. He was arrested for aggravated assault with a motor vehicle and aggravated assault with a firearm. He will apply for a pretrial intervention—a way for first-time offenders to avoid a trial and a criminal record and a way for him to keep his concealed-carry permit. Permits are revoked only when an arrest is followed by a conviction.

Herbert C. has three alcohol-related arrests on his criminal record: a conviction for driving under the influence and two more arrests last year—a wife-beating charge that was later dropped and a disorderly intoxication charge to which he pled guilty that stemmed from a bar fight during which he brandished a knife. Since none of these arrests resulted in a felony conviction, he legally retains his concealed-weapons permit. Herbert says, "I always enjoyed having a gun. I'm a good guy." While the arrests should have led to license suspension (but not revocation), Florida's Office of the Secretary of State only was aware of two of Wayne and Herbert's five arrests.

Compared to any other high-income country, gun carrying is relatively common in the United States. Much of this gun carrying, including that done by self-professed law-abiding citizens, appears to be done without a license and is done against the law. In recent years, many state legislatures have made gun-carrying laws more permissive by taking discretion away from the police. The best available evidence suggests that these changes may have increased rather than reduced violent crime.

SUMMARY

A gun in the home is a risk factor for suicide, homicide, and unintentional firearm fatality. It is also a risk factor for nonfatal gunshot injury. It even appears that a gun in the home is more likely to be used to threaten intimates than to protect against intruders. Other forms of home self-defense are often as effective and are far less dangerous.

Inappropriate gun storage is common and is most dangerous when children are living in the household. Formal firearm training does not appear to improve storage practices. There is evidence that current educational programs that focus on the child rather than the adult, such as the NRA's Eddie Eagle program, are not protective; if they give parents a false sense of security, they may well be counterproductive. A 2002 Packard Foundation report concluded,

> The potential of education approaches aimed at children and adolescents appears to be limited, making it critical that parents understand the risks that guns pose to their children, and take action to shield their children from unsupervised exposure to guns. (K. Reich, Culross, and Behrman 2002, 14)

One location with high-profile gun violence in the late 1990s was public schools. Though the frequency of school shootings has not increased, recent incidents have been unusual in that they did not occur so much in urban settings as in generally more peaceful suburban and rural communities. The shootings show that lethal violence can occur anywhere and to anyone in the United States and should serve as a wake-up call for Americans to reduce this threat to their children's safety.

Reducing school violence has become a priority issue for the United States. Prevention approaches include age-appropriate discussions with students about guns and violence, conflict-resolution and anger-management training, architectural design to eliminate dark and hidden spaces where crimes can occur, visual screening techniques to spot students with weapons, random searches, and strictly enforced sanctions for bringing guns to school (U.S. Departments of Justice and Education 1998).

However, it is crucial to recognize that "no school is an island: What happens to children inside and on the way to and from school reflects what is happening in surrounding communities" (Mercy and Rosenberg 1998, 159). School violence needs to be dealt with in its larger community context (Kachur et al. 1996).

A public health approach to reducing the violence emphasizes data collection, scientific study, a multipronged strategy, and coordinated action (Mercy and Rosenberg 1998). A logical first step, particularly for adolescents, is to devise methods to better separate youth from guns (Cook and Cole 1996). For example, better storage practices and increased regulation of gun shows might have averted a number of the most lethal school shootings.

Carrying guns in public can cause many problems, and shall-issue laws make it more likely that more individuals will carry. As J. Ludwig, a leading researcher, concluded,

> Permissive gun-carrying laws invest private citizens with the discretion to judge the intentions and guilt of other parties and to potentially wound or kill another citizen on the basis of this judgment. The difficulties of making such judgments in real time, and the weight that our society places on preventing injuries to innocent parties, are evidenced by the elaborate procedures that police departments undergo when an officer draws a weapon on duty. . . . A less obvious potential cost of permissive concealed-carry laws is that some criminals may respond to the increase in gun carrying among ordinary citizens by arming themselves in response, or by resorting to violence more

quickly when dealing with their victims. Moreover, increases in permitted gun carrying may make it more difficult for police to prevent illegal gun carrying. (Ludwig 1999, 5)

Gun carrying also has benefits. The carrying of guns may help thwart some crimes, although no one knows how many have been thwarted. Increased gun carrying by citizens may also deter some individuals from even attempting a crime, although there is no solid evidence concerning the size of this effect. Indeed, there is no solid evidence about the beneficial effects of gun carrying. Instead, there is evidence that indicates that much self-defense gun use, particularly nonhome self-defense gun use, is probably inimical to rather than beneficial for society (see chap. 4).

In the United States, a recent policy issue has been between may-issue and shall-issue gun-carrying laws at the state level. Shall-issue laws are more permissive, eliminating police discretion about who should be allowed to obtain a license. The difference between shall-issue and may-issue laws is thus not whether some legal gun carrying is beneficial but whether society benefits when permits are granted to specific people to whom the police would deny such permits. The question then is: Who are these people, and why don't the police want them to carry guns? Why is it in society's interest to allow these particular individuals to carry firearms?

Surveys indicate that the large majority of Americans prefer more restrictive gun-carrying laws. Findings on the effects of permissive gun-carrying laws (shall-issue) have not been consistent, but recent studies suggest that these laws may be detrimental to public health and safety.

Based on all available evidence, arming citizens to reduce crime—in the home, in schools, or on the streets—seems likely to increase rather than reduce the level of lethal violence. Every other high-income country has opted against allowing civilians to roam the streets with lethal weapons, whether concealed or not. Their records in preventing lethal crime are far better than ours.

CHAPTER 6   DEMOGRAPHY

Firearm problems strike different groups differently. For example, suicide is more of a rural problem, while homicide disproportionately affects city dwellers. Black Americans have about half the risk of suicide of white Americans but more than five times the risk of becoming homicide victims. This chapter describes the risk of firearm injury to four vulnerable populations— young children, adolescents and young adults, women, and African Americans.

YOUNG CHILDREN

There has been a growing recognition that the developmental factors that limit a child's ability to deal with the injury environment are a reason for modifying that environment rather than a cause for blaming the child's (or the parents') injury-avoiding inadequacies.

—T. Christoffel and S. S. Gallagher

One criterion by which a country may be judged is how it protects its children. By that criterion, the United States is doing very badly with regard to firearms. Each day during the 1990s, firearms killed an average of two children between ages zero and fourteen in the United States. Firearm injuries are not a major killer of children zero to four but rank as the fifth-leading cause of death for five- to nine-year-olds and the second-leading cause of death for ten- to fourteen-year-olds (National Center for Injury Prevention and Control 1995). And many children who do not die from bullet wounds are permanently disabled, either physically or psychologically.

On an average day in the United States, one child aged between zero and fourteen is murdered with a gun. Indeed, between 1990 and 2000, almost four hundred children per year were firearm homicide victims (table 6.1). Our firearm homicide rate for children between zero and fourteen is sixteen times higher than the average of other developed nations. Our overall homicide rate for this age group is five times higher (Krug et al. 1998) (see table 1.3). Firearms are used in about 70 percent of murders of children aged five to fourteen (but in only 10 percent of murders of children aged zero to four) (CDC 1997b).

Between 1990 and 2000, an annual average of 320 children aged zero to fourteen either committed suicide with guns or were accidentally killed by guns. Our firearm suicide rate for children between zero and fourteen is eleven times higher than that of other high-income countries, while our nonfirearm suicide rate is roughly similar. Our overall suicide rate for zero- to fourteen-year-olds is twice as high as that of other developed countries. Our unintentional firearm death rate for zero- to fourteen-year-olds is nine times higher than that of other developed nations (CDC 1997b).

An international study of twelve industrialized countries for which there were comparable data on gun ownership levels from telephone surveys found that, for children aged zero to fourteen, the percentage of households with guns was strongly and significantly associated with homicide rates, suicide

TABLE 6.1. Number of Firearm Deaths of Children between Zero and Fourteen (1990–2000)

	1990	1995	2000	Average
Firearm Homicide	390	462	227	392
0–4	69	82	40	69
5–9	63	70	50	66
10–14	258	310	137	257
Firearm Suicide	144	184	110	154
0–4	0	0	0	0
5–9	2	1	0	1
10–14	142	183	110	153
Unintentional Firearm Death	236	181	86	166
0–4	34	20	19	24
5–9	56	32	18	33
10–14	146	129	49	109
Total Firearm Deaths[a]	784	853	436	730
0–4	103	105	59	95
5–9	121	107	70	102
10–14	560	641	307	533

Source: Data from CDC 2003b.
[a]Includes undetermined and legal intervention firearm deaths.

rates, and accidental gun deaths (Lester 1999). Children in countries with lots of guns (e.g., Finland, Norway, the United States) were at far greater risk of these types of violent death than children in countries with few guns (e.g., the United Kingdom, Germany, the Netherlands).

The U.S. regions and states with the most guns have the highest rates of homicide, suicide, and accidental gun deaths of children. One study of children aged five to fourteen found that in states where more households had guns, significantly more children were dying violent deaths. Children in these states were substantially more likely to be murdered and to commit suicide (and to be killed unintentionally with firearms) (Miller, Azrael, and Hemenway 2002a). The differences in violent deaths resulted almost entirely from differences in gun homicides and gun suicides. The relationship between gun prevalence and the violent death of children remained even after accounting for state levels of poverty, education, and urbanization. There was no relationship between gun ownership levels and nonfirearm homicide or nonfirearm suicide.

To help illustrate these findings, table 6.2 compares the number of violent deaths to children aged five to fourteen in "high gun" versus "low gun" states, 1991–2000. For children in the high gun states, the gun homicide rate was 2.7 times higher, the gun suicide rate was eight times higher, and the unintentional firearm death rate was twenty-four times higher. Although there were virtually the same number of children in both groups of states, 211 committed suicide with a gun in the high gun states compared to 24 in the low gun states; and 261 were victims of fatal gun accidents in the high gun states compared to 10 in the low gun states (table 6.2).

For decades, physicians have been reporting on the dangers that guns pose to children. Detroit saw a large increase in firearms and firearm injuries to children in the late 1960s and early 1970s. In a study of children with gunshot wounds who had been treated at Detroit General Hospital from 1962 to 1971, interviewers asked each child and family what had happened. The answers included: (1) a six-year-old child was lying on a sofa recuperating from an illness when a playmate brought a loaded gun for him to play with; (2) a nine-year-old picked up a loaded gun with a hair trigger that was lying on a table at a friend's house; (3) a girl was at a birthday party when a boy pointed a gun (which he did not know was loaded) at the guest's temple; (4) a man in a vacant lot was shooting at tin cans with a rifle and hit a young passerby; (5) a thirteen-year-old thought he heard a noise and went to investigate, taking his father's rifle, which he unloaded except for the round in the chamber; he fell while going downstairs, killing one sibling and wounding another; (6) a four-teen-year-old heard a noise, got his parents' gun, and checked to see if it was loaded by pulling the trigger; (7) a child thought a gun was a cap gun and pulled the trigger; (8) a man heard a noise on his porch, shot through the door, and wounded a little girl next door (Heins, Kahn, and Bjordnal 1974).

A study of gunshot wounds treated at Los Angeles's King/Drew Medical Center during the 1980s found many shootings of children. Before 1980, physicians had not treated any children under age ten with gunshot wounds; thirty-four were treated between 1980 and 1987. Of these, almost 30 percent were caused by children playing with guns. Almost 30 percent were family disputes in which the child had been shot while the gun was aimed at another family member. Twenty percent were gang retaliation against an older sibling. In only one case was child abuse the cause of the shooting (Ordog et al. 1988).

TABLE 6.2.   Child Violent Deaths
Numbers of homicides, suicides, and unintentional firearm deaths among children between ages five and fourteen in the eleven U.S. states with the most guns and the five states with the fewest guns, 1991–2000

	High-Gun States	Low-Gun States	Mortality Rate Ratio: High-Gun/Low-Gun
Total Population (person years) at Risk: 1991–2000	28.5 million	26.2 million	
Homicides			
Gun Homicides	265	89	2.7
Nongun Homicides	142	100	1.3
Total	407	189	2.0
Suicides			
Gun Suicides	211	24	8.1
Nongun Suicides	118	110	1.0
Total	329	134	2.3
Unintentional Firearm Deaths	261	10	24.0

Source: Mortality data from CDC WISQARS 2003.

Note: Gun prevalence determined by the percentage of people in each state residing in households with firearms. Gun prevalence data come from the 2001 CDC Behavioral Risk Factor Surveys for each state. Similar results are obtained if the gun prevalence index is the percentage of suicides with guns, or "Cook's Index."

The eleven high-gun states are, in order, Wyoming, Montana, Alaska, South Dakota, Arkansas, West Virginia, Alabama, Idaho, Mississippi, North Dakota, and Kentucky; the five low-gun states are, in order, Hawaii, Massachusetts, Rhode Island, New Jersey, and Connecticut.

Despite the clear evidence that guns pose a serious risk for young children, some gun owners remain unmoved. In 1999 the *Boston Globe* interviewed vendors and customers at Florida's largest gun show. One of the seven individuals highlighted was Stephen Tressler, owner of more than 150 firearms, from handguns to assault rifles, and father of three-year-old Gage, who was also at the show.

Q: Do you have safety locks on your guns?
A: No, we don't have safety locks; never did when I was growing up. We never had any accidental shooting and my whole family was involved with guns.
Q: Aren't you worried about Gage with so many firearms in the house?
A: No, because he knows already at three he's not supposed to touch them. (Grossfeld 1999)

Children can be psychologically victimized not only when they are victims but also when they are the shooters. In West Virginia in 1999, a man was accidentally shot and killed while hunting rabbits with his six-year-old grandson. The boy slipped on a steep hillside near the family home, and the shotgun he was carrying went off and hit his grandfather (*Boston Globe* 1999a).

Many children in the United States have great anxiety about guns and violence. A national study of children aged six to eleven found that through their writing, artwork, photographs, and collages, almost two-thirds depicted intense, unsettling anxieties about guns, deaths, and violence. Among nine- to eleven-year-olds, the percentage rose to three-quarters (Sesame Workshop 2001).

Guns seem to provide few health or safety benefits to children. Firearms rarely protect children against criminal attack. For example, in three national self-defense gun surveys sponsored by the Harvard Injury Control Research Center, no one reported an incident in which a gun was used to protect a child under fourteen.

Even guns other than firearms are a danger to children. For example, in one urban pediatric trauma center, between 1988 and 1995, six children per year (median age eleven) were hospitalized from air gun injuries. Thirty-eight percent of them had serious long-term disabilities as a result of their injuries (Bhattacharyya et al. 1998).

With other products, society usually shows great concern for children's safety. For example, in the 1990s, six children per year died in bunk bed accidents. In response, the Consumer Product Safety Commission (CPSC) recalled more than 630,000 beds and created new regulations that toughened spacing requirements for lower bunks and required continuous guardrails on the wall side of top bunks (*Boston Globe* 1999e).

Similarly, in the mid-1990s the CPSC identified seventeen deaths over ten years—fewer than two deaths per year—when the drawstrings on children's clothing became entangled with playground slides, school bus doors, cribs, an escalator, a fence, a farm grinder, a turn signal lever, a ski chair lift, and a tricycle. The CPSC brought manufacturers together, persuaded them to replace strings with snaps and Velcro, and advised parents to remove drawstrings from existing clothes (U.S. Consumer Product Safety Commission 1996).

These immediate and successful redesigns (often on a voluntary basis with full industry participation), along with added regulations stand in sharp contrast to the situation with firearms, which cause more than fifty times the number of fatalities for young children as these more benign products.

ADOLESCENTS AND YOUNG ADULTS

Interviewer: Why did you fire, what was the situation?
Respondent A: Well, somebody played themself in trying, try to disrespect my moms, so I had to handle my business. May he rest in peace black.

Interviewer: Did you ever shoot anyone?
Respondent B: We had this conflict, this kid, I don't know him but we was just sitting next, and he exchanged words with my friend . . . some rude boy. So he was like, I heard him, so I turned around and said "yo, what the fuck is going on, yo," the kid talking about "what you gonna do," so I said "what you mean what I'm gonna do?" so I shot 'em.

Interviewer: How is manhood defined?
Respondent C: Manhood now it's like gunhood. If you got a gun you the man [laughing]. Ain't no more manhood, it's gunhood.
(Wilkinson and Fagan 1996 [interviews with sixteen- to twenty-four-year-old men released from Rikers Island Academy])

The transition from early teen to mature adult is a dangerous time for many people. The years from fifteen to twenty-four often involve great risk taking with decreasing adult oversight. Physical abilities are reaching their peak, but social and emotional maturity, judgment, and impulse control sometimes lag behind.

Not surprisingly, adolescents and young adults are at high risk for violent injury. The leading causes of death in this age group are unintentional injuries, homicides, and suicides; disease accounts for only 23 percent of all deaths among fifteen- to twenty-four-year-olds (Sells and Blum 1996).

Motor vehicle death rates peak at ages eighteen to nineteen, followed by ages twenty to twenty-four. The motor vehicle death rate per capita is twice as great for twenty- to twenty-four-year-olds as for forty- to forty-five-year-olds. Unintentional firearm death rates peak at ages fifteen to nineteen, followed by ages twenty to twenty-four. The fifteen- to nineteen-year-old unintentional firearm fatality death rate from 1990 to 2000 was almost four times higher than the forty- to forty-four-year-old rate (CDC 2003b).

Burglary and robbery rates are also highest for the fifteen- to twenty-four-year-old age group. The decade from ages fifteen to twenty-four is typically the peak of an individual's criminal history, and many delinquents grow out of criminal activities.

By far the highest rates of homicide victimization and perpetration occur among fifteen- to twenty-four-year-olds. And compared to other age groups, a higher percentage of homicides in this age group result from gunshot wounds. For example, in 2000, 3,963 fifteen- to twenty-four-year-olds were murdered with guns, while 976 were murdered by all other means combined (CDC 2003b).

Between 1990 and 2000, an average of almost seven adolescents aged fifteen to nineteen were murdered with guns each day. For young adults between twenty and twenty-four, the figure was almost nine gun murders a day. During this period, the firearm homicide victimization rate of twenty- to twenty-four-year-olds was more than triple the rate for forty- to forty-four-year-olds and was almost nine times the rate for sixty- to sixty-four-year-olds (CDC 2003b).

Homicide perpetrators typically resemble their victims in terms of age, race, and income. In 1997, the most frequent age for arrest for murder was eighteen, the second-most frequent age was nineteen, and the third-most frequent age was twenty. Of all gun homicides in which an offender was identified, eighteen- to twenty-year-olds committed 24 percent (U.S. Departments of Treasury and Justice 1999).

Like an epidemic disease, youth gun violence often moves in waves. Gun violence among adolescents and youths has long been endemic in our society, particularly in the inner city, but from 1985 to 1993 an epidemic of youth gun violence swept through the nation. According to criminologists A. Blumstein and R. Rosenfeld, the rise in homicides resulted from the

> introduction of crack in the mid-1980s; recruitment of young minority males to sell the drugs; arming of the drug sellers with handguns; diffusion of guns to peers; irresponsible and excessively casual use of guns by young people, leading to a "contagious" growth in homicide. (1998, 1208; see also Cork 1999)

The 1985–93 homicide epidemic was caused almost entirely by two factors: increased youth homicides and increased gun homicides. Looking at victims, for example, gun homicide rates more than tripled for adolescents and more than doubled for the twenty-to-twenty-four age group. Gun homicides increased only 30 percent for the thirty- to thirty-four-year-olds and decreased for older ages (figure 6.1). Nongun homicides, meanwhile, fell for all age groups (figure 6.2).

In 1983, about one thousand adolescents aged fifteen to nineteen were murdered with guns. A decade later, in 1993, that figure had tripled to more than three thousand. By contrast, nongun homicides for fifteen- to nineteen-year-olds over the same period fell by more than 20 percent. All epidemics wane as well as wax, and 1993 marked the peak of the adolescent gun crisis. By 2000, gun homicides in that age group had fallen back to about fifteen hundred per year—still worse than 1983. The same patterns held true for twenty- to twenty-four-year-olds over the same periods (CDC 2003b).

Young people in the United States are far more likely to kill each other than are youths in any other high-income nation. Our young people kill each other with guns and, unlike people of comparable ages in other industrialized nations, have ready access to handguns. A multitude of studies of junior high and high school students as well as studies of young criminals report the same thing: adolescents in cities and even in suburbs find it easy to obtain firearms. In 2000, a national survey of high school students found that almost half said it would be easy for a teenager to obtain a handgun in their neighborhoods (Gilbert 2000).

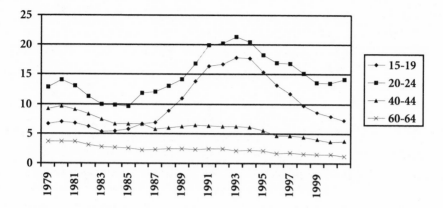

Fig. 6.1. U.S. firearm homicide death rates, 1979–2000 (per 100,000). (From CDC 2003c [accessed May 5, 2003].)

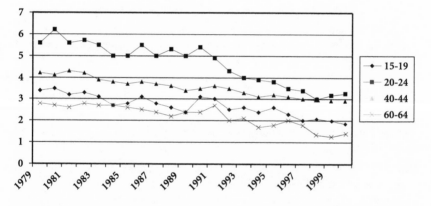

Fig. 6.2. U.S. Nonfirearm homicide death rates, 1979–2000 (per 100,000). (From CDC 2003c [accessed May 5, 2003].)

Many youths, particularly in the cities, carry guns, almost always illegally. The adolescents most likely to carry are those who engage in other high-risk, dangerous, and often illegal behaviors. These are the very adolescents we want not to carry guns. The main reason for carrying guns is protection or self-defense. The fact that many immature, high-risk individuals carry guns creates a need for others to carry (Callahan and Rivara 1992; Sheley, McGee, and Wright 1992; Webster, Gainer, and Champion 1993; New York Office of Oversight 1994; Sheley and Brewer 1995; Sheley and Wright 1995; Valois et al. 1995; Ash et al. 1996; Bergstein et al. 1996; McNabb et al. 1996; McKeown, Jackson, and Valois 1998; T. R. Simon et al. 1998; Hayes and Hemenway 1999; Luster and Oh 2001).

As an illustration of typical findings, consider an in-class survey of inner-city seventh- and tenth-graders in Boston and Milwaukee in the mid-1990s (Hemenway et al. 1996). Seventeen percent of the students reported having carried a concealed gun (which is illegal), including 23 percent of seventh-grade males. In other words, almost one in four of these inner-city males claimed to have carried a gun by age thirteen. While this type of study relies on self-report, the kids surveyed do not brag about everything. Only 9 percent reported smoking a cigarette in the past week, and 13 percent reported binge drinking; 28 percent said they had handled a firearm without adult supervision or knowledge (Bergstein et al. 1996).

Those who carried guns were more likely to smoke, binge drink, do poorly in school, and live in neighborhoods with numerous shootings. But given the small percentage of adolescents who smoke or binge drink, most of the youths who reported gun carrying were not smokers (76 percent), and most were not binge drinkers (73 percent).

The overwhelming majority gave protection or self-defense as their reason for carrying. They had reason to be afraid. Seventeen percent said there were a lot of shootings in their neighborhood. And young people are at greatest risk for being shot. Of all individuals shot in Boston in 1994, 76 percent were under twenty-five years of age (Massachusetts Weapons Related Injury Surveillance System 1996).

A contagion model is useful in understanding why so many of these adolescents were carrying guns. From their responses it appears that gun carrying made other students feel less safe, which increased the likelihood that they would in turn carry guns. Following their perceived need for protection, too many teens were carrying guns, and all were worse off than if fewer were carrying.

These youths were asked if they would prefer to live in a society where there were more guns, fewer guns, or the same number. Eighty-seven percent wanted fewer guns, and only 2 percent wanted more guns. Similarly, they were asked if they would prefer to live in a society where it was easy, very difficult, or impossible for teens to get guns. Seventy-six percent wanted it to be impossible, 19 percent wanted very difficult, and 5 percent said "easy." According to these youths, it is currently very easy for them to get guns. Even among those who had carried guns, a majority wanted it to be impossible for teens (including themselves) to obtain guns (Hemenway et al. 1996).

In a 2001 survey of twelve- to seventeen-year-olds in California, 33 percent reported that they had handled a gun, and 23 percent reported firing a gun. Yet 76 percent would prefer to live in a world where it was impossible for teens to gain access to guns, 21 percent wanted it to be difficult for teens to gain access to guns, and only 1 percent wanted it to be easy for teens to gain access to guns (Hemenway and Miller 2003).

From the late 1980s through the early 1990s, gun carrying and use by inner-city youths became increasingly common. An article on teens in inner-city New York reported that

> having a gun is normal—what's abnormal, they say, is to stay away from guns. . . . Guns are communal property among the members of a street crew, and everyone has a friend who's strapped, an older brother who's got a "swammie" and stands ready to help in the case of a beef. (Pooley 1991, 23)

Jealousy and revenge cause many shootings, but "most of the shoot-outs seem to have been caused by 'disses' and misunderstandings, paranoia and macho posturing" (27).

> For the teen gunman, the line between killer and killed is arbitrary. When teenage boys shoot it out with teenage boys, who gets buried or maimed and who gets arrested or goes on the run depends on the luck of the draw. Teenagers kill one another for the most trivial reasons: a casual insult, a careless look, an ill-timed jostle, a "dis" that leads to a "beef" that leads to a young man dead in the street. (25)

In one study of ten inner-city high schools in four states, 45 percent of the male respondents reported being threatened with guns or shot at on the way to or from school in the past few years (Sheley and Wright 1993). A longitudinal analysis of weapons use among inner-city youths concluded that, "consistent with the literature, the distinction between protective and aggressive weapon use is often a blurry one" (Tesoriero 1998, iii).

In sum, these youths

are scared—and rightly so. . . . The more kids arm themselves, the greater the chance of shootings, and the more readily kids arm themselves. Mix in youthful impulsiveness and the result is spur-of-the-moment mayhem. . . . These kids are armed and edgy. They believe they cannot walk away from a fight without irretrievably losing face. They are surrounded by violence, and feel that they have few alternatives. They cannot get out of Dodge, nor is anybody making them check their guns at the edge of town. Many of the kids involved in this life do not really want to live it. (Kennedy 1994, 78)

Rich, white suburbs are not immune to gun violence. For example, in a 1993 study of Jefferson Parish, Louisiana, a wealthy, predominantly white suburb of New Orleans, 17 percent of high school students reported that they had carried guns. More significantly, 23 percent reported that they had been threatened with guns in the past year (Sheley and Wright 1995).

More high school boys are carrying guns in states with high levels of gun ownership than in states with low levels (Wintemute 2003). How are boys in high-gun-density states getting guns? Probably from their homes or their friends' homes. Another way is theft. It is estimated that five hundred thousand guns are stolen each year (Cook, Molliconi, and Cole 1995; Cook and Ludwig 1996). In a survey of incarcerated felons conducted in the mid-1980s, about one-third had stolen their most recently acquired handguns (Wright and Rossi 1986). A grand jury in Dade County, Florida, was aghast at the ease with which youths could obtain guns, especially by theft:

Virtually every witness who appeared before us this term detailed the incredible ease with which firearms have become available to our children. They can get guns from friends, or buy them from strangers. They can get guns by stealing or even renting them from other children who have them. They can get guns through burglaries of businesses, homes, and cars.

In the personal experience of one 19 year old witness, acquiring a gun is "as easy as buying bubblegum." He was 14 years old when he stole his first gun. Another 16 year old witness was just 11 when a friend helped him steal a "38 special" from a closet during a home burglary. . . . They told us we could easily find guns in the closets and bedrooms of homes and in the glove compartment or under the seats of cars. They advised us to only look for guns in homes on weekdays during daytime hours when no one is home. They even gave us a method to determine if the home is occupied before trying to break in. Simply knock on the door first and, they said, if someone answers, apologize by saying this must be the wrong house. (Dade County Grand Jury 1997, 3)

Florida has lots of guns and fairly permissive laws concerning their purchase and carrying. By contrast, states such as New York and Massachusetts have much more stringent firearms regulations and fewer guns. Guns get into the hands of adolescents in cities such as New York and Boston not so much via intrastate theft from houses and cars as by gunrunning from states with more permissive laws.

A 1991 survey of more than eight hundred male serious offenders in six juvenile correctional facilities in four states (California, Louisiana, Illinois, and New Jersey) found that more than 70 percent reported that they would have "no trouble at all" obtaining guns after their release—most from the large, informal, inner-city street market in guns. More than half of these teenagers had stolen guns at least once in their young lives, and a third had asked someone to purchase guns for them at gun shops, pawnshops, or other retail outlets. Fifty-one percent of these boys could be described as gun dealers, having bought, sold, or traded a large number of guns. Theft was the most common way that guns were obtained for resale, but 20 percent of the inmates admitted to having gone to states "with very easy gun laws" to buy guns for resale in their neighborhoods. In other words, one in five of these teenagers were gunrunners (Sheley and Wright 1995).

In 1988, sixteen-year-old Nicholas Elliot walked into the Atlantic Shores Christian School in suburban Virginia Beach, Virginia, with a semiautomatic handgun hidden in his backpack, pulled it out, and began shooting. An article in the *Atlantic Monthly* magazine detailed how he obtained that weapon and concluded that

> a none-of-my-business attitude permeates the firearm distribution chain, from production to final sale, allowing gun makers and gun marketers to promote the killing power of their weapons while disavowing any responsibility for their use in crime. Nicholas carried a gun that should never by any reasonable standard have been a mass-market product. . . . His story describes a de facto conspiracy of gun dealers, manufacturers, marketers, writers, and federal regulators which makes

guns—ever more powerful guns, and laser sights, silencer-ready barrels, folding stocks, exploding bullets, and flame-thrower shotgun rounds—all too easy to come by, and virtually assures their eventual use in the bedrooms, alleys and school yards of America. (Larson 1993b, 49)

WOMEN

More than twice as many women are killed with a gun used by their husbands or intimate acquaintances than are murdered by strangers using guns, knives, or any other means.

—A. L. Kellermann and J. A. Mercy

Compared to men, few women in the United States are gun owners: while about 40 percent of men own firearms, only 10 percent of women own guns (Cook and Ludwig 1996; T. W. Smith 2001). When women do own guns, they likely do so for protection (Weil 1995). Although manufacturers targeted women in their marketing in the 1980s and early 1990s, the percentage of women in America owning guns did not change (Sheley et al. 1994; T. W. Smith and Smith 1995, T. W. Smith 2001).

Women are far less likely than men to be shot unintentionally; while more than one thousand men per year were killed in gun accidents from 1990 to 2000, an annual average of 143 women were killed unintentionally with guns (CDC 2003b). Not surprisingly, studies show tht women are far more likely to die unintentionally from firearms in states where there are more guns (Miller, Azrael, and Hemenway 2001, 2002b). For example, between 1991 and 2000, in the "high gun" states (where an average of 10 million women resided each year), 322 women died from unintentional gun injuries. In the "low gun" states (also where 10 million women resided each year), only 21 women died from unintentional gun injuries (table 6.3).

Women attempt suicide at least three times more often than men but succeed about one-third as often. Men are far more likely than women to use firearms in their suicide attempts, which is one reason men's attempts are so likely to lead to death. Still, guns are so lethal that although women rarely use firearms, guns are also the leading method of completed suicide among women.

Gun availability appears to substantially increase the risk of suicide among women. In states with higher levels of household gun ownership, many more women per capita die in suicides, due entirely to higher rates of firearm suicide. This result holds even after accounting for levels of poverty and urbanization (Miller, Azrael, and Hemenway 2002b). For example, between 1991 and 2000, women in the "high gun" states had over five times the likelihood of dying in a firearm suicide than women in the "low gun" states. The overall suicide rate for women in the high-gun-ownership states was 50 percent higher (table 6.3).

A subgroup analysis of the suicides of women from a large case-control study of suicide in the home in three metropolitan counties (Kellermann et al. 1992) found that having a gun in the home was a large, independent, and significant risk factor for suicide. Other factors taken into account in the analysis included age, race, neighborhood, a history of mental illness or depression, and living alone (Bailey et al. 1997).

Women are different from men in terms of homicide victimization.

TABLE 6.3.   Female Violent Deaths
Numbers of homicides, suicides, and unintentional firearm deaths among females in the eleven states with the most guns and the five states with the fewest guns, 1991–2000

	High-Gun States	Low-Gun States	Mortality Rate Ratio: High-Gun/Low-Gun
Total Population (person years) at Risk: 1991-2000	100.6 million	100.6 million	
Homicides			
Gun Homicides	2,451	659	3.7
Nongun Homicides	1,907	1,380	1.4
Total	4,358	2,039	2.1
Suicides			
Gun Suicides	2,725	510	5.3
Nongun Suicides	2,008	2,746	0.7
Total	4,733	3,256	1.5
Unintentional Firearm Death	322	21	15.3

Source: Mortality data from CDC WISQARS 2003.

Note: Gun prevalence determined by the percentage of people in each state residing in households with firearms. Gun prevalence data come from the 2001 CDC Behavioral Risk Factor Surveys for each state. Similar results are obtained if gun prevalence is the percentage of suicides with guns, or "Cook's Index."

The eleven high-gun states are, in order, Wyoming, Montana, Alaska, South Dakota, Arkansas, West Virginia, Alabama, Idaho, Mississippi, North Dakota, and Kentucky; the five low-gun states are, in order, Hawaii, Massachusetts, Rhode Island, New Jersey, and Connecticut.

Women are less likely to be murdered—females accounted for 24 percent of total homicides in 2000 (CDC 2003b). In sharp contrast to men, stranger violence is not the major threat for women. An analysis of female homicides between 1976 and 1987 found that, for deaths where the perpetrator was known, almost half of the offenders were spouses or intimate acquaintances; strangers killed only 13 percent of the women (Kellermann and Mercy 1992). A review of intimate-partner homicides in Chicago over a twenty-nine-year period concluded that "an effective prevention strategy for intimate homicide of women . . . would be to reduce the availability of firearms in the home" (Block and Christakos 1995, 522).

Women in the United States are at far greater risk of homicide than women in other high-income nations. A recent study found that less than one-third of all women in high-income countries live in the United States, but American women account for 70 percent of all female homicide victims and 84 percent of all female firearm homicide victims. Across high-income nations, countries with higher levels of gun availability had higher rates of female homicide (Hemenway, Shinoda-Tagawa, and Miller 2002).

Within the United States, women in states with higher levels of household firearm ownership are more likely to be murdered, particularly with a gun (Miller, Azrael, and Hemenway 2002b). For example, between 1991 and 2000, in the "high gun" states the gun homicide rate for women was almost four times higher than the gun homicide rate for women in the "low gun" states, and the overall homicide rate was twice as high (table 6.3).

Other evidence indicates that guns in the home pose a threat to women's lives. A subgroup analysis of female homicide victimization from a large case-control study of homicide in the home in three metropolitan counties (Kellermann, Rivara, and Rushforth 1993) found that having a gun in the home was a large and significant risk factor for homicide. Other factors taken into account in the analysis included age, race, neighborhood, a history of mental illness or depression, and living alone (Bailey et al. 1997). Most of the women were murdered by spouses, lovers, or close relatives. In those cases, 58 percent of the victims were killed with guns, and only 10 percent of the time was there evidence of forced entry. Victims were usually killed in the context of quarrels, domestic fights, or assaults. Virtually all the increased risk for homicide from having a gun in the home was attributable to the homicides in which spouses, lovers, or close relatives were the killers.

For all other murders—by other relatives (3 percent of all female murders in the study), by friends and acquaintances (24 percent of all murders), by strangers (3 percent of all murders), and other and unknown (15 percent of all murders)—there was evidence of forced entry only 25 percent of the time, and a firearm was used to kill in only one-third of the cases. Home security measures had no protective effect.

A large case-control study of women murdered by intimate partners compared to a control group of battered women found that a gun in the home was an important risk factor for being killed. A gun was present in the house for 51 percent of the case group but only 16 percent of the control group. Gun access remained a risk factor even after controlling for severity and frequency of physical violence, threats to kill, forced sex, and other abusive behavior (J. C. Campbell et al. 2001). There was no clear evidence of any protective effect of having a gun in the home—even among those women who lived apart from the abuser (Campbell et al. 2003).

One reason guns in the home constitute a threat to women is that assaults with guns are far more lethal than other assaults. A study of family and intimate assaults found that firearm assaults were three times more likely to result in death than assaults with knives and twenty-three times more likely to result in death than assaults with other weapons (Saltzman et al. 1992). An evaluation of laws restricting access to firearms by abusers under restraining orders found that such laws lead to a significant reduction in intimate-partner homicides (Vigdor and Mercy 2003).

Nonlethal as well as lethal violence against women is predominantly partner violence. For example, of adult women who are physically assaulted or raped, more than 75 percent are assaulted by a current or former husband, cohabiting partner, or date; only 14 percent are assaulted by strangers. It is estimated that 1.5 million women annually are raped or physically assaulted by their intimate partners (Tjaden and Thoennes 1998).

Guns are used against women to intimidate and wound as well as to kill. More than 6 percent of women report having been threatened with guns, and 3 percent had guns actually used against them. Most of these threats were by intimates (Tjaden and Thoennes 1998). A national survey found that gun threats in the home against women by intimates (or ex-intimates) were far more common than home self-defense gun uses by women against anyone (Azrael and Hemenway 2000).

Pregnant women are in particular danger from male intimates. Many pregnant women—estimates range as high as 20 percent—are victims of domestic violence (Gazmararian et al. 1996). And again, guns seem only to make the situation worse. In a study of abused pregnant women with incomes below the poverty level, the levels of abuse were significantly higher if the abusers had access to guns. Gun access certainly adds weight to threats of violence and harm. At a minimum, the presence of a gun can be used as a marker for a potentially more dangerous abusive relationship (McFarlane et al. 1998).

A few women strike back lethally (A. Browne 1987), and their lethal retaliation typically occurs with firearms. One study of battered women who killed their abusers found that most killed their mates with guns that belonged to the batterers; 76 percent of the battered women who used guns to kill their abusers "used the same weapon with which [the men] had previously threatened [the women]" (L. E. Walker 1984, 42).

One case-control study compared battered women in prison for killing their abusers with battered women in women's shelters who did not kill. While two-thirds of both groups had received death threats from their abusers, the death threats for nearly all (90 percent) of the homicidal battered women included a specific method, time, and/or location for their demise, compared to only 15 percent of the nonhomicidal community controls. The abused women who killed were also significantly more likely than the community sample to have experienced drug problems, to have attempted suicide by drug overdose, and to have had access to the batterers' guns (Roberts 1996).

The evidence from all these studies is compelling. For most women, living in a home and a community with many guns is an important risk factor for serious injury rather than a source of protection.

AFRICAN AMERICANS

While there are some who argue that gun control is effectively a racist policy tool designed to take the right to bear arms away from blacks [Cramer 1995; Funk 1995], there is evidence of broad-based support for gun control among blacks. In spite of historical wariness of government on the part of blacks, most blacks are willing to support gun control as a mid-level step, to restrict the availability of firearms.

—R. C. Browne

Compared to whites, blacks in the United States have a higher prevalence of most diseases (e.g., cardiovascular disease, cancer, hypertension, diabetes, renal disease) (Dreeben 2001; Sowers et al. 2002). Rates of intentional injury also show marked racial disparities. Blacks have much higher rates of homicide than whites; however, blacks have lower rates of suicide (table 6.4).

For whites, rates of homicide in the United States are typically much higher than homicide rates for residents of other high-income countries. For example, in 1995–97, our homicide rate for whites was 4.6 per 100,000, four to five times higher than the rates in France, Germany, Norway, or Spain and about 40 percent higher than the next highest country on the list (Finland) (see table 3.4). Within the United States, the black homicide rate is far higher than the white rate. In 2000, for example, the U.S. black homicide victimization rate was more than five times higher than the white rate (table 6.5), making it about twenty-five times greater than the rate of high-income countries other than the United States.

In the United States, most homicides are intraracial (i.e., whites killing whites, blacks killing blacks). For example, in 2001, considering only whites and blacks, where offenders were identified, 94 percent of the homicide victims of white offenders were white, and 86 percent of the victims of black offenders were black (U.S. Department of Justice 2002).

TABLE 6.4.   Black and White Violent Death Rates (per 100,000) by Gender, 2000

	Overall Rate[a]	Firearm Rate[a]
All Homicide	6	4
White Males	5	3
Black Males	36	27
White Females	2	1.0
Black Females	7	3
All Suicide	11	6
White Males	19	12
Black Males	10	6
White Females	4	1.7
Black Females	2	.7
Unintentional Firearm Death		0.3
White Males		0.5
Black Males		0.6
White Females		0.1
Black Females		0.1
Total Firearm Death		10
White Males		16
Black Males		35
White Females		3
Black Females		4

Source: Data from CDC 2003b.
[a]Age-adjusted

Among African Americans, young males are at particular risk for homicide victimization. In 2000, 2,501 black males aged fifteen to twenty-four were murdered, 2,243 of them with firearms (CDC 2003b). National surveys find that black youths (aged eighteen to twenty-four) are no more likely to report having been physically assaulted (punched, hit, or beaten) than their white counterparts. However, black youths are far more likely than whites to report having been threatened with or shot at with a gun. Black youths are less likely to have long guns in their homes but equally likely to have handguns, the type of gun used most often in assaults (R. C. Browne 1999b). And even inner-city black youths who currently do not own handguns have easy access to them.

The causes for the large racial disparities in U.S. homicide rates are not completely understood. Possible explanations include blacks' lower levels of income and education and higher levels of unemployment (Council of Economic Advisors 1998). Sociologist Leonard Beeghley (2003) argues that along with guns, "racial discrimination constitutes one of the variables explaining the high American homicide rate. No explanation of the American anomaly can be complete without taking this issue into account" (71). Blacks face discrimination in the labor market (Darity and Mason 1998; Bertrand and Mullainathan 2002), in criminal justice (Human Rights Watch 1999), and elsewhere. One study of domestic homicides in Atlanta found that when rates of household crowding were taken into account, the relative risk of homicide in black populations was not significantly elevated (Centerwall 1995). Other studies suggest that black segregation and isolation are important predictors

TABLE 6.5. Black and White Homicide and Suicide Rates (per 100,000) by Age Categories, 2000

	Black		White	
	Overall Rate[a]	Firearm Rate[a]	Overall Rate[a]	Firearm Rate[a]
Homicide				
15–24	48.4	41.8	6.5	4.7
65+	6.9	2.2	2.0	0.7
All ages	21.0	14.8	3.7	2.1
Suicide				
15–24	8.2	5.3	10.9	6.2
65+	5.2	3.5	16.4	12.1
All ages	5.6	3.2	11.5	6.6

Source: Data from CDC 2003b.
[a]Age-adjusted

of black urban homicide rates (Rosenfeld 1986; R. D. Peterson and Krivo 1993; Shihadeh and Flynn 1996).

In sharp contrast to homicide, African Americans are less likely than whites to commit suicide, though the racial disparity among black and white adolescents and young adults has been decreasing because of an increase in firearm-related suicides among young black males (Shaffer, Gould, and Hicks 1994; Joe and Kaplan 2002). Overall, the black suicide rate is currently about half that of the white suicide rate. However, for fifteen- to twenty-four-year-olds, the white rate of suicide was only 30 percent higher than the black rate in 2000. By contrast, for those aged sixty-five and over, the white rate was more than three times higher. A majority of the suicide deaths for both blacks and whites are gun suicides (table 6.5). Compared to whites, a higher percentage of fifteen- to twenty-four-year-old black suicide victims used firearms (64 versus 57 percent); a lower percentage of elderly black victims used firearms (68 versus 74 percent) (CDC 2003b).

Overall, blacks are at substantially higher risk for death from firearms compared to whites (table 6.4), and blacks are more likely than whites to favor gun control policies (Lipman 1997; R. C. Browne 1999a). While firearm owners are less supportive of gun control and fewer black households contain firearms, even after controlling for firearm ownership and other factors, blacks in the United States are more likely than whites to favor gun control (R. C. Browne 1999a).

SUMMARY

In the United States in the 1990s, two children per day under the age of fourteen died from firearms, and many more were seriously injured. Our rate of child firearm fatalities is far greater than that of any other developed nation. We have more guns and more suicides, more homicides, and more accidental gun deaths of children.

Across U.S. regions and states, where there are more guns, children are at significantly greater risk for dying. They are at greater risk for victimization because of (1) an accidental gunshot wound; (2) a gun suicide; (3) a suicide by all methods combined; (4) a gun homicide; and (5) a homicide by all methods combined. They are not at increased risk for nongun suicide or nongun homicide.

The greatest risk of gun violence is to adolescents and young adults. Young people in the United States are far more likely to be murdered than are youths in other high-income countries. In U.S. regions and states with more guns, youths are at higher risk for accidental gun injuries, suicide, and homicide.

Women in the United States are five times more likely to be murdered as women in other high-income countries. In U.S. regions and states with more guns, women are more likely to die violent deaths—from murder, from suicide, and from accidental shooting.

Women are at much higher risk of violence from male intimates than from strangers. Guns may commonly be used as threats in violent domestic relationships. When guns are used to intimidate, the violence can become more severe. While women rarely perpetrate gun violence, a gun in the home increases the likelihood that a battered woman will kill her abuser. When women kill, the outcome is also terrible. The men are dead, and the women often are sent to prison.

Guns may occasionally have some beneficial effect for some women at some times, but the net effect is clearly quite negative. No study has shown that a gun in the home reduces the likelihood of burglary, robbery, home invasion, abuse, or any other crime against women.

Blacks in the United States have lower rates of suicide than whites but much higher rates of homicide and gun homicide, in part because of differences in education, poverty, housing, employment, and treatment based on racial characteristics.

Many policies can reduce the danger of guns to children, youths, women, and blacks. For example, to reduce the dangers to children, states might enact safe gun-storage requirements, which are mandatory in most other developed nations. America probably needs a new social norm that makes it common for parents to ask other parents if guns are in their homes and whether they are stored securely.

Numerous policies can reduce gun possession and carrying among youths (U.S. Department of Justice, OJJDP 1996). Some policies focus on the demand side. Programs such as "Hands-Without-Guns" provide media messages about the dangers of adolescent gun carrying (Hemenway et al. 1996). Other programs teach violence prevention and provide after-school activities that reduce the lure of gangs and keep youths off the streets. Youths who are at greatest risk for perpetrating gun violence should be referred to psychological and social services, including drug and alcohol treatment.

Other policies focus on the supply side. For example, national one-gun-per-month laws combined with waiting periods can reduce gunrunning across state lines. Increased tracing of guns used in crimes, combined with strong enforcement against scofflaw dealers, can also decrease the supply of guns on the street. Elimination of secondary sales through nondealers, such as at gun shows, can also limit teens' access to guns. Supply-side restrictions can have an immediate effect (Cook and Leitzel 1996)—tracing data show that a third of guns used in crime by juveniles are quite new, having been manufactured within three years of the crime, and half of all guns illegally acquired by young people involved straw buyers. A study of incarcerated adolescent males found that two of the main factors that prevented them, on at least one occasion, from acquiring or carrying firearms were the inability to find a source for a gun and the lack of money for its acquisition (Freed et al. 2001).

The public health approach to preventing gun violence suggests multiple policies. Punishing the "bad guys"—the kids who use the guns—is important, but punishment alone is neither good parenting nor an effective societal response to problem behavior. Women and women's organizations need to take a stronger stand on firearm issues to help create a society that is less dangerous for children, youths, and women. Fewer than one in ten women owns a firearm. Compared to men, women are more likely to favor reasonable firearm policies that will promote the public health.

One woman who had lost a child to guns was on her way to testify at a state firearms hearing when progun demonstrators began to heckle her. She responded, "We love our children more than you love your guns" (Tapper 1999).

CHAPTER 7   SUPPLY

The ultimate fact is that the gun industry is simply a business, and nothing more.
It is neither a national trust nor a repository of American values.

—T. Diaz

In a gun's life span, four main opportunities exist for legal interventions or regulations to be imposed: (1) the time of manufacture; (2) the time of sale; (3) the period of possession or carrying; and (4) the period of use (Baker, Teret, and Dietz 1980). A comprehensive policy approach to reducing gun injuries includes sensible regulations concerning all four of these periods, but most regulatory resources have gone into the latter two time periods. This chapter examines the first two: the time of manufacture and the time of sale. Put another way, many individuals and institutions can help reduce the problems caused by firearms; this chapter examines two such groups—the manufacturers and the sellers (both licensed and unregulated) of these weapons.

MANUFACTURERS

The gun industry is a business, making a consumer product, but the product is more lethal and its manufacture less regulated than that of almost any other consumer product. Sleepwear, toys, automobiles, vitamins—virtually all products—are subject to oversight by the Consumer Product Safety Commission, the National Highway Traffic Safety Administration, the Food and Drug Administration, and other national regulatory agencies. The actions of these agencies have helped lead to a marked decrease in injuries and deaths in the United States. But guns and ammunition are largely free of such federal safety and health regulation.

Surprisingly little is known about the companies that manufacture most guns for the U.S. market. All but one of the major domestic manufacturers

(Sturm, Ruger, and Company) are privately held companies. A number of other major domestic manufacturers are subsidiaries of foreign companies, like Beretta (Italy), Browning (Japan), and Smith and Wesson (England). Imports are a major component of the U.S. market. Almost all the manufacturers "vigorously conceal information that most other U.S. industries routinely reveal" (Diaz 1999, xvii). Neither Congress nor any other national authority has ever comprehensively examined the firearms industry.

The ownership, sales, and profits of these firms are not publicly available. The number of guns sold, by caliber or by product line, is a closely held secret. The wholesale value of all firearms and ammunition manufactured in the United States was estimated at $1.7 billion in 1995; the retail value of all firearms sold, including imports, was about $9 billion (Diaz 1999). To put this in perspective, the retail value of alcohol sold in the United States in 1995 was $80 billion, and new car dealership sales were about $500 billion.

> Because nearly all of the major manufacturers are privately held and shrouded in secrecy, little is publicly known about their revenues, profits, lobbying, or inner workings. But for at least a decade, the domestic firearms market, while highly cyclical, has been in a slow retreat, largely because of a decline in hunting. U.S. gun production peaked at 5.7 million guns in 1980; it averaged around 4 million units annually between 1995 and 1997, the most recent years for which federal data are available. "We are a mature industry and we are fighting for a very finite amount of business," explained one CEO. (*Business Week* 1999, 67)

More importantly for injury prevention, the health and safety records of these companies' products are not available.

Like most firms, gun manufacturers are primarily interested in sales and profits. A problem for the industry is that, given reasonable care, guns last a very long time. In the past few decades, with fewer young people growing up into the markets for traditional hunting and sport shooting, the industry has tried to convince people that they need new guns.

They succeeded, to some extent, through innovation and fear-inducing advertising. Instead of innovating in the direction of safety (e.g., childproof guns) the industry has developed weapons with greater lethality. Manufacturers have made guns that hold more rounds, increased the power of the rounds and the speed with which the bullets can be shot, and made guns smaller and more concealable (Diaz 1999). These changes all increased the public health risk from firearms.

Ammunition and accessories with "Rambo" appeal—bipods, flash suppressors, grenade launchers, laser sights, and expanding bullets—have been increasingly offered to civilians. Ammunition has come on the market with such names as Eliminator-X, Ultra-Mag, Black Talon (whose razorlike talons can tear protective gloves, exposing surgeons to infectious diseases), and Starfire (advertised as "the deadliest handgun cartridge ever developed for home or personal defense," with "fast knock-down" because of the "massive wound channel" it can create [Diaz 1999, 151]).

Public health has not been a prime manufacturer concern. Indeed, the industry often seems to go out of its way to circumvent the public safety intent of the few regulations that Congress has passed. For example, in 1994 the federal government banned many assault weapons. A detachable ammunition magazine, which allows for clips with hundreds of rounds, was central to the definition of an assault weapon. The law as enacted specifies that, to be banned, a gun must have at least two additional characteristics, such as a flash suppressor or a folding stock. When the manufacture of Colt's AR-15, the civilian version of the U.S. Army's M-16 rifle, was made illegal by the ban, Colt replaced it with the Colt Sporter, which differs from the AR-15 only in that the Sporter lacks a flash suppressor and a bayonet, thereby circumventing the law's intent (Fortgang 1999).

In 1993, a crazed California mortgage broker used two TEC-DC9s to kill eight people and wound six others in a San Francisco law office. Advertised as being as "tough as your toughest customers" and as having "excellent resistance to fingerprints," the gun was one of nineteen banned by name in the 1994 federal law. The TEC-DC9 (reportedly named for the District of Columbia) is based on a model (the TEC-9) originally designed for South African police to brutally control riots. Street gangs liked the gun, which was regularly carried by drug lords on the popular 1980s TV show *Miami Vice.*

The 1994 federal law made preexisting assault weapons and accessories legal to own, sell, and buy. Before the law went into effect, Navegar, the manufacturer of the TEC-DC9, increased its production levels. Then in 1994, it released a new version of the gun, the AB-10. Carlos Garcia, Navegar's owner, seemed to treat the law cavalierly: Garcia said the AB stood for "after ban." The only changes made to the gun were the removal of both the threaded barrel (which can hold a silencer) and the option of a barrel shroud. In 1997, Navegar's three sister guns, the TEC-9, the TEC-DC9, and the AB-10, were traced to more than fourteen hundred crime scenes (Fortgang 1999). A California study found that young adults purchasing assault-type handguns were more likely than other young adult gun purchasers to have criminal histories and to be charged with subsequent crimes (Wintemute, Wright et al. 1998). A 1999 California law set limits on copycat assault weapons (*Boston Globe* 1999b).

In the late 1960s, a surge in firearm violence was attributed in part to the easy availability of Saturday night specials. These guns—small, cheaply made, generally low-caliber handguns—were mostly imported and were mostly revolvers. The 1968 Gun Control Act effectively eliminated the importation of these guns by requiring that imported handguns exceed minimum size requirements and pass a series of design and performance tests. Domestically manufactured handguns were exempt from these criteria.

Domestic manufacturers quickly picked up the slack, producing precisely the type of handgun associated with the violence that led to the Gun Control Act. In the 1980s and 1990s, the majority of these domestically manufactured handguns were pistols produced by Southern California manufacturers, who collectively came to be known as the "Ring of Fire" companies. Compared to the earlier imported revolvers, the pistols were smaller and thus easier to conceal and had greater ammunition capacity. They were also poorly made: most could not pass the import performance tests (Wintemute 1996). In the early 1990s, more than 60 percent of guns traced in crimes by the Bureau of Alcohol, Tobacco, and Firearms (ATF) came from the Ring of Fire companies (Wintemute 1994).

A scathing June 1996 PBS *Frontline* piece on Lorcin Engineering, along with subsequent newspaper articles, demonstrated a multitude of public health problems caused by this small Ring of Fire company. Although President Jim Waldorf claimed to cater to law-abiding folks of limited means, for four years running in the 1990s, Lorcin's top seller, the L380 pistol, was the gun most often traced at crime scenes. Aside from being a gun of choice for criminals, shoddy security resulted in the theft of thousands of firearms from the firm's Mira Loma, California, plant; the ATF arrested four men for the theft and the subsequent sale of the guns from the trunks of their cars (*Los Angeles Times* 1997).

Design and construction defects seemingly caused many additional unintentional injuries. Between 1994 and 1997, some thirty-five wrongful death or injury claims were filed against Lorcin, involving people killed or wounded when their Lorcin pistols accidentally discharged. In a critique of the 1996

Lorcin L-22 pistol, *Gun Tests* magazine, the *Consumer Reports* of the firearm industry, wrote, "We wouldn't pay any amount of money for a gun that self-destructs in a couple of hundred rounds. Stay away from this one." Of the Lorcin L-25, *Gun Tests* wrote that the gun's "best attribute was that it didn't bite the shooter's hand" (*Los Angeles Times* 1997).

In the firm's best year, sales hit $14.7 million, and Waldorf and his partner took home a combined $1.85 million. But their liability coverage was minuscule, and because of the lawsuits, they filed a petition to reorganize under chapter 11 of the U.S. Bankruptcy Code. Creditors forced Waldorf and his partner to scale back their salaries to about $250,000 (*Los Angeles Times* 1997).

The 1997 *Los Angeles Times* article ends with this cheery international note: "Waldorf, ever the super-salesman, is tapping a new market where urban crime is on the rise: South Africa. Lorcin's sales there have climbed to about 25,000 guns a year and are expected to rise" (*Los Angeles Times* 1997). By July 1999, reports from Johannesburg indicated that "hundreds of thousands of cheap, poor quality firearms have flooded South Africa in the past five years," making it less likely that the national crime prevention strategy could be effective (*Business Day* 1999).

As a group, manufacturers have been accused of marketing their products to children (Langley 2001), making misleading claims about the safety benefits of firearms (Vernick, Teret, and Webster 1997), and maintaining lax distributional policies that allow criminals and adolescents easy access to guns (*Wall Street Journal* 1999). Manufacturers were named as defendants in dozens of recent lawsuits filed by city, state, and other organizations (e.g., the National Association for the Advancement of Colored People).

Firearms manufacturers can do much to help reduce the levels of gun violence and injuries from guns in America. For example:

(1) *Manufacturers can help increase the efficiency of law enforcement efforts, reducing the likelihood of further gun-related injury and death.* As each motor vehicle has a unique serial number, each firearm should also have a unique serial number. (Guns from different manufacturers currently can have the same serial number.)

Manufacturers can make the serial numbers harder to obliterate. The Boston police and the ATF found that almost one in five guns seized from Boston street gangs between 1991 and 1994 had obliterated serial numbers, and an additional 4 percent had no serial numbers (Kennedy, Piehl, and Braga 1996). Massachusetts law now requires manufacturers to sell only handguns with improved tamper-resistant serial numbers. Manufacturers can put the serial number inside the gun or on the outside in a manner that it can be read only with an optical enhancer, such as an infrared light. The new law helps police not only in investigating handgun crimes but also in returning stolen weapons (Commonwealth of Massachusetts 1996).

Manufacturers can make firearms that would mark or "fingerprint" each bullet as it is fired. That would permit the matching of the bullet and gun with a high degree of accuracy. Marking could be done by the firing pin or by an idiosyncrasy in the rifled bore. Improved bullet identification would be a great help to law enforcement (Karlson and Hargarten 1997). The potential benefits of ballistic fingerprinting received media attention in 2002 when random sniper killings terrorized the Washington, D.C., area over a three-week period. A national database of ballistic fingerprints might well have helped catch the killers sooner.

Manufacturers can do more to ensure that their dealers are not acting unlawfully or irresponsibly. In 1999, Smith and Wesson, the nation's top handgun manufacturer, made a good initial step, requiring its dealers to sign a code of ethics—to agree to conduct thorough checks of individuals purchasing handguns, to avoid buying or selling firearms known to be stolen, and to avoid selling firearms to straw purchasers. Dealers who fail to sign the agreement are not allowed to sell Smith and Wesson products. The key now is implementation—how actively the company enforces the code, cooperates with federal and local law enforcement, and stops selling to dealers who violate the terms of the agreement (ABCnews.com 1999).

(2) *Manufacturers can increase the safety of guns, reducing the likelihood of unintended injury.* For example, a grip safety, which has been available on some handguns for years, allows a firearm to be fired only when the safety is pushed in, as it would be if the gun were being held to be fired. The concept is similar to a locomotive's "dead man's throttle," which requires positive pressure on the throttle or the engines will stop. The grip safety was designed in 1884 by the son of one of the founders of Smith and Wesson. According to the story, D. B. Wesson heard of a child who was injured while shooting a handgun and commissioned a childproof design from his son. The grip safety, like a childproof safety cap, generally cannot be worked by very young children. It was manufactured on models of Smith and Wesson guns from 1888 to 1937 (Karlson and Hargarten 1997).

In many accidental firearm injuries, the shooter does not know the gun is loaded. A loaded-chamber indicator shows whether there is a round in the firing chamber. Not all guns have such indicators—in one study, of 259 pistol models identified, only 10 percent had loaded-chamber indicators (Vernick et al. 1999)—and people who are unfamiliar with a particular gun model have difficulty using many indicators. All pistols should have easily recognizable loaded-chamber indicators as standard equipment (Karlson and Hargarten 1997).

A magazine safety prevents a pistol from being fired if the magazine is removed, even if there is still a cartridge in the firing chamber. An inexperienced user may not realize or remember that removing the clip does not completely unload the weapon if a cartridge has already been fed from the clip into the chamber. While some semiautomatic pistols come equipped with magazine safeties, many do not (Karlson and Hargarten 1997). In a study of 259 pistol models, only 14 percent had magazine safeties. Yet patents as early as 1903 recognized the importance of both magazine safeties and loaded-chamber indicators in preventing injury (Vernick et al. 1999).

Some guns go off when dropped. For example, the Strum Ruger replica of the Colt 1873 Peacemaker reportedly caused some forty deaths and six hundred injuries resulting from unintentional discharges when the gun was dropped. In contrast to other consumer products, there was no recall. No governmental regulatory agency has authority to require the recall of firearms, even when they have hazardous designs. And the manufacturer and sellers of the firearm did not keep sufficient records to know who had bought the firearms and consequently could not notify purchasers about the problem (Larson 1993a).

The current trigger-safety mechanisms on many firearms can be improved. The safeties on many pistols are released by a simple flick of a switch. In fact, revolvers typically are manufactured without any safeties. When there are safeties, they are not always uniform across firearms. For example, on some handguns the action is locked when the manual thumb safety is in the up position, and on others it is locked when the switch is in the down position (Karlson and Hargarten 1997). There should be industrywide standards for safety switches and other components (Hemenway 1975).

(3) *Manufacturers can resist the temptation to develop new products that pose a danger to public health.* In the 1980s, some manufacturers began to make guns with more plastic and less metal; such guns are more likely to be mistaken for toys, and, when disassembled, such guns are more difficult to detect with metal detectors in courtrooms, prisons, airports, and elsewhere. A 1988 federal law required that all guns sold in the United States contain a minimum amount of metal. There is now little profit to be made by further devel-

opment in this area, and it is unlikely that an all-plastic firearm will be produced or made available anywhere in the world.

A new product, tiny nubu guns, resemble key chains but can be lethal. In 1995, Tokyo police confiscated more than one thousand such guns that had been imported by a Japanese jeweler (*New York Times* 1995b). Another new gun, with four bullets, resembles a cellular telephone. It is difficult for law enforcement to monitor illegal possession of such firearms, and they may pass through metal detectors (*Boston Globe* 1998d).

The higher-caliber "pocket rockets" of the 1990s made the gang warfare in U.S. inner cities more lethal (Caruso, Jara, and Swan 1999), and the reduced cost and increasing popularity of laser sights is increasing projectiles' accuracy. Recoil-compensated handguns are making even larger-caliber handguns more manageable to shoot, and .50-caliber rifles are receiving increasing publicity.

Sniper rifles firing .50-caliber rounds are now available in gun shops and over the Internet. The rifle was originally designed to take out armored personnel carriers, fortified bunkers, and helicopters. John L. Plaster, author of *The Ultimate Sniper,* offers this description of .50-caliber performance: "Here's a bullet that even at 1.5 miles crashes into a target with more energy than Dirty Harry's famous .44 Magnum at point-blank" (Vobejda and Ottaway 1999; Violence Policy Center 1999). The rifles are expensive, heavy (some weigh one hundred pounds), and cumbersome (more than five feet long), so most criminals will not use them. But the guns can be used for assassinations and other singular criminal acts. One of the rifles was found at the Branch Davidian compound in Waco, Texas, and another in the arsenal amassed by John C. Clark, a mentally disturbed man who killed a Traverse City, Michigan, police officer. Another concern is the possible use of these firearms to shoot down civilian airplanes. "The .50 caliber can continuously fire and get off a large number of shots even at an airplane going over a hundred miles an hour" (*New Republic* 2003, 18).

Not surprisingly, the Secret Service lobbied to outlaw the rifle when it was introduced into the civilian market. The social benefits of a .50-caliber "tactical rifle" are unclear; the social problems it could cause are enormous. At the very least, the sale of armor-piercing and incendiary ammunition for these rifles, currently banned for handguns, should be outlawed.

Other potentially dangerous innovations include: (a) the glaser safety slug, embedded with lead shot, which breaks apart on impact (and thus does not ricochet) but, like a shotgun shell, inflicts tremendous tissue damage; (b) the fléchette, a cartridge with a dart-shaped projectile that can penetrate deep into the body; and (c) caseless ammunition, cartridges with no case or primer, which means that law enforcement officials will be unable to identify crime weapons by the cartridge left on the scene (Karlson and Hargarten 1997).

Which firearms will become popular in the twenty-first century depends on many factors, including cost, advertising, taste, liability laws, and governmental regulations. The problem is that, unlike the case of food or motor vehicles, in the firearms area we have no institutional or regulatory structure to deal quickly or definitively with new technologies that may threaten public safety.

(4) *Manufacturers can embrace technological innovations that enhance gun safety and public health.* An appropriate regulatory authority not only could prohibit dangerous new technologies but also could require or encourage safety improvements. Some manufacturers are developing "smart" or "personalized" guns that cannot be fired except by authorized users. These guns can help prevent unintentional injury to children and adolescents as well as the criminal use of stolen guns (which will also reduce the likelihood of firearm theft) (Teret and Webster 1999).

The federal government began providing some funds for the development of smart weapons in the mid-1990s, and by 1998 more than one hundred patents had been issued (*Boston Globe* 1998a). The technologies that prevent shoplifters from sneaking T-shirts out of malls and enable cash registers to read credit cards could become the next weapon of choice in the fight against gun violence. Some of the cities suing gun manufacturers have demanded that the industry set aside some of its gross revenues for smart-gun development (Barrett and O'Connell 1999). A smart gun might also help police, who are sometimes killed with their own service firearms.

Less lethal weapons could be beneficial to police and private citizens. Police officers need a more diverse arsenal of weapons than a baton and a handgun. Too often, police shoot and kill suspects when less deadly force would be sufficient. Less lethal weapons could benefit police, bystanders, and even potential criminals.

In 1985, the U.S. Supreme Court ruled that police cannot use deadly force to prevent the escape of an apparently nonthreatening suspect (e.g., an unarmed burglar fleeing the scene) (*Tennessee v. Garner* 471 U.S. 1 [1985]). That ruling led to the formation of a small less-than-lethal-weapon develop-

not a consumer product

ment program, which has been exploring electrical, chemical, impact, and light technologies (Hayeslip and Preszler 1993).

In 1999, a man on Massachusetts' Cambridge Common appeared crazed. He had a weapon and threatened suicide. Cambridge police arrived and shot the individual, knocking him down. The police quickly retrieved his weapon and put him in custody. The individual was unhurt, for the projectile with which he was shot was a beanbag. Baltimore police began using beanbag ammunition, fired from a twelve-gauge shotgun, in 1997. The first use was during a family disturbance, against a man standing behind a screen door wielding a large knife. The beanbag hit him in the stomach, causing him to double up and drop the knife. When captured, he reportedly said, "Thank you for not killing me" (Rivera 1997).

Unfortunately, most police officers at most times have only their lethal handguns. A 1999 story from Los Angeles presents the police dilemma:

> A police officer shot and killed a naked, blood-covered 16 year old boy. . . . Officers Karen Thiffault, 38, and Daniel Palma, 22, arrived at an intersection about 4:30 A.M. Saturday when they saw a boy without clothes, covered in blood, and "acting in a bizarre manner." . . . The boy fixated on Thiffault after she tried to calm him by talking. He then charged the officer while screaming unintelligibly. Fearing her weapon would be used against her, Thiffault shot the boy, police said. (*Boston Globe* 1999d)

Less lethal firearms could also be beneficial for private citizens. A primary motive for handgun ownership is self-defense, but handguns as currently designed are poor weapons for home and self-protection. Handguns are often difficult to shoot accurately, yet only an extremely accurate shot will immediately incapacitate an assailant. And handguns are so dangerous to the family—from accidents, arguments, or impetuous suicide attempts—that virtually all experts advise that guns be stored in a locked area separate from ammunition.

An ideal handgun for self-defense would be less prone to accident and less lethal when used intentionally but quick to stop an attacker without requiring a precise shot. Much of the basic technology needed to design more effective yet less lethal weapons is already available. For example, bullet material, construction, and consistency could be modified to reduce the likelihood of fatal injury. Wax and plastic bullets could be used in place of the conventional round-nosed bullet. Another option is increased reliance on spherical bullets, which limit bullet penetration and tissue damage (Hemenway and Weil 1990a).

A more fundamental approach is the redesign of guns to shoot electricity, tranquilizers, or anesthetics. Such projectiles have the potential to render an attacker harmless, without the need for either deadly force or great accuracy. Police departments have had some success using electronic guns to subdue individuals believed to be high on phencyclidine (PCP). Farmers sometimes immunize cattle with biodegradable, freeze-dried vaccine bullets shot out of an air gun (Hemenway and Weil 1990b).

Perhaps it is even worth looking to science fiction for a model. Weapons in the popular television series *Star Trek* were highly powerful, befitting the hostile universe in which they were used. Handheld phasers, for example, were far more destructive than today's handguns. But with the flick of a switch, a phaser could be turned into a completely nonlethal weapon. With phasers on stun, a hit left the victim immobilized but unhurt. Similarly, zookeepers today use tranquilizer guns to render dangerous animals helpless but hopefully unharmed. There may be lessons to be learned here. While Captain Kirk and the crew of the *Enterprise* explored the universe without the benefits of seat belts, air bags, or even a crashworthy interior, they were fortunate enough to possess the stun phaser. Real-world government policies should help bring to fruition such effective but less-than-lethal weapons.

Government can help create an improved nonlethal handgun by providing increased resources to underwrite private research and development efforts or by undertaking the research itself. Scientists at the National Institute of Standards and Technology or in the armed services, for example, could do much of the technical work. Once such a weapon is developed, government can educate the citizenry about the benefits. Government purchases of the new weapon would help encourage private demand since many gun buyers imitate police purchases (Hemenway 1989). Finally, government authorities could tax the sales of the current lethal handguns or subsidize production of the less lethal weapons.

Safer, less lethal weapons are not a panacea for our gun problems. But since many citizens are apparently determined to purchase and use handguns, increased attention to weapon redesign might bring great public health benefits.

SUPPLY

LICENSED DEALERS

You'd think, you'd hope, that a business as deadly as dealing guns would be regulated closely. It's not. Almost anyone can get a federal gun dealer's license and
then get away with almost anything. Even when a gun is sold illegally and someone is shot, the government often lets the dealer go about his business.

—D. Olinger and B. Port

There are two types of gun sellers at the retail level: federally licensed firearms
dealers, and everyone else. Federally licensed dealers may have guns shipped
to them across state lines. They may also sell handguns across state lines,
though only to another dealer. The original retail sale of every gun must be
through a federally licensed dealer.

Almost anyone can become a licensed dealer in the United States. As
recently as 1993, there were more than 270,000 dealers—more than the number of gas stations. In large part because of administrative reforms by the
Clinton administration and Public Law 103-159 (that included the Brady Bill),
which raised the annual license fee from thirty dollars to two hundred dollars,
that figure decreased to about 100,000 in 2000—still an enormous number of
dealers. The larger dealers, who operate from stores, are known as "stocking
dealers"; the smaller dealers—still the majority—who sell guns out of their
homes or other casual premises are known as "kitchen table" dealers.

The Brady Law requires licensed dealers to check the background of each
prospective purchaser, to keep specific records about each gun sale, and to
make the information available to the ATF. The records are useful mainly for
tracing the sale of firearms that are later linked to crime and reported to the
ATF for tracing. However, federal laws also contain elaborate restrictions to
prevent the ATF from using these records to set up any kind of national database of gun ownership (Diaz 1999).

The ATF is also forbidden from making more than one inspection per year
of any licensed dealer. Since there are so many dealers and so few ATF inspec-
tors, a typical dealer is inspected about once every seven years. The bureau's
small size—between 1973 and 1999 the number of agents remained basically
unchanged—limits its effectiveness. So too do the minor penalties for dealer
misconduct. The federal Firearms Owners' Protection Act of 1986 reduced
record-keeping violations by a dealer from a felony to a misdemeanor, a dis-
incentive for federal prosecutors in cases where a dealer has forged or

destroyed records to hide evidence. The law also requires prosecutors to prove that dealers who sold guns to criminal or straw purchasers did so "knowingly and willfully," and proving someone's state of mind is a nearly insurmountable legal hurdle. In addition, ATF agents are not allowed to pose as felons to make undercover purchases (a tactic commonly used by drug agents) but must use convicted felons in undercover operations, which makes prosecution more difficult because juries are reluctant to believe convicted felons (Butterfield 1999a).

An example of an extremely successful ATF operation illustrates some of the enforcement problems. B&E Guns in Cypress, California, had long aroused the suspicions of ATF agents. In 1990 the ATF revoked the owner's license because he was found to be forging records. The owner simply transferred the license to his wife. In the mid-1990s, more than two hundred guns that the ATF had traced to B&E Guns began showing up in murders, robberies, and shootings in southern California. Other guns traced to B&E were smuggled into Japan and Australia.

The bureau raided the firm and found that it had illegally sold nine thousand guns in less than two years: three thousand guns were listed as having been sold to other dealers who were unaware of the transactions, and another six thousand guns had no records of any kind. Agents claim this latter procedure was especially lucrative because a gun with no paper trail could be sold to criminals for double the normal markup. Because such actions are only misdemeanors, prosecutors allowed the store manager to plea-bargain, and he was sentenced to a year in prison (Butterfield 1999a).

Sting operations in Chicago and Detroit demonstrate the ease with which felons can obtain firearms directly from dealers. In 1998, police officers from Chicago (where possessing a new handgun is illegal) posed as local gang members and went firearms shopping in the suburbs. In store after store, clerks willingly sold powerful handguns to these agents, who made it clear that they intended to use the guns to "take care of business" on the streets of Chicago. Dealers also sold handguns to undercover officers who were obviously making illegal straw purchases for colleagues who could not legally buy them. The clerks even offered the undercover buyers unsolicited advice about how to evade state and federal laws—for example, by splitting up purchases to avoid reporting requirements concerning sales of multiple guns at one time (Daley 1998a, 1998b).

Authorities in Detroit and surrounding Wayne County conducted a similar sting operation in 1999. Ninety percent of the dealers sold guns to undercover officers standing in as straw purchasers for prohibited buyers. It did not matter whether the dealers were those with high numbers of gun traces or were selected randomly. Virtually all fell for the sting. In one videotaped transaction, a dealer told an officer that if he wanted to buy a gun for his friend, he had to sign a required federal form and take the risk if the ATF discovered the ruse: "You want to tell me you are buying the gun and you want to lie on the sheet, I don't care. This question here says, 'Are you buying this gun for yourself?' All of us know you are not" (Meier 1999a). A national study of firearm dealers in twenty cities found that the majority were willing to sell a handgun even when they were told it was being purchased for another person "because s/he needs it." Dealers in the Northeast were least likely to be willing to make such illegal sales (Sorenson and Vittes 2003).

In the past few years the ATF has stepped up its tracing program in an attempt to reduce illegal gun trafficking. Because most states do not have either licensing or registration requirements, tracing does not mean following a gun as it changes hands. All that can typically be determined is the original sale by a federally licensed firearm dealer. Unfortunately, serial number obliteration and inadequate record keeping mean that many guns cannot even be traced to the original dealers. In 1998, of the two hundred thousand firearm serial numbers sent to the bureau, only about 50 percent could be successfully traced to the original dealers (Meier 1999a). Still, the increased bureau emphasis on tracing data has shown that (a) a small number of dealers account for most of the guns that are used in crime, and (b) many guns used in crime are quite new, recently purchased from licensed dealers (Cook and Braga 2001). These two facts suggest that concerted action against scofflaw dealers can have a substantial impact on reducing gun-related crime.

ATF tracing data show that 389 dealers—less than 0.5 percent of all dealers—accounted for more than half of all crime guns traced in 1996–98 (Butterfield 1999a). One hundred and thirty-seven dealers in 1998 each accounted for, on average, approximately one hundred guns that were used in crime during the preceding two years. For example, a dealer in West Milwaukee, Wisconsin, sold 1,195 guns used in crime and recovered during that period; a dealer in Riverdale, Illinois, a Chicago suburb, was the source of 1,176 crime guns; and a dealer in Carson City, Nevada, supplied 326 guns used in crime in 1998 alone—and 324 of the crimes were committed outside of Nevada (Butterfield 1999c).

Many of the guns used in crime are quite new. Of the criminal handguns seized by police in seventeen cities in 1996–97, 49 percent of those that were traced had been purchased from a federally licensed dealer within the prior three years (ATF 1997; Butterfield 1999a). Similarly, a 1999 ATF report on criminal firearms seized in twenty-seven cities found that 49 percent of the guns used by eighteen- to twenty-four-year-olds had been purchased within the past three years, often by intermediaries acting on behalf of the real buyers (ATF 1999; Butterfield 1999b). In Chicago, for example, 83 percent of the thirty-five Bryco .380 semiautomatics used in homicides in 1996 were less than three years old; 76 percent of the thirty-four Lorcin .380s used in homicides were less than three years old (ATF 1999).

"The data are hugely significant, because it shows that there is a stream of guns, especially semiautomatic handguns, that are moving very rapidly out of gun stores into the hands of criminals," says David Kennedy, a Harvard researcher and the director of the Boston Gun Project, which has helped reduce juvenile gun violence in Boston in part by trying to identify and crack down on gun dealers and intermediaries who sell to minors. "It means this is something we can fix" (Butterfield 1998).

Nationwide, the dealer with the most guns traced to it in 1998 was Badger Guns and Ammo in West Milwaukee. In 1999 it posted a billboard proclaiming that it had been "Voted number one by the *Milwaukee Journal*," referring to the store's ranking in the sale of traced crime guns as reported by that newspaper. The owners said the ranking and advertising had helped their business (McBride 1999).

The ATF needs more resources and more enforcement authority to help it crack down on scofflaw gun dealers. Like local police, ATF agents need to be allowed to pose as felons in sting operations. Serious dealer misconduct should be upgraded from a misdemeanor to a felony. And the congressional restrictions that bar the bureau from computerizing many of its records should be lifted.

The ATF needs to continue to work closely with local authorities. Many urban police chiefs have begun to shift their enforcement emphasis. Instead of focusing solely on locking up criminal gun users, these officers are putting more effort into stopping guns from reaching criminal hands. For many years, most police forces attached little importance to tracing a gun or trying to halt the supply of guns to criminals and juveniles. When the police seized a gun, they put it in an evidence locker and often later resold it through a gun dealer. This procedure contrasted sharply with police work on drugs, where investigators routinely reduced charges to low-level street dealers in an effort to track down kingpins (Butterfield 1999d).

Many cities, including New York, Minneapolis, Indianapolis, Baltimore, and St. Louis, are emphasizing tracking guns and cracking down on illegal gun transfers. St. Louis Mayor Clarence Harmon, who served as police chief during the early 1990s, issued an order to trace every gun the police found. His officers discovered that a handful of corrupt gun dealers in rural areas were selling to straw purchasers or gun traffickers, who then resold the guns out of the trunks of their cars. He "came to believe that the gun manufacturers had to know that certain dealers were selling to guys on the street, or ought to know" (Butterfield 1999d).

The recent increase in gun tracing by urban police has shown that, in most cities, the biggest source of crime guns was the network of licensed dealers operating within their home states. "The most important effect was to replace the hopelessness of the late '80s and early '90s with a confidence that the right measures aimed at the right targets could interrupt the flow of guns to the bad guys. Suddenly the seemingly intractable debate over gun control became a debate over 'gun-crime interdiction'" (Larson 1999, 36).

Not only the police but also the public health community can play a role in reducing availability of firearms to inappropriate users. In California, for example, the prevention program in Contra Costa's Health Services Department found that in the early 1990s, most of the county's gun dealers were not complying with state and local laws. For example, two-thirds did not have the required state certificate of eligibility, meaning that they were selling guns without reporting their sales to state authorities; were not performing the necessary background checks on prospective customers; and were probably avoiding the state sales tax. More than 80 percent of the county's dealers were operating in residentially zoned areas, and 73 percent lacked the required local business licenses. The publication of such information led to increased enforcement, further local ordinances, and a dramatic reduction in the number of licensed dealers in that county from 700 in 1995 to 144 in 1997 (Contra Costa County Health Services Department 1995).

Gun manufacturers could do more to police their dealers and reduce illegal transactions. In a 2003 affidavit filed in a case against the manufacturers brought by twelve California cities and counties, Robert Ricker, the former chief lobbyist and executive director of the American Shooting Sports Council (then the main gun industry trade association), testified that gun manufacturers knew that some dealers corruptly sold guns to criminals but pressured one another into remaining silent for fear of liability. "Leaders in the industry have long known that greater industry action to prevent illegal transactions is possible," particularly through a network of manufacturers' representatives who stay in close touch with dealers. But industry officials have "resisted taking constructive voluntary action." From 1992 through 1997, the industry convened annual meetings at which manufacturers discussed whether they should take voluntary action to better control the distribution of guns. Unfortunately, "the prevailing view was that if the industry took action voluntarily, it would be an admission of responsibility for the problem." Such a "see no evil, hear no evil" approach encouraged "a culture of evasion of firearms laws and regulations" (Butterfield 2003).

THE UNREGULATED MARKET

Eric Harris and Dylan Klebold had gone to the Tanner gun show on Saturday and they took me back with them on Sunday. While we were walking around, Eric and Dylan kept asking sellers if they were private or licensed. They wanted to buy their guns from someone who was private and not licensed because there would be no paperwork or background check. It was too easy. I wish it had been more difficult. I wouldn't have helped them buy the guns if I had faced a background check.

—Robyn Anderson, testifying before the House Judiciary
Committee investigation of the Columbine school killings, January 27, 2000

The biggest loophole in the retail market is that private sales—which do not involve licensed dealers—are effectively unregulated. It is estimated that 40 percent of retail gun sales occur between private individuals, at flea markets and gun shows, in backyards, and over the Internet. Criminals and terrorists can readily obtain guns in these places. And terrorists have gone to gun shows to obtain weapons (*USA Today* 2001; Lebowitz 2002). There is no federally mandated record keeping when two private individuals make a private firearms sale (*Washington Post* 1999).

No federal rules exist requiring individuals who make "occasional sales" (an undefined phrase) to check on the backgrounds of would-be purchasers or keep records of the sales, although a few states, including Pennsylvania and Maryland, have imposed requirements. Under federal law, unlicensed sellers are required only not to sell knowingly to felons or minors.

Many private transfers of firearms occur at gun shows; on average, more than one hundred gun shows take place every weekend, attended by up to five million people a year. Some visitors claim that it is not unusual to see signs at the shows that say "No Questions Asked" or obviously stolen military firearms being sold. Branch Davidian leader David Koresh, Oklahoma City bomber Timothy McVeigh, and serial killer Thomas Lee Dillon all bought firearms at gun shows. Buford Furrow, the racist killer who shot children at a Jewish community center in Los Angeles in 1999, bought several of his weapons at gun shows. And the guns used by the teenage shooters in the Littleton high school massacre in 1999 were purchased at a gun show (Fortgang 1999; Meier 1999b).

The boom in gun shows began with the passage of the 1986 Firearms Owners' Protection Act, which allowed licensed dealers to sell at gun shows in their home states, allowed unlicensed private individuals to sell their personal guns in much greater quantities, and restricted the ATF's inspection authority. The consequence of this loosening in the laws was described in a May 1993 letter from Bill Bridgewater, then executive director of the National Alliance of Stocking Gun Dealers, to a U.S. House subcommittee:

> There are literally hundreds of "gun shows" around the country where you may rent tables, display your wares, sell what you please to whomever you please and once again the sale that is made with no records, no questions and no papers, earns the highest sales price. . . . There are wide open "gun shows" the length and breadth of the United States, wherein anyone may do as he chooses, including buy firearms for children. (Diaz 1999, 32)

An executive of a major hunting organization is quoted as saying, "Gun shows used to be fun, full of real good hunting rifles. Now you go in and they're selling pamphlets that tell you how to make pipe bombs and how to make your semiautomatic gun into an automatic. These people are not concerned about hunting pheasants" (Bai 1999, 38).

Licensed dealers sometimes sell illegally at these shows. They may claim to be collectors but are actually full-time dealers motivated by profit to avoid the taxes, paperwork, and background checks of licensed sellers (*Roanoke Times* 1999). It is also illegal for dealers to sell handguns to anyone under age twenty-one and long guns to anyone under age eighteen. But the age limit for handguns sold in private sales is eighteen, and there is no age limit for the private sale of long guns (U.S. Code, title 18, section 922).

The solution to these various problems is simply to require that all gun sales go through licensed dealers so that teenagers cannot buy handguns, background checks can be performed on all sales, and guns used in crime can be traced from purchaser to purchaser. Currently, many secondary sales do not go through dealers, so the ownership path of a gun is rarely known. For example, after more than three months of intensive work, investigators had managed to trace only one of the guns used at the Littleton school massacre through all its buyers and sellers. Royce Spain, a former gun store owner and dealer who at one time owned the TEC-DC9 used at Littleton, says that "the gun shows have monopolized the market. The stores just can't make it. . . . If I were a gangster I would go to a gun show. People with AK-47s walking up and down the aisles. . . . It's just a fester spot" (Olinger 1999a). "If you're not a licensee," ATF Special Agent S. H. McCampbell said, "you're only governed by your conscience. And many of these people have no conscience" (*Roanoke Times* 1999).

In 1999, the nation's major police organizations, including the International Brotherhood of Police Officers and the International Association of Chiefs of Police, unequivocally called on Congress to close the "gun show loophole" (Handgun Control 1999).

It is not just gun shows that can be a problem. Criminals can also obtain firearms by answering classified ads. For example, a federally licensed dealer denied Benjamin Smith a firearm when a background check showed that a restraining order had been issued against him. Smith turned to the classified section of the *Peoria (Illinois) Journal Star* to purchase a .380-caliber semiautomatic handgun and a .22-caliber pistol from a private seller. Smith used the guns in an interstate shooting spree, killing two and wounding nine before killing himself. Gun control proponents are pushing for newspapers to stop running classified ads for guns (Join Together 2002).

The Internet is becoming an increasingly popular source for both legal and illegal gun sales. "Hundreds of merchants on the Internet are selling rifles, revolvers and semiautomatic pistols and they can get you one as quickly as Amazon.com can send you a book, only with less paperwork" (Reuters 1999). While it is illegal to ship a firearm across state lines to anyone other than a federal firearms dealer, most of the online sellers contacted by one journalist were willing to sell him a gun directly, without even asking his age (Orr 1999). Again, to limit sales to felons, we need regulations mandating that all sales go through dealers, new laws that give the ATF better enforcement power, and appropriations that give the agency more resources for enforcement.

Finally, theft and gunrunning are also responsible for a large portion of the illegal gun trade. For example, between 1989 and 1996 in Florida, the Metro-

Dade County Police Department received more than ten thousand reports of firearms stolen in burglaries. Each report is for an incident of burglary, so the total number of firearms stolen is far greater. A Dade County grand jury concluded,

> We have reached one inescapable and shameful conclusion. When we legally arm ourselves for our own protection, we may be inadvertently arming the very persons we are seeking to protect ourselves against. The statistics from the Metro-Dade Police Department prove that a substantial number of stolen firearms come from our homes, our cars, and our businesses. . . . A necessary component of any right to lawfully possess a firearm should be the requirement that we do so in a responsible manner. . . . Any firearms we keep in our homes must be maintained in a safe or other secure container to prevent their theft, especially when we are not at home. Any firearms we choose to legally keep in our cars must be secured in a locked compartment stronger than a glove box to prevent their theft, especially when we are not seated in that car. (Dade County Grand Jury 1997, 11)

As discussed in chapter 6, many youth and criminals in restrictive gun states obtain their firearms through gunrunning followed by secondary-market sales. Available tracing data show the influence of gunrunning from permissive to more restrictive states. Florida has very permissive gun laws, while New York has very restrictive gun laws. In Miami, 70 percent of guns used in adolescent crime and 77 percent of guns used in young adult crime originally came from Florida. By contrast, in New York City, only 6 percent of guns used in adolescent crime and 10 percent of guns used in young adult crime originally came from New York state. It is difficult to think of any other common consumer item that 90 percent of the time was originally sold at retail in some other state. The majority of guns used illegally by fifteen- to twenty-four-year-olds in New York City came from five southern states—Virginia, North Carolina, South Carolina, Georgia, and Florida (ATF 1999).

Analysis of the data from communities that have been involved in the ATF tracing program indicate that, as expected, (a) the percentage of guns traced to out-of-state sources is greater for juveniles than adults (since most adults can legally purchase guns in most communities), and (b) the percentage of guns traced to out-of-state sources is greatest in states with the most stringent gun control laws (Donenfeld 1999; Cook and Braga 2001). The problem lies not only with scofflaw dealers but with the entire secondary market, including trades at gun shows and other private transfers.

SUMMARY

Gun manufacturers are more interested in profits than in public health and safety. And although firearms are one of the most dangerous consumer products, the safety of guns is less regulated than virtually any other commodity.

As the National Highway Traffic Safety Administration and the Environmental Protection Agency regulate automobiles, a federal agency should be responsible for ensuring that guns are manufactured with public safety in mind—by helping to increase the efficacy of law enforcement and decrease the danger from firearms. The history of firearm manufacturers in the United States makes it clear that government efforts are needed to ensure that every gun has a unique, tamper-resistant serial number; that firearms mark or fingerprint each bullet as it is fired; and that caseless ammunition does not become the ammunition of choice for criminals. Government regulation is also needed to ensure that guns meet minimum safety requirements (e.g., they should not fire when dropped). Like medicine bottles, guns should be childproof, and like cameras, guns should have loading indicators. Magazine safeties should be standard equipment for pistols to prevent guns from firing when the clips are removed, and safety features should be standardized across manufacturers.

A federal agency is needed to provide quick regulatory oversight for new technology. The agency's goal would be to promote innovation in the direction of public safety rather than public endangerment.

Serious problems also exist in the distribution of firearms. Currently—as inner-city youth know—it is far too easy for juveniles and felons to obtain guns. An encouraging sign is that many urban police departments are taking a preventive (public health) approach to reducing gun violence. Instead of focusing exclusively on locking up criminal gun users, police have begun to put more systematic effort into stopping guns from reaching criminal hands. Gun tracing has shown that a relatively small number of dealers are responsible for supplying most of the guns used in crime and that many of the guns used in crime are quite new. These facts suggest that interdicting the illegal supply of firearms might substantially reduce gun-related crime. The ATF needs more power and more resources to effectively enforce the laws dealing with the illegal distribution of firearms.

SUPPLY

New laws are needed to reduce the flow of guns to criminals through the secondary market. Most private sales at gun shows, flea markets, over the Internet, and so forth currently occur without background checks or government oversight. This enormous regulatory loophole needs to be closed. Virtually all firearm transfers should be required to go through licensed dealers to allow proper background checks of purchasers and provide some government control.

CHAPTER 8   POLICY BACKGROUND

> For more than 200 years, the federal courts have unanimously determined that the Second Amendment concerns only the arming of the people in service to an organized state militia; it does not guarantee immediate access to guns for private purposes. The nation can no longer afford to let the gun lobby's distortion of the Constitution cripple every reasonable attempt to implement an effective national policy towards guns and crime.
> —Former U.S. Attorneys General Nicholas Katzenbach, Ramsey Clark, Elliot L. Richardson, Edward H. Levi, Griffin B. Bell, and Benjamin R. Civiletti

Prescribing reasonable and feasible firearm policies for the United States requires understanding the context in which American firearms policy is set. The starting point for any discussion of this topic must be the U.S. Constitution—specifically, the Second Amendment, which is sometimes claimed to limit possible policy alternatives. After examining these arguments, the chapter turns to U.S. public opinion concerning various policy options. Finally, the chapter describes the empirical literature on the evaluation of past firearm regulations.

THE SECOND AMENDMENT

Debates about gun policy typically include a discussion of the Second Amendment of the U.S. Constitution. The large majority of Americans (60 to 90 percent) believe that the U.S. Constitution provides for the right of private gun ownership, and the majority of gun owners (55 percent) believe that stricter gun measures would violate that perceived right (Chafee 1992; Blendon, Young, and Hemenway 1996). The media perpetuates these views (Byck 1998), but they are incorrect.

Many of the members of the Continental Congress, which adopted the

Articles of Confederation in 1777, distrusted centralized government. The Articles specified that every state "shall always keep up a well regulated and disciplined militia, sufficiently armed and accoutred" to be ready for action, but did not include a proviso on any private right to bear arms (DeConde 2001).

Similarly, the Second Amendment of the U.S. Constitution focused on the militia. The amendment reads, in its entirety, "A well regulated Militia, being necessary to the security of a free State, the right of the people to keep and bear Arms, shall not be infringed." When the National Rifle Association (NRA) placed the words of the Second Amendment near the front door of its former national headquarters, it omitted the first thirteen words.

When the U.S. Constitution was adopted, each state had its own militia, an organized military force comprised of ordinary citizens serving as part-time soldiers. The purpose of the militia was to secure each state against threats from without (e.g., invasions) and threats from within (e.g., riots).

It has been claimed that the Second Amendment provides individual Americans with a constitutional right to have firearms for personal self-defense; some people also argue that this right is crucial to allow individual Americans to rise up to combat government tyranny. While the intellectual and historical records are not completely clear, they seem to provide little support for these positions. Like the Tenth Amendment, the Second Amendment appears to focus on the relationship between the federal government and state governments.

Neither the natural rights tradition of John Locke nor the English constitutional tradition of William Blackstone provides much evidence for an individual rather than a collective interpretation of the Second Amendment. Locke emphasized the importance of the social contract: when an individual enters civil society, "he gives up" his power "of doing whatsoever he thought fit for the preservation of himself." The very notion of political society is that rights should be determined and disputes resolved not through private judgment of each individual backed by private force but rather by the public judgment of the community. By contrast, the unrestrained use of force according to one's own private judgment leads to a war of all against all, which actually undermines rather than furthers the goal of self-preservation (Heyman 2000, 243).

As for resisting tyranny, Locke focused on the right of revolution, which he said belongs to the community, or the people as a whole. Blackstone also rejected a view that would "allow to every individual the right of determining [when resistance is appropriate] and of employing private force to resist even private oppression." Such a doctrine is "productive of anarchy, and in consequence equally fatal to civil liberty as tyranny itself" (Heyman 2000, 258).

Some historians, but not all (Malcolm 1994), also believe that English history provides little support for the individual right to own weapons. The ancient constitution did not include it; it was not in the Magna Carta of 1215 or the Petition of Rights of 1628. No early English government would have considered giving the individual such a right. The Game Act of 1671 limited the right to have a gun to wealthy individuals. Article VII of the Declaration/Bill of Rights of 1689 also restricted the right to the upper classes: "That the Subjects which are Protestants may have Arms for their defence suitable to their Condition and as allowed by Law," with the phrase "suitable to their condition" serving as a euphemism for socioeconomic status. Historian L. G. Schwoerer (2000) concludes that Article VII was a gun control measure drafted by upper-class Protestants. In 1693, the Whigs did introduce a rider to the Game Act "to enable every Protestant to keep a musket in his house for his defence, not withstanding this or any other act" (50). However, the rider was defeated 169 to 65.

The history of the writing of the Second Amendment also provides little support for an individual-rights interpretation. The Constitutional Convention was called because of the failure of the national government under the Articles of Confederation. The delegates at the Philadelphia convention feared a weak government incapable of repelling foreign invasions or suppressing domestic insurrections. The Federalists, who dominated the convention, wanted a strong central government, including a standing army, which could be supplemented by a trained, well-regulated militia (Finkelman 2000).

At Pennsylvania's ratifying convention, the Antifederalists were soundly defeated. After the convention, they published their reasons for dissent, which included fourteen proposed amendments to the U.S. Constitution. Some of these were later incorporated, almost word for word, into the Bill of Rights. Others were not. One, for example, asserted that "the inhabitants of the several states shall have liberty to fowl and hunt in seasonable times . . . and in like manner to fish in all navigable waters." Another provided "that the people have a right to bear arms for the defense of themselves . . . or for the purpose of killing game . . . ; and as standing armies in the time of peace are dangerous to liberty, they ought not to be kept up." A third declared "that the power of organizing, arming and disciplining the militia . . . remain with the individual states" (Rakove 2000, 134–35).

The same men who wrote the Constitution also wrote the Bill of Rights. The Federalists completely and totally dominated the Congress of 1789. They were not interested in creating or protecting the right to kill game, to hunt in seasonal times, to fish in all navigable waters, or to bear arms for the defense of themselves. The demands for these explicit rights were on the table and could easily have been put into the Bill of Rights. They were not. However, the Federalists were willing to assure the Antifederalists that the national government would not dismantle or disarm the state militias (Finkelman 2000).

Federalist James Madison's first draft of the proposed amendment read, "A well-regulated militia, composed of the body of the people, being the best security of a free state, the right of the people to keep and bear arms shall not be infringed; but no person religiously scrupulous shall be compelled to bear arms." This language clearly concerns the militia. It starts with the militia, it talks about the "body of the people" rather than individual inhabitants, and it excludes conscientious objectors from the requirement of joining the militia. Indeed, much of the debate over the amendment concerned the propriety of exempting religiously scrupulous persons from the obligation to bear arms if summoned to do so (Rakove 2000). Nowhere in the debate concerning this amendment was there the slightest hint about a private or individual right to own a weapon (Finkelman 2000).

The underlying debate concerning the Second Amendment was about limiting the powers of the proposed national government, not about limiting the police powers of individual states. At issue was where the boundaries between national and state responsibilities would lie. Many Americans feared standing armies and hoped that the maintenance of a well-regulated militia would eliminate the need for a substantial national military establishment (Rakove 2000).

The militia was an institution created by government. One of the Antifederalists' fears was that the national government would disarm the state's citizenry, not by confiscating weapons but by failing to provide citizens with military arms, which they rarely possessed or maintained. Antifederalist George Mason argued for an express declaration that the state governments might arm and discipline the militia should Congress fail to do so. Madison argued that the power to arm the militia would in fact remain a concurrent one, shared between federal and state governments (Rakove 2000).

The debate over the Second Amendment also dealt with the role of the militia in suppressing insurrection, and again what was at stake was the question of which level of government—state or national—would be empowered to use the militia. But to all it was clear that the militia was to be used to help defeat insurrections; there was no plan for an armed citizenry, independent of government, acting as a main deterrent against despotism (Rakove 2000). While some of the early state constitutions, written during the revolution, not surprisingly endorsed the right of revolution, the framers of the Constitution did not endorse such a right for their own democratic republic. Every two years there would be an opportunity to participate in an orderly process to replace the existing government (Finkelman 2000).

With the exception of one recent case (*United States v. Emerson*, 270 F. 3d 203 [5th Cir. 2001]), the federal courts have consistently ruled that the Second Amendment concerns a well-regulated (or organized) militia—which the courts currently define as the National Guard—and does not guarantee or protect an individual's right to own or possess a firearm (Vernick and Teret 1993; Henigan, Nicholson, and Hemenway 1995).

In the *Emerson* case, a federal judge in Texas did something that no federal court had done for more than sixty years—he held that the Second Amendment protects an individual's right to keep and bear arms. His decision that an individual under a domestic violence restraining order had a right to own a gun was reversed at the superior court level, but two of the judges expressed their view that the Second Amendment protects an individual's right to possess firearms. Some have argued that this view is dicta—unnecessary to the outcome of the case and not binding on other courts. In 2002, Attorney General John Ashcroft pushed further, reversing Justice Department precedent by proclaiming that the Second Amendment did confer an individual right.

Later in 2002, in *Silveira v. Lockyer*, (312 F. 3d 1052 [9th Cir. 2002]), the Ninth Circuit Federal Court of Appeals unanimously upheld California's strict assault weapons ban and rebutted the idea of a constitutionally protected individual right to bear arms. "The [Second] Amendment was not adopted to afford rights to individuals with respect to private ownership or possession."

The U.S. Supreme Court's last word on the Second Amendment came in 1939 (*United States v. Miller*, 307 U.S. 174 [1939]). Defendants in the case had been convicted of transporting an unregistered sawed-off shotgun across state lines. They appealed under the 1934 Firearms Act, claiming that it violated the Second Amendment and was therefore unconstitutional. The Supreme Court rejected that argument, holding that the purpose of the Second Amendment was "to insure the viability of state militias." The unanimous Court stated,

> In the absence of any evidence tending to show that possession or use of a shotgun having a barrel of less than eighteen inches in length at this time has some reasonable relationship to the preservation or efficiency of a well-regulated militia, we cannot say that the Second Amendment guarantees the right to keep and bear such an instrument. (id. at 176)

In subsequent years, the Supreme Court has consistently refused to reopen the issue. In 1983, for example, it let stand a decision upholding a Morton Grove, Illinois, ordinance that banned the possession of handguns within its borders (*Quilici v. Morton Grove*, 695 F.2d 261 [7th Cir. 1982], *cert. denied* 464 U.S. 863 [1983]). The policy measures to be suggested in the remainder of this book are not nearly as restrictive as the Morton Grove ordinance.

In June 2002, the Supreme Court refused to review the *Emerson* case. It also refused to review a 2001 Oklahoma case (*United States v. Haney*, 264 F. 3d 1161 [10th Cir. 2001]) in which the Tenth Circuit Court of Appeals in Denver ruled, consistent with case law, that a gun control law does not violate the Second Amendment "unless it impairs the state's ability to maintain a well-regulated militia." The militia, it added, is "a governmental organization"(id. at 1165); it is not individuals possessing their own guns. The U.S. Supreme Court may eventually have to weigh in on these recent conflicting interpretations.

A flavor of the previous consistency and definitiveness of the courts' interpretation of the Second Amendment is provided by some recent rulings:

> "As the language of the [Second] Amendment itself indicates, it was not framed with individual rights in mind. . . . Reasonable gun control legislation is clearly within the police power of the State and must be accepted by the individual though it impose a restraint or burden on him" (*Burton v. Sills*, 53 NJ 86, 106 [1968]).

> "Since the Second Amendment right 'to keep and bear arms' applies only to the right of the state to maintain a militia, and not to the individual's right to bear arms, there can be no serious claim to any express constitutional right of an individual to possess a firearm" (*Stevens v. United States*, 440 F. 2d 144, 149 [6th Cir. 1971]).

"Appellant's theory . . . is that by the Second Amendment to the United States Constitution he is entitled to bear arms. Appellant is completely wrong about that" (*Eckert v. City of Philadelphia*, 477 F. 2d 610, 610 [3d Cir.], *cert. denied*, 414 U.S. 839 [1973]).

"It is clear that the Second Amendment guarantees a collective rather than an individual right" (*United States v. Warin*, 530 F. 2d 103, 106 [6th Cir.], *cert. denied*, 426 U.S. 948 [1976]).

"The Second Amendment guarantees no right to keep and bear a firearm that does not have some reasonable relationship to the preservation or efficiency of a well regulated Militia" (*Lewis v. United States*, 445 US 55, 66 [1980]).

"Construing [the language of the Second Amendment] according to its plain meaning, it seems clear that the right to bear arms is inextricably connected to the preservation of a militia. . . . We conclude that the right to keep and bear arms is not guaranteed by the Second Amendment" (*Quilici v. Village of Morton Grove*, 695 F. 2d 261, 265 [7th Cir. 1982]).

"Considering this history, we cannot conclude that the Second Amendment protects the individual possession of military weapons" (*United States v. Hale*, 978 F. 2d 1016, 1019 [8th Cir. 1992]).

"The [Second] Amendment protects the people's right to maintain an effective state militia, and does not establish an individual right to own or possess firearms for personal or other use" (*Silveira v. Lockyer*, 312 F. 3d 1052, 1066 [9th Cir. 2002]).

Indeed, even including the *Emerson* case, no federal firearms legislation has been struck down on Second Amendment grounds. When the gun lobby brings cases against federal gun restrictions, it rarely uses the Second Amendment and instead claims unconstitutionality based on the Tenth Amendment, which deals with the separation of powers between the federal and state governments, or other constitutional provisions (Vernick and Teret 1999).

Expert interest groups have clearly stated positions in support of the collective interpretation of the Second Amendment. The American Civil Liber-

ties Union (ACLU), the organization that is probably the staunchest sup-
porter of the Bill of Rights, believes that the constitutional right to bear arms
is primarily a collective one, designed to protect states' right to maintain militias to assure freedom and security against the central government. "In
today's world that idea is somewhat anachronistic and in any case would
require weapons much more powerful than handguns or hunting rifles." The
ACLU thus believes that the Second Amendment does not prohibit "reasonable regulation of gun ownership, such as licensing and registration" (ACLU
1999). The ACLU's Policy 47 states, "The ACLU agrees with the Supreme
Court's long-standing interpretation of the Second Amendment that the
individual's right to bear arms applies only to the preservation or efficiency of
a well-regulated militia. Except for lawful police and military purposes, the
possession of weapons by individuals is not constitutionally protected.
Therefore, there is no constitutional impediment to the regulation of
firearms" (ACLU 1999).

The American Bar Association, which represents more than four hundred
thousand attorneys, has a long-standing position on the Second Amendment
that is consistent with the courts' interpretation.

> Few issues have been more distorted and cluttered by misinformation
> than this one. There is no confusion in the law itself. The strictest gun
> control laws in the nation have been upheld against Second Amend-
> ment challenge. . . . Yet the perception that the Second Amendment is
> somehow an obstacle to Congress and state and local legislative bodies
> fashioning laws to regulate firearms remains a pervasive myth. . . . As
> lawyers, as representatives of the legal profession, and as recognized
> experts on the meaning of the Constitution and our system of justice,
> we share a responsibility to "say what the law is." . . . The argument that
> the Second Amendment prohibits all State or Federal regulation of cit-
> izens' ownership of firearms has no validity whatsoever. (American Bar
> Association 1999)

In the past two decades, many legal scholars have claimed that the courts
have misinterpreted the intent of the Second Amendment (e.g., Kates 1983;
Levinson 1989; Malcolm 1994; Van Alstyne 1994). Other scholars claim to
refute the revisionists (e.g., Henigan 1991; Williams 1991; Wills 1995; Dorf
2000; Finkelman 2000; Heyman 2000; Rakove 2000; Schwoerer 2000; Uviller
and Merkel 2000). Perhaps the most interesting new thesis argues that Madi-

son wrote the Second Amendment to assure the southern states that Congress would not undermine the slave system by disarming the militias, which were the principal instruments of slave control throughout the South (Bogus 1998).

Courts have the power of reinterpreting the law, and the Constitution can be amended. For at least the previous sixty years, courts in the United States have generally held that the U.S. Constitution does not provide individuals with any right to own or carry a firearm, apart from its connection with the "preservation or efficiency" of the militia. Owning a gun is a privilege. Most important, the Constitution does not prevent reasonable gun policies. As summarized by American Bar Association President R. W. Ide III,

> It is time we overcome the destructive myth perpetuated by gun control opponents about the Second Amendment. . . . Federal and state courts have reached in this century a consensus interpretation of the Second Amendment that permits the exercise of broad power to limit private access to firearms by all levels of government. (1994)

Even in the aberrant *Emerson* case, the courts ruled that an individual under a restraining order does not have a right to possess a firearm.

It is sometimes claimed that the Second Amendment helps guarantee that an armed citizenry will be able to overthrow potential tyranny of the federal government. However, this notion appears largely ahistorical. American Revolutionary leaders were never of a mind to permit armed rebellions against their governance. For example, in 1786, when debt-ridden farmers, led by Daniel Shays, rose up in arms to demand that the Massachusetts state government reduce their taxes, the federal Congress authorized troops to help suppress the rebellion. Similarly, in 1794, when western Pennsylvania farmers rose in arms to block collection of a federal tax on distilled liquor, the uprising was crushed by troops headed by Generals George Washington and Light Horse Harry Lee.

On both occasions, self-styled patriots were objecting to what they saw as acts of tyranny. The Second Amendment was not about instigating insurrection—as a Timothy McVeigh might plan—but about enabling government to combat it. In the absence of an organized police force in the eighteenth century, it was expected that the militia's primary responsibility would be internal security rather than defense against invasion (Dorf 2000).

The governmental response to the Whiskey Rebellion, like the earlier Shays uprising, revealed "the establishment's lack of respect for the idea that dissatisfied citizens could keep firearms and use them against the will of the government, even if the insurgents considered the regime tyrannical" (DeConde 2001, 41).

When the Bill of Rights was added to the Constitution, every state had some form of firearms regulation. In the debate about the Second Amendment, no one argued that its passage might hinder the state's authority to regulate firearms, because the Second Amendment was not about individual rights. In 2000, a group of more than forty historians and law professors signed a letter to the NRA president, Charlton Heston, publicized in an advertisement in the *New York Times,* stating that "the law is well-settled that the Second Amendment permits broad and intensive regulation of firearms" (Bogus 2000).

PUBLIC OPINION

Public support for the regulation of firearms is strong and widespread.... In general, people endorse measures to regulate guns, increase gun safety, and reduce gun violence, except for policies that entail a blanket prohibition on owning guns.

—T. W. Smith

The American public has been polled for more than sixty years about firearms, and the large majority has consistently supported stronger gun regulations. Year after year, every independent national polling firm—whether Gallup, Roper, Harris, Yankelovich, the National Opinion Research Center (NORC), CBS, ABC, or CNN—reports the same findings. Most Americans and even most gun owners favor more government control over firearms.

Some questions have been asked on national surveys for decades. Since 1959 Gallup and NORC have asked a random sample of adults, "Would you favor or oppose a law which would require a person to obtain a police permit before he or she could buy a gun?" Few states or localities have such a requirement. Yet every year, between 69 and 81 percent of respondents have answered "yes" to this question (Young et al. 1996). The results are amazingly consistent year after year.

When asked about specific gun control measures that have been mentioned in policy discussions, Americans favor virtually every one except for the banning of handguns or long guns. Consider the results from three surveys conducted by NORC between 1996 and 1998 (Smith 1999). Although none of these measures is currently mandated by federal law,

1. 95 percent of Americans favor safety and quality standards for domestically manufactured handguns comparable to those that imported handguns must meet;
2. 90 percent support mandatory gun safety training before a person can buy a gun;
3. 90 percent favor requiring that serial numbers on guns be tamper resistant;
4. 88 percent back having all new handguns be designed so that they "cannot be fired by a young child's small hands";
5. 85 percent want both a five-day waiting period and a background check before a handgun can be purchased;
6. 85 percent endorse mandatory registration of handguns;
7. 82 percent support a requirement that pistols have magazine safeties;
8. 82 percent support requiring a police permit before a gun can be purchased;
9. 80 percent want owners to be liable if a gun is not stored properly and is misused by a child;
10. 79 percent favor requiring background checks for sales between private individuals;
11. 79 percent favor making manufacturers liable for any injuries that result from defects in the design or manufacturing of guns;
12. 78 percent back the requirement that guns be stored unloaded;
13. 77 percent back the requirement that trigger locks be used;
14. 77 percent believe that the sale of handgun ammunition should be regulated in the same manner as the sale of handguns;
15. 75 percent want the federal government to regulate the safety design of guns;
16. 75 percent think Congress should hold hearings to investigate the practices of the gun industry, much like the tobacco industry hearings;
17. 73 percent want to ban the sale of all high-capacity gun magazines;
18. 73 percent favor having all new handguns come with an indicator to show whether the weapon is loaded;

19. 72 percent want mandatory registration of long guns (rifles and shotguns);
20. 70 percent back requiring that all new handguns be personalized so that only a weapon's owner will be able to fire it;
21. 69 percent want to exclude from the American market imported guns that cannot be bought by citizens in their country of origin;
22. 60 percent favor allowing concealed-carry permits only for those with special needs, such as private detectives; and
23. 54 percent want a ban on the domestic manufacture of "small, easily concealed, and inexpensive handguns."

By contrast,

24. only 39 percent support restricting the possession of handguns to "the police and other authorized persons"; and
25. only 16 percent want "a total ban on handguns."

The groups most likely to support these new policies are women and non-gun owners. Still, a majority of men support all of the first twenty-three policies. And even among gun owners, who represent only 25 percent of the adult population, a majority favor twenty-one of the first twenty-three policies listed (only 49 percent favor the mandatory registration of rifles and shotguns and 37 percent favor restricting concealed gun carrying to police and those with special needs).

The NORC's 2001 survey gives largely similar results (Smith 2001). And it is not just the NORC surveys that obtain such results. All polls show strong popular support for new governmental regulations, short of a ban on handguns or all firearms. For example, a 1999 random national poll conducted by CNN/Gallup/*USA Today* found that 83 percent of respondents favored "a law which would require background checks before people—including gun dealers—could buy guns at gun shows," 79 percent favored "the registration of all handguns," and 68 percent favored "a ban on the manufacture, sale and possession of semi-automatic assault guns, such as the AK-47" (National Journal's Cloakroom 1999).

A 1999 ABC News/*Washington Post* national poll found that 90 percent of respondents supported background checks at gun shows, 79 percent favored mandatory trigger locks, 75 percent favored registration of handgun owners, and 66 percent favored a ban on Internet gun sales. Majorities favor such policies, even among men, Republicans, and gun owners. Americans were split evenly on a ban on concealed-weapon carrying, while only 32 percent favored a ban on all handgun sales (Merkle 1999). A subsequent poll by the same group largely duplicated these results (*National Journal* 2000).

Whenever a question has been asked on independent national polls over the past decades, a sizable majority of Americans has favored "stricter gun control laws" as well as the registration of handguns and long guns, the Brady Bill, assault weapons bans, and the ban on plastic guns (Young et al. 1996). For example, a 1998 Harris national poll found that 76 percent of respondents favored "stricter laws relating to the control of handguns." Even among gun owners, two-thirds wanted stricter controls (National Journal's Cloakroom 1998).

Polls that also ask about membership in the NRA find that even among self-identified NRA members, a majority favor most moderate gun control measures such as handgun registration and mandatory safety training before purchasing a firearm. Most NRA members supported the Brady Bill, and less than half want to repeal the assault weapons ban (Weil and Hemenway 1993; *Time*/CNN poll 1995).

National surveys show that the public wants to severely punish criminals who use guns and to prohibit individuals convicted of various crimes from purchasing handguns (Teret et al. 1998). Although the vast majority of Americans want to make such purchases illegal, most states currently allow persons convicted of the following crimes to legally buy handguns:

1. publicly displaying a firearm in a threatening manner (95 percent of adults, including 91 percent of gun owners, support preventing people convicted of such crimes from having guns);
2. possession of equipment for illegal drug use (92 percent of adults, including 89 percent of gun owners);
3. domestic violence (85 percent of adults, including 80 percent of gun owners);
4. assault and battery that does not involve a lethal weapon or serious injury (85 percent of adults, including 75 percent of gun owners);
5. drunk and disorderly conduct (84 percent of adults, including 73 percent of gun owners);
6. carrying a concealed weapon without a permit (83 percent of adults, including 70 percent of gun owners);

7. driving under the influence of alcohol (71 percent of adults, including 59 percent of gun owners);
8. shoplifting (68 percent of adults, including 56 percent of gun owners); and
9. indecent exposure (61 percent of adults, including 48 percent of gun owners).

Some progun writers claim that gun control is inherently racist, a policy tool designed to take away from blacks the right to bear arms (Kates et al. 1995). Yet minorities tend to be the strongest supporters of proposed gun control policies. In spite of blacks' historical wariness of government, general support for gun control appears higher for blacks than for whites, even after holding constant a large variety of factors, including gun ownership, income, education, urban residence, and church attendance (Browne 1999a). Since minorities are at the highest risk for being victims of gun violence, minorities will be among the largest beneficiaries of reasonable gun policies.

D. B. Kopel, an attorney who has written widely on the benefits of firearms, titled a 1988 article "Trust the People: The Case against Gun Control." But if politicians actually trusted the people, we would have much more stringent and rational gun policies than we do. Every independent poll indicates the same thing—the large majority of the populace wants more governmental action to regulate guns, to make guns safer, and to keep guns out of the hands of dangerous people.

EVALUATING REGULATION

> Gun control does not work in America, because it barely exists.
> —*The Economist*

A crucial step in the public health approach to injury prevention is the after-the-fact evaluation of public and private policies. It is important to know what has and what has not worked. Unfortunately, sufficient scientific policy evaluations have not occurred in the areas of violence prevention in general and of firearms policy in particular (Reiss and Roth 1993).

Part of the problem results from insufficient funding for research and evaluation. Another major limitation has been the lack of a good data (surveillance) system for firearms. Detailed and disaggregate information on firearm ownership or firearm injuries is rarely available. In trying to evaluate interventions, researchers are often forced to rely on crude proxies and aggregate measures.

For example, to determine the effect of right-turn-on-red laws on pedestrian injuries, it is usually insufficient to have data on the total number of automobile fatalities. It is crucial to have data on the number and circumstances of pedestrian injuries, those struck at intersections, and especially those injured by vehicles making right turns at red signals. Social scientists rarely have the ability (the statistical "power") to detect small effects, such as 1–2 percent changes in injury levels. A right-turn-on-red law may not have a statistically detectable impact on total automotive fatalities, but it may have a sizable and detectable effect on one component of the problem—pedestrians struck at intersections.

Minimum legal drinking age laws have been shown to reduce traffic fatalities. The evaluations did not have the statistical power to show that the law reduced the overall number of crashes, traffic injuries, or traffic fatalities. However, the evaluations were able to demonstrate that the intervention worked in the sense that raising the drinking age reduced fatal injuries to the age group affected, eighteen- to twenty-year-olds, and that the effect occurred when these young people would most likely have been drinking and driving—at night, especially on the weekend.

Most firearm policies in the United States have been quite modest, with expected modest effects. State and local policies are often undermined by the easy flow of guns across political boundaries. Still, a policy that reduced firearm injuries by 0.5–1 percent—percentages too small to be detected by aggregate data—if applied to the entire U.S. population in the mid-1990s would amount to an overall decrease each year of 75–150 homicides and 90–180 suicides.

One study attempted to assess the individual effects of nineteen separate local and state gun policies on citywide violence rates, broken down into homicides, robberies, aggravated assaults, and so forth (Kleck and Patterson 1993). Policies included prohibiting gun possession by alcoholics, prohibiting gun possession by drug addicts, prohibiting gun possession by minors, a state constitutional provision allowing the right to bear arms, a ban on the sale of Saturday night specials, and restrictions on open handgun carrying.

The model had serious structural problems (see appendix A) and few measures of the level of policy enforcement. It also had insufficient statistical power to detect small changes at an aggregate level. For example, it did not examine the effect of the laws against drug addicts' possession of guns on the lethal violence perpetrated on or by drug addicts or the effect of prohibiting gun possession by minors on the violence inflicted on or perpetrated by minors. It tried to find an effect of these individual policies on the overall levels of homicide, robbery, and burglary. Not surprisingly, few of these firearm laws by themselves had a statistically significant effect on these aggregate crime rates.

Nonetheless, the analysis concluded that

> there do appear to be some gun control laws which work, all of them relatively moderate, popular and inexpensive. Thus, there is support for a gun control policy organized around gun owner licensing or purchase permits (or some other form of gun buyer screening), stricter local dealer licensing, bans on possession of guns by criminals and mentally ill people, stronger controls over illegal carrying, and possibly discretionary add-on penalties for committing felonies with a gun. On the other hand, popular favorites such as waiting periods and gun registration do not appear to affect violence rates. (Kleck and Patterson 1993, 283)

In all areas of policy, it is often quite difficult to effectively evaluate the impact of particular laws. The evaluator is trying to contrast actual events to a counterfactual—that is, what would have happened had the law not been passed. The latter is in some sense unknowable.

Two main study designs that have been used to evaluate firearm policies are cross-sectional studies (comparing localities with and without various laws at a point in time) and longitudinal studies (before- versus after-the-law evaluations, sometimes called interrupted time series). One academic review of the firearms evaluation literature found that all the cross-sectional studies were problematic for several reasons (Cook 1991). For example, "the results are sensitive to the specification of the model to be estimated. There are many plausible variables that may influence interstate variations in the rates of personal violence, and the decision of which of these variables to include in the analysis is subject to a large and unquantifiable degree of uncertainty" (1991, 48). The reviewer concluded,

> It appears that the intrinsic difficulties with this [cross-sectional] approach virtually ensure against generating reliable, persuasive results that will be a useful guide to state legislators. (48–49)

A second academic review of the firearms evaluation literature argued that time series analyses had fatal problems (Kleck 1997b). For example, in before-after studies, "it is very difficult to tell exactly *when* the effect of a new law is supposed to become evident" (353). Kleck concluded that "univariate time series research on the impact of individual laws is virtually worthless" (377).

While one need not entirely agree with either claim, formal evaluations of gun control laws have had many problems, and the results need to be taken with a grain of salt. For example, supposedly sophisticated econometric studies that combine the cross-sectional and time series approaches can suggest that middle-aged and elderly black females are the source of much criminal activity (Lott 1998a) or that when Indiana closed its gun show loophole, a 102 percent reduction in the state's auto theft rate occurred (Lott 2003). Such results are just one piece of evidence that indicates that the author's models are misspecified and the findings should not be accepted as valid.

Nonetheless, careful studies have been conducted, and a review of the empirical literature of the past thirty years of the effect of gun control laws on suicide shows a strong and significant effect (Miller and Hemenway 1999). For example, cross-sectional studies find that suicide rates in 1970 (Medoff and Magaddino 1983), 1980 (Yang and Lester 1991), and 1985 (Boor and Bair 1990) were significantly lower in those U.S. states with stricter gun control laws. Time-series (longitudinal) studies also often find an effect on total suicide rates. In 1978, Canada tightened restrictions on gun ownership, virtually outlawing handguns; a nationwide educational campaign about safe use and storage of firearms was also undertaken. It appears the law led to a onetime drop in both the firearm and total suicide rates but not the nonfirearms suicide rate (Lester and Leenaars 1993, 1994; Carrington and Moyer 1994; Leenaars et al. 2003).

In 1976, the District of Columbia adopted a very restrictive handgun law. A time-series analysis covering 1968–87 found that the adoption of the law coincided with an abrupt and sustained 23 percent decline in firearms suicide rate. There were no parallel increases in suicide from nonfirearm methods, nor were similar declines in firearm suicide rates seen in adjacent metropolitan areas of Maryland or Virginia, to which the legislation did not apply (Loftin et al. 1991). The abruptness of the localized decline after the law suggests that many of the handguns used in these urban suicides may have been of recent vintage.

A 1998 synopsis of the impact of gun control legislation on suicide concluded,

POLICY BACKGROUND

[This] literature review of the effectiveness of gun control legislation indicates that restricting access to firearms through gun control legislation diminishes suicide. Reducing the availability and accessibility of means appears to decrease suicide rates, and substitution of other means does not appear to offset the benefits of restrictions. (Lambert and Silva 1998, 132)

Gun laws can also reduce unintentional firearm injuries. Canada's 1977 Criminal Law Amendment Act appears to have reduced accidental shootings. Results from a before-after study of the law "indicate that the passage of [the measure] was accompanied by a decrease in the accidental mortality rate from firearms" (Leenaars and Lester 1997, 121).

Across U.S. states, some researchers also find an effect of gun control laws on fatal gun accidents (Geisel, Roll, and Wettick 1969; Lester and Murrell 1981, 1986), while others do not (Murray 1975; DeZee 1983). A study examining the effect of state laws holding adults criminally liable for children's deaths resulting from negligent storage estimated that the laws significantly reduced accidental shooting deaths among children aged zero to fourteen (Cummings, Grossman, Rivara, and Koepsell 1997), but this result is due to the effect of one state (Webster and Starnes 2000).

It has been more difficult to find an effect of U.S. gun laws on crime levels than it has been to find such an effect on suicide or accidental firearm injury. Most studies do not find a substantial, statistically significant impact of U.S. firearm laws on crime rates (Kleck 1997b). We should not expect that most gun laws would have a discernable beneficial effect on assaults, burglaries, rapes, or robberies. The vast majority of these crimes are committed without guns. The principal effects of gun control laws on crime will typically be on gun robberies and on homicides.

In addition, crime guns currently move easily across state lines. While most guns used in suicide and in accidental injury are probably legally owned by the individuals involved and come from the state where the incident occurred, recent tracing data show that crime guns used in states with strict gun control laws usually come from more permissive states (Webster, Vernick, and Hepburn 2001). Crime gun movement reduces the effect of most local firearms laws on local crime.

There are other reasons to expect that it will be difficult to detect current gun policies' effects on aggregate crime levels. Many state and local firearm regulations are relatively minor and are often not well enforced. One study examining gun laws in different nations concluded that the evidence indicated that major gun laws reduced deaths due to crime, but no effect of minor gun control laws could be detected (Podell and Archer 1994). A recent study of a strong state law, the 1990 Maryland ban on Saturday night specials, found that the law probably led to a 9 percent drop in handgun-related murders, with no effect on the rate of murders with other weapons (Webster et al. 2002). One of the most restrictive pieces of local legislation, the handgun licensing law for Washington, D.C., begun in 1976, was associated with a reduction in the fraction of assaults and robberies committed with a gun (Jones 1981) and a 25 percent reduction in homicides (Loftin et al. 1991). However, the district's restrictions on handgun transfers proved ineffective in stopping the tide of drug-related lethal violence beginning in the mid-1980s.

For national firearms laws, it is often difficult to evaluate the effects of regulations because of the lack of good comparison groups. By contrast, for local laws, it is possible to compare communities that did not enact local ordinances to those that did. In other words, for national laws it is often more difficult to determine the counterfactual—what would have happened without the law.

The 1993 Brady Bill mandated background checks and, for a few years, a five-day waiting period before a handgun could be purchased from a licensed dealer. It would seem, at first blush, to have been an amazingly effective law. As the criminal-records database has become more complete and readily available to law enforcement officials, more and more prospective gun purchasers have been denied because they had criminal histories. For example, in the seven months between November 1998, when the "instant check" system came on line, and June 1999, an estimated one hundred thousand convicted criminals, fugitives, and people with histories of mental illness were stopped from buying guns (Butterfield 1999b).

The Brady law also helped eliminate many kitchen-table dealers, reducing the number of licensed firearms dealers from more than 270,000 to fewer than 100,000. The reduction allows for better oversight by the Bureau of Alcohol, Tobacco, and Firearms (ATF) and reduces the likelihood of prospective criminal purchasers finding careless or scofflaw dealers. The Brady law also appears to have quickly and dramatically reduced the trafficking of handguns from previously permissive states, such as Mississippi, into jurisdictions with stringent handgun controls, such as Chicago (Cook and Braga 2001). Finally, crime peaked in the United States in 1993. Since the passage of the Brady law in that year, gun homicide, overall homicide, and gun robberies have declined substantially—just what would be expected if the law were effective.

But is the Brady law responsible for all, some, or even any of these crime reductions? We don't know. The problem for the scientific evaluator is that U.S. crime, particularly crime involving firearms, is very volatile. Gun crime seems to move in waves or cycles, and there are no good models that explain those waves. Many other factors certainly changed during the 1990s (e.g., the decline in crack cocaine markets in inner cities and different police practices) and might help explain the decline in gun crime.

One way to evaluate the Brady law is to compare those states that already had background checks and waiting periods before the Brady law was passed to those that did not. In theory, the law might have had a differential and greater impact on states that had not previously required background checks on gun purchasers. However, since guns currently move easily across state lines—from states with permissive firearm laws to states with more stringent laws—making it harder for criminals to buy guns from Florida dealers can affect not only Florida crime but also New York crime. Examining only the differential impact of the Brady law might overlook a large part of its effect. A careful study that examined the Brady law found little evidence for a differential effect (Ludwig and Cook 2000).

Some recent U.S. studies provide suggestive evidence about the (possible) effect of four types of firearm policies: (1) disarming batterers; (2) prison enhancements; (3) one-gun-per-month laws; and (4) firearm purchase denials.

1. *Disarming batterers.* A number of states have laws preventing individuals who have restraining orders issued against them from owning or purchasing firearms. A careful analysis suggests that these laws may have reduced intimate-partner homicides. The effect appears to be largest for women killed by firearms and to be confined to states that have a searchable database of restraining orders. The study's main limitations are that it could not control for variability of enforcement or for certain other statewide programs, such as the availability of victim services (Vigdor and Mercy 2003).

2. *Sentence enhancement.* Project Exile, a sentence-enhancement program combined with an advertising campaign stressing zero tolerance for gun offenses in Richmond, Virginia, has been touted as a highly successful enforcement policy, resulting in a 40 percent

decline in homicide between 1997 and 1998. However, a careful analysis finds that the policy had little effect. The program went into effect in February 1997, and Richmond's 1997 homicide rate was 30 percent higher than the city's 1996 rate. U.S. crime rates fell from 1997 to 2000, most steeply in high-crime places such as Richmond. Project Exile focused on adults, yet adult homicide arrest rates increased relative to juvenile arrest rates after the program was enacted. The law may have been a sensible approach to punishment, but the evaluation found that the program's effects, if any, were too small to detect (Raphael and Ludwig 2003).

3. *One-gun-per-month laws.* The ATF's increased gun tracing has provided a wealth of provocative information. Gun traffic moves one way, from states with weak gun laws to states with strong gun laws. Indeed, in states with strong gun laws, criminals obtain the majority of their guns from states with weak laws; where laws are weak, criminals obtain the majority of their guns locally (Schumer 1997).

Virginia had long been a major source of crime guns for other states. In 1993, a Virginia law took effect limiting handgun purchases by an individual to one gun in a thirty-day period. The law appears to have had a dramatic effect on interstate gunrunning. Tracing data showed that Virginia dealers were the source for 35 percent of crime guns purchased in New York, New Jersey, Connecticut, Rhode Island, and Massachusetts before the law's enactment . For criminal firearms purchased after the law, only 16 percent of the guns traced by police in these northeastern states came from Virginia. The law was an effective means of disrupting the illegal interstate transfer of firearms (Weil and Knox 1996). However, if only a few states have one-gun-per-month laws, gunrunners may just take their business to other states.

4. *Firearm purchase denials.* A series of studies concerning firearm background checks in California suggests that stopping individuals with felony convictions from purchasing firearms reduces violent crime and that even more categories of individuals should be prevented from buying guns.

One study of more than three thousand individuals who had been denied handgun purchases in California in 1991 found that 91 percent were denied because of prior criminal activity. These individuals were nearly twice as likely as other handgun purchasers to select small, inexpensive handguns, which are easily concealed and disproportionately used in crime (Wintemute, Wright, et al. 1999).

A second, more pertinent study looked at prospective gun purchasers in 1977 and followed them over time. The subsequent criminal histories of individuals who were denied purchase of handguns because of prior felony convictions were compared with individuals who had prior felony arrests but no convictions and were allowed to buy handguns. It might be expected that the former group of convicted criminals would continue to perpetrate more crimes. But after adjusting for prior criminal history, those who had been arrested but not convicted and thus were easily able legally to obtain handguns had more subsequent per capita gun and violent offenses. These "findings suggest that denial of a handgun purchase is associated with a reduction in risk for later criminal activity of approximately 20% to 30%" (Wright, Wintemute, and Rivara 1999, 89).

Results of a third study suggest that individuals with prior misdemeanor convictions, especially for violence, probably should not be allowed to purchase handguns. The subsequent criminal histories of handgun purchasers with prior misdemeanor convictions were compared with handgun purchasers who did not have prior criminal histories. Those with misdemeanors were seven times more likely to be subsequently charged with crimes, and those with at least two prior convictions for misdemeanor violence were fifteen times more likely to be charged with murder, rape, robbery, or aggravated assault. Nearly one in five handgun purchasers with prior misdemeanor convictions were charged with new crimes within a year of the purchase, compared to fewer than one in fifty handgun purchasers without prior convictions (Wintemute, Drake, et al. 1998). The evidence does not prove that allowing gun acquisition worsened criminal activities, but it does show that a misdemeanor conviction is a strong predictor of the potential for subsequent illegal behavior—that these are individuals most people would not want to see given easy access to firearms.

SUMMARY

On the subject of the Second Amendment, the U.S. legal system has spoken clearly and nearly unanimously. According to the courts, the Second Amendment does not provide an individual right to own a gun, and, most important, there is no constitutional barrier to reasonable gun policies in the United States.

As conservative former judge Robert Bork wrote,

> The Supreme Court has consistently ruled that there is no individual right to own a firearm. . . . The Second Amendment was designed to allow states to defend themselves against a possibly tyrannical national government. Now that the federal government has stealth bombers and nuclear weapons, it is hard to imagine what people would need to keep in the garage to serve that purpose. (1996, 16)

Meanwhile, the public supports virtually all reasonable gun policies. Indeed, the public's position on gun policy has remained remarkably stable: a large majority favor most policies short of an outright ban on handguns or all guns. A majority of gun owners and even self-described NRA members also favor most such policies, which are not currently in place in the United States.

Three comprehensive surveys on popular preferences with respect to gun policies, conducted in 1996, 1997, and 1998 by the NORC, which is affiliated with the University of Chicago, have quite consistent findings. The 1998 survey, for example, found that

1. the public supports the regulation of guns as consumer products (e.g., 95 percent of the public, including 92 percent of gun owners, support holding domestically produced handguns to the same federal safety and quality standards as imported handguns);
2. the public supports further restricting gun purchases by criminals (e.g., 95 percent of the public, including 91 percent of gun owners, support denying firearm purchase for those convicted of "publicly displaying a firearm in a threatening manner");
3. the public supports stricter laws regarding the sale of firearms (e.g., 80 percent of the public, including 66 percent of gun owners, want private sales to be subject to the same background checks as those required for dealer sales);
4. the public supports the registration of handguns (85 percent of the general public and 75 percent of gun owners); and
5. the public supports an increase in restrictions on who may carry concealed firearms (e.g., 60 percent of the general public wants

licenses to carry concealed weapons to be issued only to those with special needs, such as private detectives).

Those who "trust the public" should favor such policies. Unfortunately, the power of the gun lobby has prevented many reasonable policy proposals from being enacted into law.

An important issue is whether firearms policies, however well meaning, actually work to reduce crime and firearm injuries. Unfortunately, there exist few convincing evaluations of past firearms laws (Ohsfeldt and Morrisey 1992; Kleck 1997b). Major impediments include the lack of funding for evaluations and the lack of good disaggregate data. Good data exist for motor vehicle injuries, permitting researchers to conduct good studies—for example, to determine the impact of motorcycle helmet laws on motorcycle injuries rather than to try to discover an effect on all transportation injuries. Researchers can look for the impact of increased highway speed limits on injuries occurring on those specific highways with higher speed limits. By contrast, in the firearms area, researchers are often reduced to trying to find an effect of laws making it illegal for mentally ill persons to own a firearm by examining data only on overall rape, robbery, or aggravated assault rates (Kleck and Patterson 1993).

The evidence that does exist suggests that gun laws may have been effective in reducing suicides and fatal gun accidents. There is also an indication that one-gun-per-month laws may reduce gunrunning, that background checks on gun purchasers can reduce violence, that disarming batterers can reduce intimate partner homicides, and that additional categories of individuals (e.g., those with violent misdemeanor convictions) should be prohibited from buying handguns.

It has usually been difficult to find a statistically significant effect of local gun laws on violence and crime. Indeed, there may be little such effect, probably because it is easy for criminals in the United States to obtain guns in areas with permissive laws and transport the guns to areas with stricter controls. Also, crime often moves in waves, and we lack good models to explain or predict those waves.

Various mid-1990s law enforcement initiatives in Boston, New York, and elsewhere have received a great deal of media attention, in part because they have been associated with rapidly falling crime. The Boston Gun Project, for example, which started in 1995, is a collaboration of researchers, police, prosecutors, the probation and parole system, social services, and the ATF. The group began by getting detailed information about the city's firearms problem and discovered that even in the most dangerous neighborhoods, those caught up in violence were a small minority of juveniles and young adults. They were often chronic offenders with robust criminal histories. Their violence was not about drugs but about respect, romantic matters, and standing vendettas—the origins of which were often unclear even to the participants (Kennedy, Piehl, and Braga 1996).

By debriefing offenders, the Boston Gun Project found that most of the guns used by these youths were trafficked illegally rather than stolen. The city police and the ATF cracked down on the traffickers. Police, clergy, gang-outreach workers, and community groups worked with the gangs. The message was: the violence stops today. If anyone in your gang commits a violent crime, law enforcement will come down hard on the entire gang. Conversely, if you want help—job training, drug treatment—it is available. Never before had so many agencies shared intelligence and cooperated so fully.

The goal was to make it safe for gang members to put down their guns. And the initiative seemed to be wildly successful—Boston homicides, which averaged about one hundred per year before the initiative, fell to forty-three in 1997 and thirty-five in 1998 (Kennedy 1999). This public health approach makes good sense and is rightfully touted as a model for other cities to follow. But it is also true that homicide rates fell during this same period in other Massachusetts cities without this initiative. An evaluation suggests that the Boston policy initiative may have had a substantial impact (Braga et al. 2001), but it is not easy to determine the counterfactual—what would have happened in Boston without the intervention.

CHAPTER 9   POLICY LESSONS

You know, terrorism against freedom isn't just practiced with bombs and box cutters. Anti-freedom elitists in academia, the media, rich foundations and government can do permanent damage to individual freedoms just as real as an insurrection or coup. Together they form a sort of Taliban, an intolerant coalition of fanatics that shelter the anti-freedom alliance so it can thrive and grow. ... The Constitution is pristine and inviolate. And those who promote that we be less free are political terrorists. If you consider the Constitution less relevant, if you ignore or distort the Second Amendment, if you conspire to make lawful firearms less accessible to lawful citizens. . . . The fact that you were born on American soil won't mask the fact that you're an enemy of freedom and a political terrorist.

—Wayne LaPierre (National Rifle Association)

The public health approach is optimistic, flexible, and pragmatic and has succeeded in many areas. It emphasizes the wide array of policies that can be used to improve the nation's health. By contrast, gun advocates sometimes appear pessimistic, inflexible, and doctrinaire, seemingly unable to visualize more than a narrow range of punitive policy alternatives. Gun advocates also make constant claims about the benefits of firearms, claims that are not supported by the empirical literature. This chapter discusses the limitations of the gun advocates' approach and the inaccuracies of their claims. It also discusses the lessons for U.S. firearms policy that can be derived from examining the public health approach used for other products (e.g., tobacco and alcohol), the approach of other developed nations toward regulating firearms, and the effects of our permissive firearm policies on other nations.

PRIVATE GUNS, PUBLIC HEALTH

THE WRONG ARGUMENTS

In 1994, Wayne LaPierre, executive director of the National Rifle Association (NRA), wrote a book about guns and gun policy. The book contains many inaccuracies, but most telling are the omissions. For example, the book contains only one sentence on suicides, even though more than half of gun deaths are suicides. Of twenty policy proposals concerning firearms, all twenty aim to increase the likelihood and severity of punishment for criminal gun users. Not a single proposal deals with the manufacture of firearms, the distribution of firearms, or even the safe storage of firearms. Other progun writers commonly advocate only those policies that concern the criminal use of firearms (Kates 1990). A usual argument is that policy should be aimed solely at "controlling criminals, not guns" (Kopel 1993, 8).

Everyone agrees that we should punish criminals, particularly violent criminals. An issue is whether we need even more severe punishments. The United States already leads the developed world in punishment. While our criminal victimization rates resemble those of other developed countries (except for homicide, which is primarily murder with firearms), we have far higher rates of imprisonment. California's NRA-backed "three strikes and you're out" law succeeded mainly in locking up large numbers of nonviolent offenders (Browne and Lichter 2001). Getting even tougher is probably not the answer (Walker 1994).

No one suggests that we should not punish violent offenders, particularly those who use guns. But as criminologist Gary Kleck explains,

> [Get-tough policies] have been tried, carefully evaluated, and found to be either ineffective in producing significant crime reductions or hopelessly expensive. These failed strategies include longer prison terms, mandatory prison terms, use of capital punishment, "selective incapacitation" of career criminals, increasing police manpower, and reducing procedural restraints on police and prosecutors. While there are many promising alternatives to gun control for reducing violence, the "get tough" approach is not one of them. (1997b, 15)

Whether or not Kleck has accurately summarized the literature, he points out that many other policies besides punishing "bad guys" can reduce our firearm injury problem. This book focuses on those other policies that directly involve guns.

If we want to reduce lethal violence and injury—if we want to prevent violence rather than just assign blame or punish individuals after it has occurred—we must consider a wide variety of policies. For motor vehicles, for alcohol, for chainsaws, or for any other potentially dangerous commodity, it would be stupid (and irresponsible) for policymakers to refuse to consider ways of changing the product and the environment to reduce morbidity and mortality.

Gun proponents are often blind to any policies that don't deal with the gun user. If making gun assaults illegal and severely punishing the "bad guys" who use guns in assaults doesn't work, they are left with no other policy recommendations.

Attempts to reduce drive-by shootings by restricting access to firearms are doomed to failure. It must be borne in mind that in *all cases of drive-by shooting, the weapons themselves and the use to which they are put are already illegal and carry heavy penalties.* . . . The prospect of all these penalties appears not to deter drive-by shooters, and why should it? They are, after all, on their way to commit first-degree murder, punishable by no less than a death penalty. Further gun control laws could hardly be expected to offer more deterrence than that. (Polsby and Brennen 1995, 9–10)

Yet we can pursue many policies—along with punishing misuse—that will substantially reduce the likelihood of drive-by shootings. Since many of the shooters (e.g., urban teenagers) obtain guns illegally, we can interdict the distribution of guns. For example, we can reduce gun availability for potential drive-by shootings (1) by passing a national one-gun-per-month law that will reduce gunrunning; (2) by requiring all firearm transactions to go through licensed dealers with the required background checks (thus plugging the secondary-market loophole); (3) by tracing all guns used in crime and by giving the Bureau of Alcohol, Tobacco, and Firearms (ATF) stronger enforcement authority and more resources to be deployed against scofflaw dealers who supply the firearms; (4) by improving gun storage practices and producing personalized firearms to reduce gun theft; (5) by licensing gun owners and registering all handguns so that fewer unauthorized users will gain access to firearms.

The lesson from every other high-income country is that we don't need to accept our level of drive-by shootings or any other type of gun violence as a normal part of life. All other industrialized nations have enacted firearm policies that effectively reduce the likelihood of such untoward events.

In other injury areas, policymakers have rejected the argument that since something is already illegal, we can do little more to prevent the unlawful activity. For example, even though it's already illegal to speed, we do more to reduce speeding than simply increasing the likelihood and severity of punishment. Speeding is often effectively curtailed by the judicious placement of speed bumps, raised intersections, neckdowns, chicanes, textured pavements, traffic circles, and other "traffic calming" roadway techniques that reduce speeding around pedestrians (Ribadeneira 2000; Bunn et al. 2003). Similarly, although it is already illegal to drink and drive, we do more to reduce drunk driving than simply increase the likelihood and severity of punishment. Many policies such as server training, dramshop liability, and designated-driver campaigns reduce the incidence of such unlawful behavior; collapsible steering columns and automatic air bags reduce the harm from motor vehicle crashes caused by drunk drivers.

Gun proponents often argue that no firearm policies can ever be effective and claim that criminals will always get guns:

> There is and will continue to be a market demand for handguns. Criminals will be able to obtain guns whether or not regulations are passed or not. It is the ordinary citizen who will unfairly have his or her rights restricted if handgun regulations are enacted. (Seal 1999)

The evidence completely contradicts this claim. We can learn not only from other high-income countries but from states such as Hawaii, which has stringent gun regulations and few (but not zero) gun-crime problems. Few criminals use guns when guns are difficult to obtain.

The same claim, with slightly different rhetoric, is that determined criminals will always get guns. However, the most fundamental law of economics is that raising the price of an object—reducing availability or making access more difficult—will reduce (though usually not eliminate) the number of objects demanded. Perhaps determined yacht buyers will always buy yachts, but sufficiently raising the price will drastically reduce the demand. In particular, making it more difficult for inner-city teens to obtain firearms will reduce firearm use. And since firearm use among youths is, in effect, contagious (i.e., one gang obtains guns largely because other gangs have guns), making it more difficult to get guns can have a multiplicative effect. The

POLICY LESSONS

"Boston miracle"—the enormous reduction in that city's gun homicides in the late 1990s—appears to have resulted in part from efforts to interdict and restrict young people's easy access to firearms and to increase the likelihood and severity of punishment for gun use (Piehl, Kennedy, and Braga 2000).

A related argument against gun policies is "that criminals are fundamentally different than non-criminals" (Funk 1995, 771). Certainly, criminals as a group have, on average, different characteristics than noncriminals. One could equally well say that drunk drivers are fundamentally different from nondrunk drivers or that people who drive at excess speeds are fundamentally different from motorists who drive at more reasonable speeds. But we can still have multiple policies, including punishing bad behavior, that will reduce the problem. In the motor vehicle arena, such policies include making cars more crash resistant, making roads safer so that leaving the highway is less likely to result in death, improving emergency medical care, restricting availability to alcohol for problem drinkers, and providing access to alcohol rehabilitation. Some injury experts want to design cars so that they can't exceed speeds of eighty miles per hour.

Many policies can reduce the likelihood of gun use by criminals and reduce the likelihood of death when criminals use guns. We can make it harder for criminals to get guns and make the guns they obtain less lethal. No studies show that U.S. criminals differ fundamentally from criminals in other high-income countries, yet our murder rates are often an order of magnitude higher. No study shows that criminals in states with few firearms differ fundamentally from criminals in states with many firearms. Yet murder rates are lower in states where firearms are less readily available.

Sometimes the argument for the futility of any firearms policy is that "the 200 million guns now in circulation would be sufficient to sustain roughly another century of gun violence at the current rates" (Wright 1995, 64). Fortunately, careers in violent crime are often quite short; each new cohort of violent youths must obtain its own guns—either new guns from licensed dealers or used guns from current owners (Cook 1996). Gun interdiction can have a substantial impact against inner-city gun use, especially since young criminals prefer new firearms.

A recent mantra of the gun lobby is that we don't need new gun laws, we just need to enforce the existing laws. But this is a false dichotomy. Actually, we need both better laws and better enforcement. A main reason that the ATF does not enforce the laws against scofflaw dealers more effectively is because the NRA has lobbied successfully to limit the bureau's ability. New laws, such as increasing the penalty for deliberately falsifying information sent to the ATF, are needed to allow the ATF to successfully enforce the law. What is not needed are NRA-backed state "preemption" initiatives, which take away cities' and localities' ability to deal effectively with their gun problems.

Gun proponents tend to neglect firearm accidents and suicides, whose combined death toll is always higher than homicides. Or gun advocates make inappropriate comparisons to imply that the firearm injury problem is not a serious one. Kleck (1997a, 295), for example, compares unintentional firearm fatalities with all fatalities from motor vehicles. For this comparison, he excludes all firearm suicides and all firearm homicides. His measure of exposure to risk is the number of households with guns versus the number of households with motor vehicles. He concludes that deaths per motor vehicle are greater than unintentional gun deaths per gun, implying that the gun problem isn't terribly serious and that guns aren't terribly dangerous. But the time Americans spend using their cars is orders of magnitudes greater than the time spent using their guns. It is probable that per hour of exposure, guns are far more dangerous. Moreover, we have lots of safety regulations concerning the manufacture of motor vehicles; there are virtually no safety regulations for domestic firearms manufacture.

Between 1991 and 2000, firearms killed more than thirty-four thousand Americans annually, and an estimated three times that number were nonfatally wounded. Drowning is one of the leading causes of injury fatality in the United States, but it pales in comparison to firearms. In the same decade, under five thousand Americans drowned annually. It is, of course, possible to find some groups in which more people drowned than were shot. Kleck (1997a, 296) compares the drowning death rate for zero- to four-year-olds from swimming pools with the unintentional firearm injury death rate for this age group. Again the implication is that not guns but swimming pools are dangerous. Pools are indeed dangerous for children, but kids have much more exposure to pools than to guns. Children between zero and four commonly swim in pools; they tend not to hunt, target shoot, use guns in self-defense, or clean household guns. In contrast to a swimming pool, most children zero to four ought not even to know that there is a firearm in the house or where it is stored. Their exposure for firearm injury ought to be close to zero. The fact that an average of twenty-three children aged zero to four were killed with firearms each year in 1991–2000 and that many more were nonfatally wounded should be completely unacceptable.

When two children (aged fourteen or younger) per year died from being locked in automobile trunks in the mid-1990s, car manufacturers added safety latches to the trunks' interiors. Yet in the same period, when some 150 children the same age died each year from unintentional firearm deaths, manufacturers did virtually nothing to make their guns safer.

It is common for gun proponents to mischaracterize the firearms literature. For example, Kleck (1997b) summarizes the aggregate studies of gun ownership levels and crime as follows: "The studies are split between studies that support the idea that higher levels of gun ownership are associated with higher crime rates and those that do not" (249). Yet six of the seven cross-sectional studies he cites find a statistically significant direct correlation between areas with high gun density and homicide rates. Not surprisingly, there are far fewer statistically significant results from studies looking at the effect of guns on the total robbery rate, the violent crime rate, or the index crime rate, because gun levels should have little discernable effect on these crimes. The large majority of robberies and other crimes of violence do not involve firearms.

Kleck often uses the lack of statistical significance in a study to imply, incorrectly, the lack of any association between the variables in question. To claim that a study shows that the correlation between two variables is statistically significant, social scientists generally require that the odds be at least nineteen to one that the correlation did not result from chance. Thus, finding a statistically significant correlation means one is quite sure that the association is a real one. But the converse is not true. A result that is not statistically significant does not imply that there is no real association—only that this particular study did not yield highly convincing evidence. It is quite easy for a study not to find statistically significant correlations between variables that are actually highly associated, just by using too small a number of observations or by measuring the variables inaccurately.

For example, Kleck summarizes the case-control literature on firearms and suicide, saying that "only 2 case-control studies of adults claim that gun ownership is associated with an increased risk of suicide, while a third study found no increase in suicide risk" (Kleck 1998, 474). It sounds like there is not much evidence, and the evidence is mixed. But five overlapping case-control studies (120 cases) have found a statistically significant relationship between guns in the home and suicide of adolescents (Brent et al. 1994). Focusing on adults only, Kleck does not inform the reader that the one study without statistically significant results ($p > .05$) did not involve the United States but New Zealand, where extensive background checks for gun ownership are common, gun storage requirements are strict, and there are virtually no hand-guns. The study had only twenty cases of gun suicide, but even so, in homes with guns, the odds for suicide were 40 percent greater than in homes with-out guns ($p < .10$). In other words, the study was too small to have the power to show that the 40 percent increase in suicide was "statistically significant at the 5% level"; it was just large enough to find that the odds were better than nine to one (but not nineteen to one) that the relationship between guns and suicide did not result from chance (Beautrais, Joyce, and Mulder 1996).

John Lott claims, "In the U.S. the states with the highest gun ownership rates also have by far the lowest violent crime rates" (2003, 76). He provides no evidence, no citations, and no discussion for this assertion. By contrast, in a sworn affidavit in 1997, Canadian academic and gun advocate Gary Mauser claimed, "The prevalence of firearms has been shown to be unrelated to crime." Mauser also did not provide evidence or citations for this conclusion. In fact, of course, many studies have shown a strong positive relationship between gun prevalence and gun crimes. For example, a 1992 review of the lit-erature found that most studies concluded that gun prevalence was positively associated with overall homicide rates (Ohsfeldt and Morrisey 1992). Even Kleck (1991) concluded that the following generalizations were consistent with the best available evidence on guns and robbery: (1) gun ownership lev-els positively affect the rate of gun robberies; (2) murder of the victim is more likely in gun robberies; (3) guns enable robbers to tackle more lucrative and risky targets; (4) robbers armed with guns are more likely to complete their crimes.

Gun proponents make many claims about the advantages of a heavily armed society, with almost no empirical support. For example, there are con-tinual assertions about the beneficial effects of guns on burglary. "Gun con-trol has not reduced crime; in fact it has encouraged burglary" (Kopel 1992, 431). "A significant reduction in the number of Americans keeping loaded guns in the home would, if the experience of other countries is a guide, lead to a large increase in the burglary rate, and to many more burglaries being perpetrated while potential victims are present in the home" (Kopel 1992, 418). "The potential defensive nature of guns is further evidenced by the dif-ferent rates of so-called 'hot burglaries,' where a resident is at home when a criminal strikes" (Lott 1998a, 5). The only citation is to a comparison of four locations—one city and three countries (Kleck 1997b). No study is referenced that compares a large sample of cities, states, or nations.

However, real evidence exists about guns and burglary rates. An international compilation of victimization surveys in eleven developed countries found that the United States, which is first among high-income nations in gun prevalence and last in terms of gun control, was fourth in terms of the percentage of households in which a completed burglary had occurred in the previous year and fourth in terms of burglary attempts that were not successful (table 9.1). Relative to other high-income countries, our guns do not seem to prevent burglary attempts or stop burglars in the act. Using Cook's index as a proxy for gun availability, the relationship between gun availability and burglary is nonsignificant and negative, and the relationship between gun availability and the percentage of attempted but unsuccessful burglaries is nonsignificant and negative. Such international results at the very least provide no evidence suggesting that guns either reduce attempted burglary or make it less likely that attempted burglaries will succeed.

A study across U.S. counties using data from the National Crime Victimization Surveys found that higher gun prevalence increased the likelihood of burglary victimization and did not change the proportion of hot burglary, so that the total number of hot burglaries per capita was higher in areas with more guns. The researchers suggested that guns are attractive loot for burglars, who often target houses with many guns (Cook and Ludwig 2003). State-level analyses also indicate that more guns lead to more burglaries (Duggan 2001; Cook and Ludwig 2003).

TABLE 9.1. Burglary Rates in Eleven Industrialized Nations from Victimization Surveys (percentage of households in each country, 1995)

	Completed Burglary	Attempted Burglary	Attempted or Completed Burglary	Percentage of Attempts Not Completed
Canada	3.4	2.8	5.3	45
England	3.0	3.4	6.1	56
Netherlands	2.6	3.3	5.1	55
United States	2.6	3.0	4.9	53
France	2.4	2.2	3.9	48
Scotland	1.5	2.5	3.6	65
N. Ireland	1.5	1.1	2.5	42
Switzerland	1.3	1.1	2.2	46
Sweden	1.3	1.1	2.0	46
Austria	0.9	0.5	1.3	36
Finland	0.6	0.7	1.2	52
Average excluding United States	1.9	1.9	3.3	49

Source: Data from Mayhew and van Dijk 1997.

One study purports to show that permissive gun-carrying laws reduce crime (Lott 1998a). However, the study also yields results contrary both to common sense and generally accepted social science; for example, this study shows that increasing unemployment and reducing income both reduce violent crime and that reducing by one percentage point the percentage of the population that is female, black, and aged forty to forty-nine will reduce homicide by 59 percent. Technically superior studies using better models (Black and Nagin 1998; Dezhbakhsh and Rubin 1998; Ludwig 1998) as well as more recent data (Donohue 2003; Hepburn et al. 2003) find that permissive gun-carrying laws may increase violent crime.

Gun proponents often make bold claims about the benefits of self-defense gun use. Yet no study indicates that a gun in the home makes one safer, no study indicates that a gun in the home will be used more often against intruders than against family members, no study shows that a loaded gun in the home increases safety relative to an unloaded gun, and no study shows that using a gun in self-defense reduces the risk of being murdered. Moreover, reliable studies do find that a gun in the home increases the risk both for homicide and suicide (Brent et al. 1991; Kellermann et al. 1992, 1993; Cummings, Koepsell, and Grossman et al. 1997), that guns in the home are used more often by former or current intimates against women than by anyone in self-defense (Azrael and Hemenway 2000), and that a loaded rather than unloaded gun in the home increases the risk of suicide (Brent et al. 2000). The preponderance of the evidence is clear: guns in the home, on average, increase one's chances of death or nonfatal injury.

Kleck (1997a) claims that guns are used more often in self-defense than in criminal gun use. Again, no study has ever shown this. Indeed, every survey that asked similar questions both about self-defense gun use and criminal gun use against the respondent finds far more cases of criminal gun use. Twice a year, year after year, the National Crime Victimization Survey shows that "firearm self-defense is rare compared with gun crimes" (McDowall and Wiersema 1994, 1982). Many different private (nongovernmental) surveys yield the same result (Hemenway and Azrael 2000).

Self-defense gun use is continually presented as a socially desirable act. But the data tell a different story. Three national surveys of self-defense gun use reveal that the majority of such uses are probably illegal (Hemenway, Miller, and Azrael 2000) and not in the public interest (Hemenway and Azrael 2000).

Given the emphasis placed on the supposed benefits of self-defense gun use by the gun lobby and progun writers, the paucity of data showing any real benefits of self-defense gun use is amazing. One study mainly of career criminals that is cited continually by gun advocates found that 34 percent of imprisoned felons said that they had "been scared off, shot at or captured by an armed victim" (Wright and Rossi 1986, 154). However, that study did not ask for any specifics about these gun uses or even for a breakdown among the three categories. We do not know whether those shot at were prevented from committing the crime, whether the armed victims were armed with guns, the percentage of these attempted crimes that occurred at residences, whether it was a "law-abiding citizen" who used the gun against the criminal, and so on. We do know that many of the 34 percent responded "no" when asked if they had "ever run into a victim armed with a gun" (Wright and Rossi 1986).

That study also found that, when contemplating criminal activity, more felons worried regularly that (1) they might get caught, (2) they might go to prison, (3) their families might look down on them, (4) they might hurt or kill someone, or (5) they might get shot at by police than worried about getting shot at by victims (Wright and Rossi 1986). The majority of criminals with guns got them for protection, not for use in crime. They probably needed protection against other criminals rather than prospective victims. Half of the respondents who used guns had gotten into bar fights, 40 percent had been stabbed, and 70 percent had been assaulted. The study seems to indicate the dangers of an armed society, not the benefits.

There may be individual benefits from having a gun and using it in self-defense, but there exists no evidence to suggest any general societal benefits. On the contrary, many studies suggest a large net public health cost from an armed society. Homes with guns and states with more gun owners have more violent deaths (Miller, Azrael, and Hemenway 2001, 2002a, 2002b, 2002c, 2002d). And states with high levels of household firearm ownership have lower levels of social capital and mutual trust (Hemenway et al. 2001).

Still, it is important to point out that whatever the evidence regarding the actual benefits of self-defense gun use, most reasonable firearm policies would have little or no effect on the possibility of legitimate self-defense gun use by nonfelons. Such policies should help reduce gun accidents, gun suicides, gun robberies, gun homicides, and gun intimidation. Perhaps that is why polls show that the overwhelming majority of Americans favor the passage and implementation of such policies.

PRIVATE GUNS, PUBLIC HEALTH

LESSONS FROM OTHER PRODUCTS

Like firearms, cigarettes and alcohol provide some benefits to consumers but also cause major public health problems (McGinnis and Foege 1993). The public health approach to reducing the negative health effects of these two products while maintaining Americans' ability responsibly to buy, own, and use these goods provides lessons for an approach to reducing firearm injuries.

Tobacco

Consider the difference between asking, "Why do large numbers of people continue to smoke cigarettes?" and asking "Why do these particular people continue to smoke?" The first question directs attention to the tobacco culture in which everyone lives: the growing of tobacco, the advertising of cigarettes, the meaning of smoking. The second question directs attention to the psychology and physiology of individual people within that culture. Prevention concerned solely with these individuals conceals an endorsement of the structure. It also—not to lose sight of what really counts here—is simply less effective than prevention that changes the conditions of the tobacco culture.

—S. N. Tesh

Like firearms, cigarettes are a widely used consumer product, enjoyed by millions of Americans in all walks of life and romanticized in advertisements and on film. Like gun control, the history of smoking control "is one of ongoing struggle with an implacable foe" (Nathanson 1999, 429). However, in the United States, the social movement to reduce the harm caused by cigarettes is further along than the movement to lessen the harm caused by firearms. In most other high-income countries, the opposite is true.

In the first half of the twentieth century, cigarettes were often advertised as beneficial to health. Thanks in large part to improved data about smoking and smoking-related illness, medical studies accumulated throughout the 1950s. As a result, in 1959 the U.S. Public Health Service proclaimed that "the weight of the evidence at present implicates smoking as the principal etiological factor in the increased incidence of lung cancer" (Burney 1959, 1835). The 1964 surgeon general's report concluded, "Cigarette smoking is a health hazard of sufficient importance to the U.S. to warrant appropriate remedial action" (U.S. Department of Health, Education, and Welfare 1964, 33). The science was not without controversy, as the protobacco forces incessantly attacked the medical studies and continually touted the few results that did not find a cigarette-cancer connection (Kellermann 1997). However, the surgeon general's report on tobacco had sufficient influence that Congress imposed warning labels for cigarettes in 1965.

Data and research were crucial in the tobacco area. More and more studies found a strong connection not only between smoking and cancer but also between smoking and heart disease. More important, while it was long known that smoking could be annoying to others, scientific evidence began to show that it was also a health hazard to nonsmokers. Tobacco use could no longer be viewed solely as an issue of the smoker's health—it was also one of nonsmokers' rights. The exposure of innocent victims—nonsmokers, fetuses, and children—made it clear that governmental action was needed to help those at risk from the "polluting" smoker (Bayer and Colgrove 2002).

The nation's first grassroots organization against smokers' pollution was formed in Maryland in 1971. The Group against Smokers' Pollution (GASP) emphasized nonsmokers' rights and attempted to make smoking unpopular so that smokers would quit. In 1973, due to the dangers of involuntary smoking (sometimes called passive smoking, secondhand smoke, or environmental tobacco smoke), the Civil Aeronautics Board required no-smoking sections on airlines, and Arizona became the first state to ban smoking in some public places. By 1995, smoking was banned on all commercial flights, forty states regulated smoking in state government work sites, and thirty states restricted smoking in restaurants (Nathanson 1999).

The public health approach emphasizes a multifaceted strategy for improving health and safety. For tobacco, that included convincing physicians to stop smoking and to start advising their patients against smoking; reducing the availability of cigarettes to adolescents (e.g., restricting the placement of cigarette vending machines), mandating warning labels, banning tobacco advertisements on radio and television, and creating antismoking ads emphasizing the health dangers of cigarettes (Lantz et al. 2000).

An important change with respect to cigarettes has been the transformation of the cigarette and smoking from symbols of modernity, autonomy, power, and sexuality to symbols of weakness, irrationality, and addiction (Brandt 1992). Cigarette smoking has become déclassé for many sophisticates, and cigarette companies are often depicted as attempting to addict children to their product.

Juries became more sympathetic to liability claims against the tobacco industry after corporate documents were unearthed showing unethical and immoral behavior (Hurt and Robertson 1998). Litigation became an important weapon for improving public knowledge, changing public opinion and even providing funds for antitobacco ads.

Although America has had some success in reducing the problems caused by tobacco use, the struggle continues. The tobacco industry markets a product of mass lethality and tries to shift the health and social costs onto the public. Protobacco forces have pushed, often successfully, to have state legislatures prevent local communities from enacting strong local measures to protect the health and safety of their citizens. The tobacco industry also tried to get Congress to prevent liability suits against cigarette manufacturers. Finally, protobacco forces have claimed that the goal of public health was to make all smoking illegal and all smokers criminals: "A widespread antitobacco industry is out to harass sixty million Americans who smoke and to prohibit the manufacture and use of tobacco products" (Dwyer 1996, 468).

The science in the firearms field is at a similar stage to the cigarette literature of the mid-1950s. For example, public health researchers are conducting many scientific studies on firearm injuries, and the large majority of studies indicate that a gun in the home is a danger for the family and probably for the entire community. But manufacturers have marketed firearms as a safety device for the home (Vernick, Teret, and Webster 1997), and the few studies that suggest some benefit from firearms are widely publicized by the gun lobby, even as they are widely discredited in the literature.

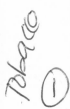

The public health struggle to reduce the harm caused by tobacco has lessons for the firearms field. For example, one lesson is the importance of federal data collection, analyses, investigations, and reports. While Congress mandated annual reports by the surgeon general on the health consequences of smoking, the gun lobby has succeeded in preventing any federal investigation or report on the gun industry. During the mid-1990s the gun lobby decimated the tiny firearms research effort that had begun at the Centers for Disease Control and Prevention (Zimmerman 1999) and arranged to make some state handgun registration files inaccessible to health researchers. Annual surgeon general reports on firearms would be immensely helpful in providing the public with updated scientific information concerning guns and public health.

A second lesson is the political importance of emphasizing the costs imposed on innocents, such as children. Guns do impose large costs on innocent victims—including those intimidated with firearms or shot accidentally or during assaults and robberies. Americans feel less safe as others in the community acquire firearms, and states with more guns have more lethal violence.

A third lesson is the importance of symbolism. While the image of the cigarette smoker and the perception of smoking has fallen in social status, guns are still portrayed as symbols of autonomy, power, sexuality, and patriotism (Kellermann 1997). Yet guns for crime or self-defense could as easily be portrayed as weapons for cowards who are unskilled at real hand-to-hand fighting or unskilled at nonviolently resolving conflict. Japan fought battles in the late sixteenth century using more guns than any European country possessed. But over the next three centuries, for a variety of reasons, the country gave up the gun. Among other things, guns were seen as removing much of the skill and beauty from combat. When it became apparent that a farmer with a gun could readily kill the toughest samurai, no true soldier wanted to use a gun (Perrin 1979).

A fourth lesson is the role of medical professionals. In the tobacco area, it was important for physicians not only to emphasize the dangers of smoking but also to stop smoking. In the firearms arena, there has been little attempt to convince physicians with young children to get guns out of their own homes, and only a small (but growing) number of physicians counsel patients to store guns appropriately.

A fifth lesson is the importance of place restrictions. Tobacco activists have succeeded in restricting smoking in many locales. In the firearms area, attempts should be made to further restrict the places where individuals can legally carry guns. Polls show that the overwhelming majority of Americans would like guns to be banned not only from airlines but also from restaurants, bars, hospitals, sports stadiums, and other public places (Hemenway, Azrael, and Miller 2001). Yet concealed gun carrying in such locations has been increasingly permitted.

A sixth lesson is the importance of grassroots activism. For example, while nonsmokers'-rights groups play an important role in tobacco policy, no similar non-gun-owners'-rights groups have been formed, although many gun control organizations and victim and survivor groups exist. In the firearms area, the discourse on rights has remained the exclusive province of the gun lobby, which claims, incorrectly, constitutionally protected status for gun owners' rights (and no rights for non–gun owners).

A final lesson from tobacco control has been the importance of tort law. In the firearms area, a host of recent liability suits led some manufacturers and dealers to put a bit more emphasis on the public's health when making their corporate policies. Smith and Wesson, for example, initially agreed to a variety of requirements in exchange for being dropped from a federal government lawsuit (ABCnews.com 1999). However, the gun industry has persuaded some state legislatures to prohibit antigun lawsuits brought by local communities. As this chapter is being written, a corporate insider is highlighting questionable manufacturer conduct at the same time the gun lobby is attempting to persuade Congress to prohibit all lawsuits against this one product. The role of tort law in improving firearm safety has yet to be played out.

As the tobacco lobby opposes regulations, arguing that they are ultimately intended to ban all smoking, the gun lobby opposes virtually every reasonable policy with the claim that it is just a thinly disguised scheme to take away everyone's firearms. Those opposed to public health research on firearms take a similar tack:

> Based on studies, and propelled by leadership from the Centers for Disease Control and Prevention (CDC), the objective has broadened so that it now includes banning and confiscation of all handguns, restrictive licensing of owners of other firearms, and eventual elimination of firearms from American life, excepting (perhaps) only a small elite of extremely wealthy collectors, hunters or target shooters. (Kates et al. 1995, 234)

Public health research is designed to bring science to bear on important issues such as cigarette smoking and gun carrying. While the public health goal has been to eradicate certain human diseases, including polio and smallpox, making it unlawful to produce mass consumer products such as motor vehicles, tobacco, alcohol, or firearms is not on the public health agenda.

Alcohol

> In developing and applying the prevention perspective, we have been struck by, and had to resist most forcibly, the tendency to think about policy in terms of opposed pairs: dry versus wet, prohibition versus unlimited access, treatment versus prevention, good drinking versus bad drinking.
>
> —M. H. Moore and D. Gerstein

Historically, the U.S. temperance movement was a moralistic rather than a public health movement. But like public health practitioners, Prohibitionists strove to avoid putting complete blame on the victims for their problems.

And Prohibition, while causing other social problems, such as the rise of the Mob, appears to have been a striking success in some public health dimensions. Both consumption of alcohol and cirrhosis rates fell substantially (Terris 1967; Levine and Reinarman 1991).

Public health is interested in prevention, not prohibition. Prevention in the alcohol field—removed from the shadow of moralism—got its official governmental start with the establishment of the National Institute on Alcohol Abuse and Alcoholism (NIAAA) in 1971 (Beauchamp 1988). The scientific research sponsored by this agency is changing our understanding of alcohol and alcohol problems.

After Prohibition, a notion arose that the alcohol problems affected only a small minority of drinkers and that most individuals drank safely, as "social drinkers." Rather than abstention, a way to prevent alcoholism was to integrate alcohol into everyday life—such as wine with meals. Societies that had normalized alcohol use supposedly experienced few problems with alcohol. Some people argued that students should learn to drink at school, much as they learn to drive automobiles (Chafetz 1967).

The proalcohol forces have vigorously promoted the claims that most ordinary people's drinking is perfectly harmless, that regular drinking is good for you, and that education is the most effective way of combating "the excessive drinking we all deplore." A policy prescribed is extensive treatment of alcoholism by experts in group psychotherapy in expensive inpatient units (Kendell 1995, 181).

In the mid-1970s and again in the mid-1990s, with sponsorship from the World Health Organization, a large international group of alcohol researchers—"the leading scientists of the alcohol world" (Kendell 1995, 181)—produced reports on sound policy prescriptions from the results of the scientific literature that refuted the claims of the increasingly powerful international alcohol industry (Bruun et al. 1975; Edwards et al. 1994). A strong link was demonstrated between high levels of societal drinking and high levels of alcohol problems. Where alcohol use was normative and alcohol was widely used—and especially where wine was treated as a food and commonly served at meals—the result was a very high rate of alcohol consumption, disease, and alcohol-related deaths and injuries. The more alcohol was restricted (e.g., via taxes or age restrictions) the lower the rates of cirrhosis, highway fatalities, and other alcohol-related problems (Beauchamp 1988).

The alcohol industry likes to present the world as one of alcoholics and sensible drinkers. But the world is a continuum: alcohol-related problems go beyond alcohol dependence (Pacurucu-Castillo 1995). While heavy drinkers contribute disproportionately to alcohol-related problems, there are many more low-level alcohol consumers. Low-level consumption impairs cognitive and physical functioning, and the individual is often unaware of the effect. In addition, occasional binge drinking causes serious social problems. For many alcohol problems (though not cirrhosis), the highest-risk group is so small it accounts for only a fraction of the total amount of damage. Light and moderate drinkers—and particularly those light drinkers who occasionally drink immoderately—generate the bulk of alcohol-related problems (e.g., impaired driving, family dysfunction) (Kreitman 1986).

Scientists in the alcohol field concluded that a population-based strategy is most effective for reducing alcohol-related problems. "Entirely risk-free drinking exists only as a fantasy," and "any attempts to put across a message which encourages drinking on the basis of hoped-for gains in coronary heart disease prevention would be likely to result in more harm to the population than benefit" (Edwards et al. 1994, 209).

Education appears at best to have an indirect effect on prevention by creating heightened political and public awareness of the issues. Research does not support the deployment of school-based education, public education, or advertising restrictions as lead policy choices. Conversely, "environmental measures which influence physical access to alcohol can make a significant contribution to the prevention of alcohol problems." Such measures include minimum legal drinking ages; restrictions on the hours of sale and on "happy hours"; policies on the number, type, and location of sales outlets; server training; increased taxation; random breath tests; and rules concerning specific situations (e.g., alcohol at baseball games) (Edwards 1997).

Public health experts advocate such specific policies as outlawing the sale of alcohol at gas stations to reduce drinking and driving, keg registration and home delivery restrictions to help prevent underage drinking, and limits of sales at community events to reduce unruly behavior and other associated alcohol-related problems. Many nongovernmental organizations can also institute policies to help reduce the harm caused by alcohol. For example, alcohol merchants can provide incentives for their employees carefully to check age identification, the media can portray responsible alcohol use, work sites can restrict alcohol at work events, colleges can establish alcohol-free dormitories, insurance companies can provide premium discounts to outlets that train their servers, and religious institutions can stop using alcohol as door prizes (Toomey and Wagenaar 1999).

Abundant evidence shows the effectiveness of one specific policy, alcohol taxation, which reduces the overall population level of alcohol consumption and alcohol-related problems. In addition, evidence shows that young drinkers, heavy drinkers, and dependent drinkers are all influenced by price (Edwards 1997). The effects of price can be large. It has been estimated that if beer had been taxed at the rate of distilled spirits since 1951 and no erosion of the beer tax had been allowed to occur, the number of youths killed in traffic crashes would have been reduced by 54 percent (Coate and Grossman 1987).

The alcohol lobby has political clout and fights such initiatives. A decade ago, a statewide proposition in California to raise alcohol prices by a nickel a drink met with fierce industry opposition. Representatives of the wine industry declared a jihad and unleashed the dogs of war—tens of millions of dollars in advertisements that helped to confuse the electorate and defeat the tax initiative (McGuire 1990).

Public health successes in the alcohol field have not been as visible as in tobacco. But in most industrialized Western countries, drinking problems have declined (Single 1995). Happy hours—where people tend to drink excessively in a short period—have been banned in at least twenty states (Bethel 1999). Drunk driving deaths have fallen in the United States. But much remains to be done. Public health offers data, researchers, science, organization, a comprehensive approach, and the confident knowledge that "the level of alcohol problems which a society experiences is susceptible to amelioration by rational policy action" (Edwards et al. 1994, 2).

Public health professionals confront many similar issues when trying to address the problems caused by firearms. Both alcohol and firearms cause much damage to the health of societies, and the costs are often imposed on innocent victims. For example, alcohol problems extend well beyond the individual drinker into the lives of family members, friends, coworkers, and strangers. Alcohol increases the risk of child neglect, spousal abuse, family disruption, fires, crimes, violence, and homicide as well as motor vehicle crashes (Holder 1997). Similarly, firearm problems extend to accidents, suicides, and gun threats and intimidation, and the costs of firearm violence extend into the lives of family members and the community. Alcohol consumption has elements of contagion—the alcohol intake of one individual or one subgroup in a community typically affects the intake of others (Rehm, Ashley, and Dubois 1997). Similarly, an increase in guns in a community may lead others to acquire guns out of fear or because of conformity.

The struggle to reduce the harm caused by alcohol has lessons for the firearms field. One lesson is the importance of federal funding for research: NIAAA research funding is currently far in excess of federal support for firearms research. A second lesson is the potential benefit from the use of international conferences to reach consensus concerning research findings. While there have been occasional conferences about suicide research, such an approach has not generally been used in the firearms area.

Another lesson is that opponents will try to depict the world as dichotomous, composed of a tiny percentage of problem users on one side and everyone else on the other. The progun advocates talk continuously about criminals and "decent, law-abiding citizens." For the "good guys," gun possession can only increase rather than reduce the safety of everyone. The gun lobby claims that socialization into the gun culture would reduce firearm accidents and injuries. However, the empirical evidence shows that where gun possession and use are normalized, more gun-related problems arise.

Like the alcohol industry, the gun lobby advocates two narrow policy prescriptions. Gun manufacturers argue for gun training (by NRA trainers) and for increased punishment of criminals. Yet the evidence suggests that more punishment and training should not be the prime solutions for our firearms problems and that a more comprehensive policy approach is needed.

Overall, firearms, like alcohol, provide some societal benefits, including direct health benefits (medical and public health researchers have documented the beneficial effects of small amounts of alcohol on coronary heart disease). Like alcohol policy, firearms policy is a contentious arena beset by vested interests; in both areas, public health research tries to provide science where passion and prejudice have too often ruled the day (Edwards 1997).

An important milestone in the attempt to change the U.S. vision concerning the prevention of alcohol problems was the 1981 National Research Council Report that suggested a wide array of alcohol policies (Moore and Gerstein 1981). For the report's three main conclusions, we might almost be able to replace the word *alcohol* with *firearms*.

1. "Alcohol problems are permanent because drinking is an important and ineradicable part of this society and culture."
2. "Alcohol problems tend to be so broadly felt and distributed as to be a general social problem, even though they are excessively prevalent in a relatively small fraction of the population."
3. "The possibilities for reducing the problem by prevention measures are . . . real, and should increase with experience." (116)

POLICY LESSONS

LESSONS FROM OTHER COUNTRIES

[The] fixation of Americans on guns is an inexplicable and horrific aspect of American culture to people in other countries.

—Lawrence Stone

The United States has more guns than any other high-income nation. For example, a 1989 telephone survey of twenty-eight thousand randomly selected individuals in fourteen industrialized countries found that the United States led all other nations in terms of households with civilian firearms (Killias 1993); more recent surveys confirm that ranking (Killias, Van Kesteren, and Rindlisbacher 2001) (table 9.2). More importantly, we have far more handguns than other countries. While Canada and New Zealand have almost comparable levels of long gun ownership to the United States, those countries have few handguns, the gun of choice for criminals. In the movie *Bowling for Columbine*, Michael Moore implies that U.S. and Canadian citizens are equally armed. With respect to handguns, he is very much mistaken. The Canadian government estimated that in 1998 there were 1.2 million handguns in Canada, compared to 76 million in the United States (Canadian Firearms Centre 1998).

TABLE 9.2. Households with Civilian Firearms (in percentages)

Country	Households with Civilian Firearms[a]
United States	48
Switzerland	35
Norway	31
Canada	26
Finland	25
France	25
Australia	16
Belgium	15
Spain	13
Northern Ireland	9
Germany	9
Scotland	5
England and Wales	4
The Netherlands	2

Source: Data from Killias, Van Kesteren, and Rindlisbacher 2001.
[a]Years reported range from 1989–96.

U.S. gun control laws are also weaker than those of other industrialized nations. For example, almost all other high-income countries have a licensure system for gun ownership (United Nations 1998) (table 9.3). Virtually all of these countries also require registration of all firearms, both handguns and long guns (Cukier 1998). For those individuals with firearms, almost all countries have mandatory storage requirements. The large majority of high-income nations also require a training certificate before one can legally obtain a firearm. And the majority does not consider "protection" a legitimate reason for obtaining a handgun. The United States is clearly an outlier in terms of firearm regulations.

In Canada, for example, handguns are restricted and heavily regulated weapons. There is a twenty-eight-day waiting period to purchase a firearm and a requirement for firearms training before firearm purchase; furthermore, would-be purchasers are also required to provide references. All firearms are registered, and licenses are required for firearm ownership. Gun advertising cannot depict or extol violence against another person. None of

TABLE 9.3. Firearm Regulations

Country	License System	Storage Regulations	Training Certificate Needed for Purchase	Handgun Ownership Permitted for Protection
Australia	Yes	Yes	Yes	No
Austria	Yes	Yes		Yes
Belgium	Yes	Yes	Yes	Yes
Canada	Yes	Yes	Yes	No[a]
Denmark		Yes		No
Finland	Yes	No		No
France			Yes	Yes
Germany	Yes	Yes		Yes
Japan	Yes	Yes	Yes	No
Luxembourg	Yes	No		No
New Zealand	Yes	Yes	Yes	No
Norway	Yes	Yes	Yes	Yes
Spain	Yes	Yes	Yes	Yes
Sweden	Yes	Yes		No
Switzerland	Yes	Yes	No	Yes
United Kingdom	Yes	Yes		No[a]
United States	No	No		Yes

Source: Data from United Nations 1998.
Note: A blank indicates no response.
[a]In exceptional cases, permits may be issued.

these requirements hold for most states in the United States, even though gun advocates have long claimed that guns in the United States are heavily regulated—that there are "20,000 laws concerning firearms" (National Rifle Association 2002). Gun proponents provide no source for this number, and if it is true, they must be counting many local laws, such as zoning laws, laws against firing guns in cities, and so on. Yet the trend has been for state governments to enact "preemption laws," which forbid local governments from enacting gun laws (Vernick and Hepburn 2003). But the key point is that the number of laws is not the criterion for judging permissiveness of regulations. All knowledgeable international experts agree that the United States has the most permissive gun laws of any industrialized nation.

The U.S. level of lethal violence is also far out of line with those of other industrialized nations. The fact that most of our lethal violence involves firearms lends credence to the generally accepted (outside the United States) hypothesis that the prevalence of guns is a prime reason U.S. homicide rates are so high. An international study of the fourteen developed countries with valid and comparable measures of gun ownership levels found that gun ownership was significantly and positively associated with gun homicide and total homicide rates but not with rates of homicide without a gun (Killias 1993). Using a validated proxy for firearm ownership levels (Azrael, Cook, and Miller 2004), it has been shown that, across the twenty-six developed nations, gun ownership was positively and significantly correlated with gun homicides and total homicides (Hemenway and Miller 2000). (See appendix A.)

It is often claimed that Switzerland, which has a heavily armed population but a low homicide rate, disproves the gun–lethal violence connection. "Across the Atlantic, England's low crime rate is invariably highlighted by gun control proponents. Switzerland, which entirely disproves the 'guns cause crime' thesis, is of course, ignored" (LaPierre 1994, 174).

But good international studies examine all high-income countries for which data are available, not just one or two nations. Furthermore, the U.S. crime rate is not high relative to England. In the mid-1990s, according to victimization surveys, assault, robbery, burglary, and motor vehicle theft rates were higher in England and Wales than in the United States (Langan and Farrington 1998). But their murder rate was much lower.

For Switzerland, the guns available are not typically handguns, and most are not personally owned by the civilian population—only about one-third of Swiss households have privately owned firearms. Most Swiss guns are military weapons assigned to a militia for use in event of war. In Switzerland, gun possession comes with a burden of responsibility. Every able-bodied male goes through regular military training for twenty-two years, from age twenty to forty-two. Privates and lower-ranking noncommissioned officers are issued 5.56 assault rifles, which they store at home along with gas masks and twenty rounds of ammunition. Weapons and ammunition must be kept in a sealed container and be stored under lock and key. The guns must be presented for regular inspections, where it is also determined whether the ammunition is still properly sealed. Ammunition cannot be purchased and is inspected regularly, and every bullet must be accounted for. Misuse of military weapons as well as failure to store them securely is severely punished by military justice (Switzerland Embassy 1999).

By contrast, a large proportion of guns in private U.S. households are handguns. These guns are not for national defense but are truly personal weapons, primarily designed for use against other citizens. They are under the domain of the individual owner and are owned for personal gratification, with no obligation to the state. The number and nature of the guns and the attitude toward gun ownership clearly differ greatly between Switzerland and the United States.

Israel is also often touted as a high-gun, low-crime country. Given Israel's security problems, it is not surprising that there are large numbers of armed soldiers and security forces in the streets and that many civilians carry firearms. Yet even though private firearm ownership has risen sharply in Israel in recent decades, its civilian firearm ownership rate still appears to be well below that of the United States (Williams 2000). Relatively few Israelis own handguns (Zimring and Hawkins 1997b).

The Israeli government strictly controls firearm possession among its citizens. A license is required for each firearm owned, and the number of firearms a citizen may possess can be restricted. Applicants face waiting periods of up to three months while police, medical, and psychological checks are conducted. Prospective owners must also pass gun competency tests. "Despite Israel's image abroad as a firearm-friendly society, eligibility for a gun license is determined after thorough criminal-and-medical history checks, and then on a show-need, case-by-case basis" (Williams 2000).

Israeli homicide rates are about average for high-income countries. What differentiates Israel from other developed nations is its security situation, which drives Israeli citizens' demand for firearms. The very tough licensure laws help stop the massive proliferation of civilian firearms. Still, a leading Israeli criminologist, S. F. Landau, reports that most recent homicides were

committed by licensed firearms owners and that "there are many more innocent victims of licensed firearms than persons protected by them from terrorist or criminal attack" (2003, 140).

While every country has its own distinct history and culture, the experience of other developed countries puts to the test many unsubstantiated
claims in the American gun debate.

1. Kleck suggests that "much social order in America may precariously
   depend on the fact that millions of people are armed and dangerous
   to each other" (1988, 17). Yet all other high-income countries have far
   fewer civilian guns than the United States, and most maintain as
   much or more "social order." Indeed, throughout the world and in
   our own historical West, having more armed citizens who pose a
   danger to each other invariably means less social order.
2. While gun proponents hail the permissive U.S. gun regulations as a
   hallmark of freedom, civil libertarians in other countries often favor
   stronger gun control measures. Viewed from abroad, America's so-
   called freedom is portrayed as the freedom to sit behind the door
   with a gun. Australian civil libertarians argue that handguns in society increase the dangers of violent crime and that the fear of crime
   makes people hostages in their own homes and thus less free. Civil
   libertarians in Australia also see the fear of crime as leading to the
   creation of repressive criminal laws and more police authority, further reducing real freedom (Kopel 1992).
3. The gun lobby claims that it is not possible to have a licensing system
   without police abuse of authority and that severe regulations of
   handguns will quickly lead to equally severe regulations of long guns.
   Yet virtually every other developed country has a licensing system,
   and police abuse does not appear to be common. In addition, while
   countries such as Great Britain and Japan strongly restrict both
   handguns and long guns, many developed nations have very strict
   laws only concerning handguns. The other frontier countries—Australia, Canada, and New Zealand—have many long guns but few
   handguns (Kopel 1992).
4. The gun lobby's most popular slogan has long been, "When guns are
   outlawed, only outlaws will have guns." Yet the twentieth-century
   experience of Japan and Great Britain has instead been, "When guns
   are outlawed, very few outlaws will have guns." Gun crime in En-

gland and Japan, which have virtually outlawed guns, is extremely rare by American standards. And in England, 60 percent of the time a "firearm" is used in a robbery, it is in fact a harmless replica or a bluff that involved no firearm at all (O'Donnell and Morrison 1997).

5. Kleck (1997b) claims that if handguns are outlawed, a sizable percentage of criminals will switch to long guns, which are more lethal. The end result can be an increase in homicides. Yet many high-income countries severely restrict handguns but not long guns; their violence rates are often no different than ours, but they have far lower rates of gun violence and homicide. In New Zealand, for example, 20 percent of households have at least one long gun, and handguns are rare. Our murder rate in the 1990s was six times higher than New Zealand's (and our unintentional firearm death rate was also six times higher). Not surprisingly, gun use in robberies and murders is far lower in New Zealand (Newbold 1999).

Historically, the United States has often required strict gun control for people under our protection. After the Spanish-American War, for example, we followed a general policy of trying to place firearms out of the reach of the people, largely restricting their possession to law-enforcement officers; strong regulations requiring licensing and registration for gun ownership were mandated in the Philippines (DeConde 2001).

After the Philippines gained independence from the United States, the proliferation of firearms produced a reign of terror. This disorder, sometimes labeled gun pollution, prompted or provided the excuse President Ferdinand Marcos needed to declare martial law in 1972 and impose a dictatorship (DeConde 2001). Whereas the American gun lobby claims that civilian gun ownership prevents tyranny, in this instance, guns in private hands seem to have enabled rather than prevented a tyrant from eliminating democratic liberties.

INTERNATIONAL EFFECTS OF
OUR PERMISSIVE POLICIES

Most of the guns in Mexico were bought in the United States, then smuggled across the border, and officials of both governments say little can be done to stop that traffic. . . . These firearms are utilized by the narcotraffickers and organized crime groups.

—T. Weiner and G. Thompson

The people and policymakers of other industrialized countries cannot understand how Americans tolerate such high levels of lethal violence. Virtually all foreigners understand that the root of the distinctive American crime problem is the easy accessibility of firearms.

From an international perspective, the United States is viewed as the prime example of what not to do in terms of gun policy. Indeed, the out-of-control U.S. gun situation provides ammunition for gun control forces in other nations; they appeal to the constant fear that American gun culture, like other aspects of our culture, might be spreading to their countries. In the past few years, most other developed nations have tightened their already tough (by American standards) gun control laws.

In Japan, seventeen people were killed with guns in all of 1996; more are killed in the United States on a slow afternoon. Japan has some of the toughest gun laws in the world (e.g., handguns are illegal, and police can inspect homes to make sure that hunting rifles are under lock and key). Yet,

> as strict as the laws are, the public is clamoring for the government to make them tougher. Although this is still one of the least violent societies in the world, and the vast majority of violence is committed by yakuza gangsters against one another, many people feel the "American disease" of guns is spreading here. (Jordan 1997)

In Canada, federal Justice Minister Anne McLellan said that Ontario's overwhelming support of the 1995 gun control law showed that the province rejects the culture of violence that surrounds firearms use in the United States.

> The people of Ontario get it. People have legitimate concerns about their safety, about their security. One of the things they don't want to have is our big cities, like Toronto, becoming like big American cities where so many people have concealed weapons and handguns. (Vienneau 1998)

In Australia in 1998, Conservative Prime Minister John Howard, who helped push for stronger and more uniform gun legislation, said,

> The gun culture is something that is abhorrent to Australians and I will do all in my power to stop it coming into this country, and I don't care who criticizes it. (*Sydney Morning Herald/The Age* 1998)

Our enormous stock of firearms and the lack of reasonable controls make the United States a bad neighbor. For example, while the U.S. government complains about illegal drugs being smuggled through Mexico, our neighbor to the south is concerned that smuggled American firearms are flooding that country and exacerbating the violence there. A 1996 report by the Mexican federal attorney general's office found that the routes used to ship guns south to Mexico were the same ones drug gangs use to ship drugs north to the United States. A Mexican Foreign Ministry official stated that "what makes drug-related crimes so violent is the firepower the narcotics traffickers can gather. It's more than the local police can handle." Most guns seized by Mexican police are made and sold in the United States (Thomas and Anderson 1996; Weiner and Thompson 2001).

Caribbean legislators claim that the United States is glaringly inconsistent for failing to stem the flow of guns into their countries while demanding maximum effort by the island nations to stop the entry of illegal drugs into the United States. The U.S. government claims there is little it can do to reduce the unlawful movement of firearms into the Bahamas or the Caribbean because there are so many guns in the United States and so many points of exit from the American mainland (The Newswire 2000).

The majority of guns smuggled into Canada come from the United States. Canada's attempts to restrict the ownership of handguns and military-style weapons are in constant threat of being undermined by the United States. Justice Minister Allan Rock declared in 1995 that "there are few countries in the world that, like Canada, live on a 5,000 kilometer border with a culture awash in guns" (Nickerson 1995). Many seized guns in Canada have been traced to dealers in Florida and Ohio (*Toronto Star* 1996). Vermont is also a common source of illegal weapons. In 1991–92 a single individual funneled 952 firearms, mostly handguns, into Canada. Fifty of the guns were linked to major crimes in Canada, including five murders and 121 robberies. In 1994 that individual was convicted in U.S. District Court in Burlington, Vermont, on violations of laws regulating the sale of guns and was sentenced to six months of home confinement. "This guy got a light slap on the wrist," said an Ontario police investigator, expressing amazement at the American tolerance for violence. "It's like you've been hypnotized by your own ultra-violent movies and TV into thinking blood on the streets is just a fact of life, like snow in the winter" (Nickerson 1995).

Smuggled American guns turn up all over the world. For example, almost a third of handguns smuggled into Japan between 1991 and 1995 were produced in the United States, the most from any country, followed by 21 percent from China, and 8 percent from the Philippines (Japan National Police Agency 1996). Gun smuggling is an international problem fueled in part by weak domestic gun control policies in the United States.

Each year it becomes clearer that domestic control of firearms is crucial to curbing international gun trafficking. The recommendations of the 1997 U.N. Commission on Crime Prevention and Criminal Justice provide minimum standards for domestic firearms legislation, including regulations on firearm storage, licensing, and record keeping. Most industrialized countries already exceed these standards. The notable exception is the United States (Cukier and Shropshire 2000).

SUMMARY

The gun lobby focuses on the hardened criminal; claims that laws will only be obeyed by decent, law-abiding citizens; extols the benefits of self-defense gun use; and proclaims that any gun policy is merely a disguised attempt to take away the guns of regular citizens whose gun rights are protected by the U.S. Constitution.

A gun lobby mantra is "Blame the criminal, not the gun." But everyone wants to incarcerate vicious criminals, and no one wants to put guns in jail. The slogan seems to mean that the gun lobby wants to focus firearms policy exclusively on criminal gun users and do nothing until after violence has occurred.

To public health professionals, it makes no sense to focus exclusively on the criminal user and ignore many cost-effective measures that can help prevent lethal violence—policies focused on manufacturers, licensed dealers, private sellers, gun owners, and gun carriers. Why should we accept having the highest homicide rate among high-income countries, year after year? Why should we let tens of thousands of Americans die each year when we can pursue reasonable gun policies that can help prevent the shootings and killings? Longer prison sentences should not be our only or our main policy response to the continuing carnage.

The gun lobby rarely talks about suicide. Yet fifty Americans a day kill themselves with firearms. It is of course true that some people who commit suicide with guns would find other means if a gun were not available. But why should we be complacent when we know that reasonable gun policies can save many other potential suicide victims who are ambivalent and impetuous?

The gun lobby rarely talks about unintentional firearm injuries. But why should we calmly accept the fact that thirty Americans each day accidentally shoot themselves and others, and two to three victims die, when we know that feasible and popularly supported policies can prevent many of these unintentional shootings?

If easy access to firearms were beneficial, the United States would be the safest country in the industrialized world rather than what it is: the least safe. States with many guns would be the safest rather than what they are: the least safe. And homes with guns would be the safest rather than what they are: the least safe.

The public health approach to reducing firearm injuries has many similarities to the approach for reducing the harm caused by tobacco and alcohol. For all three products, the goal has not been to prohibit or ban consumption but to minimize the burden on the public's health. For all three products, many of the costs are imposed on nonusers. And for all three products, there are strong and opposing commercial and vested interests whose main interest is not the public's health but increasing the product's sales and general acceptance.

The public health approach to effective consumer product regulation emphasizes accurate data collection, good science, and a population-based approach. The affected industries try to focus any prevention efforts exclusively on education and enforcement and typically portray any product-related problems as caused by a few blameworthy users. By contrast, the public health approach is interested in prevention rather than blame, science rather than moralism. The public health approach refuses to take either the product or the environment as immutable; the evidence shows that the most effective way of improving the public health is usually by modifying both.

For tobacco, alcohol, and firearms, physicians and public health professionals, both individually and collectively through their professional organizations, have been among the leaders in gathering data, conducting scientific studies, disseminating information through articles and testimony, and promoting policies that are likely to enhance the health and safety of society. The successes have been important but limited, and the struggle continues.

While the gun lobby claims that gun ownership is a right, the public health community believes that health should be a primary right for all people. Although the public health goal has been to eradicate certain germs, making illegal mass consumer products such as motor vehicles, alcohol, tobacco, or firearms is not on the public health agenda. Instead, the goal is to discover and promote those policies that cost-effectively increase public health while maintaining our true liberties.

Lessons for U.S. firearms policy also come from international comparisons of how firearms are treated in other high-income countries. Such comparisons indicate that the U.S. level of gun violence is not normal, that there are alternatives to living in communities where gun deaths are commonplace. People in the rest of the world have great difficulty comprehending America's willingness to permit appalling levels of deaths and injuries due to guns (Join Together Online 1998).

Other countries have their shares of violence and crazed individuals, but their violence is less lethal. Consider this story from London:

> A naked sword-wielding man burst into a south London church during Mass yesterday slashing and stabbing members of the congregation. Ten people were injured. . . . Six of the injured suffered stab wounds. . . . The others were hurt in a stampede to get out of St. Andrew's Roman Catholic Church. (*Boston Globe* 1999c)

In the United States, the crazed individual might well have had a gun, and numerous people would have died.

People in other high-income countries often make fun of what they see as our bizarre priorities. The Canadians describe themselves as unarmed Americans with health insurance. The British say that they live in a country where health care is a right but carrying a semiautomatic weapon is a privilege. A British magazine, *The Economist*, opines,

> No other country has chosen, like America, to turn smokers into social pariahs while making it easier and easier to own and carry guns. A society armed to the teeth but with clear lungs may be a worthy aim, though that is surely open to debate. (1998, 17)

A year before the school shooting in Conyers, Georgia, the *Edinburgh Scotsman* ran a story by a BBC reporter.

> This is the story of someone who—quite literally—went off his trolley. It happened in the small American town of Conyers, Georgia. A small accident with shopping carts in Wal-mart, the local budget department store, ended with a man being shot in the face. . . . The point of this tale

of trolley rage is not that America is especially dangerous. . . . Nor should we conclude that guns are dangerous. . . . The moral of the story is obviously that what is most dangerous in Georgia are shopping trolleys, and that the authorities should consider banning them. They were the source of the argument between these men, and unlike pistols, revolvers, machine guns, Armalite rifles and rocket launchers, there is no constitutional protection for the right to bear shopping trolleys. (Esler 1998)

International comparisons tell us that we can easily do better. We have the most guns—especially handguns—and the weakest gun control laws in the industrialized world. We have by far the highest rates of lethal violence. Yet we do not seem to be any more criminal or violent than many other developed nations. We do not need to remain the most dangerous place in the developed world to live, work, or go to school.

CHAPTER 10   POLICY ACTIONS

The United States [is] the last major democratic nation to permit private citizens
to possess guns with few meaningful restraints.

—A. DeConde

There are a wide variety of reasonable, feasible policies that could reduce the
firearms injury problem in the United States. To explore such policies, it is
first necessary to understand the history of federal firearms laws in the United
States, and this chapter begins with a brief description of these laws. The second section discusses policy prescriptions for the firearms problem. An
important first step is to increase the detailed information available about the
circumstances of violent deaths and injuries by creating a consistent national
statistical system. The last section of this chapter describes attempts to bring
such a data system into existence.

A BRIEF HISTORY OF FIREARMS LAW

Current U.S. gun laws are complicated and filled with loopholes. State and
local regulations vary greatly and are often ineffective in reducing gun crime
because firearms can be moved easily across political boundaries. Two
important federal acts dealing with firearms were passed in the 1930s. In
response to the wave of gangland violence that occurred during Prohibition,
Congress tried to stop the traffic in "gangster weapons." The 1934 National
Firearms Act appears to have reduced the use in crime of machine guns,
sawed-off shotguns, and silencers. The 1938 Federal Firearms Act began the
federal licensing of gun dealers, importers, and manufacturers. Dealers were
required to keep records of transactions, and law-enforcement personnel
were allowed to inspect these records (Sugarmann and Rand 1994).

Three decades later, following the gun assassinations of John F. Kennedy,

Robert F. Kennedy, and Martin Luther King Jr., federal laws were passed banning the interstate shipment of handguns and long guns to individuals except through licensed dealers. In addition, only licensed importers were legally permitted to import firearms or ammunition. The results of these laws were mixed, as legions of people became dealers so that they could legally buy and sell guns across state lines; by the early 1990s, the United States had more than 270,000 dealers—more gun dealers than gas stations (Sugarmann and Rand 1994). The 1968 laws also forbade the transfer of firearms to proscribed individuals, including drug users and addicts, illegal immigrants, the mentally ill, and individuals convicted of domestic violence or crimes punishable by at least one year in prison.

In 1986, the Firearms Owners' Protection Act substantially reduced the already weak federal oversight over the distribution of firearms. Among other things, the law permitted firearms dealers to conduct business at gun shows in their own states, limited the number of unannounced federal inspections of dealers to one per year, and reduced the maximum penalties for dealers who knowingly made false statements. The law also made it less likely that collectors and others who sell guns in small volume would need to become licensed dealers. The law led to a rapid increase in sales at gun shows.

The 1986 law also forbade the establishment of any system of firearms registration (common in most other developed countries). Its "relief from disability" program expanded the categories of convicted felons who could have their gun privileges restored and allocated federal funds (typically more than four million dollars per year) to help former felons (including people convicted of rape, murder, drug dealing, gun trafficking, and child molestation) legally own firearms. This amount is more than 50 percent more than the maximum the Centers for Disease Control and Prevention (CDC) was spending in the 1990s on firearms data collection and research. Funding for the "relief from disability" program was effectively ended in 1992.

The 1986 law banned the importation of gun barrels for Saturday night specials. Federal law led to the rapid growth of the domestic manufacture of inexpensive handguns by setting safety and quality standards that applied to imports but not to domestic manufacturers. The 1986 law also banned the future manufacture of machine guns for sale to other than law enforcement or military personnel, freezing the number of fully automatic weapons available to civilians.

Two other federal laws passed in the late 1980s tried to ban "cop-killer bullets" and plastic firearms. In the 1980s police were increasingly wearing new lightweight Kevlar "bulletproof" vests. Unfortunately, criminals were increasingly using armor-piercing bullets. A 1986 bill banned the sale of handgun bullets composed of specific hard metals (tungsten alloys, steel, brass, bronze, iron, beryllium, copper, or depleted uranium).

Alarmed by the increased use of plastics in firearms and the threat it could pose to airport security, in 1988 Congress passed legislation requiring that all new firearms sold be detectable by standard X-ray or metal detector security devices. The purpose of the law was prevention, since no fully plastic gun was yet on the market; the measure has seemingly been quite successful at little or no cost to society.

In 1994 the Brady Handgun Violence Prevention Law took effect in the United States. The law required background checks for purchases of handguns from federally licensed dealers. Background checks were not required for firearms purchased in the secondary market from nondealers. The law also provided for a five-day waiting period before guns could be obtained. In 1998 the waiting period was replaced by an "instant record check," and background checks for firearms purchased from dealers became mandatory for long guns as well as handguns.

Public Law 103-159 (which included the Brady Bill) raised the licensing fee for dealers from thirty dollars to two hundred dollars for three years, helping to reduce the number of licensed dealers. The law also authorized funds to help computerize criminal background information. Both of these measures are crucial components in any successful policy to keep firearms out of the wrong hands.

The 1994 Assault Weapons Ban prohibited the future production, transfer, or possession of nineteen named firearms and guns with specific assault weapon characteristics. However, the law did not apply to guns manufactured before the effective date of the bill or to copycat guns or many other firearms with somewhat similar characteristics. Perhaps the most important aspect of the law was its ban on further production of magazines with capacities greater than ten rounds.

What is most striking from this summary of federal legislation are the many crucial issues that have not been addressed at the national level. The United States has by far the most severe gun problem of any high-income country. Yet unlike most other industrialized nations, we have no national requirements for training, licensing, registration, or safe storage. We also have virtually no product safety requirements for guns, no good data collection system concerning gun injuries, and no real oversight for the entire secondary market of gun sales and transfers. The current national laws are filled with major loopholes and grandfather clauses that often impede effective enforcement.

State laws are also generally quite lax. A recent survey found that forty-three states do not require permits or registrations to purchase semiautomatic weapons; thirty-two states do not require background checks for buying handguns from private sellers; thirty-one states have no waiting period for handgun purchases; and only four states have a one-gun-per-month purchase law to reduce gun running. Six states do not even have a legal minimum age for a child to possess a handgun (Fox News/Reuters 2000). And the ease with which crime guns move across state boundaries limits the effectiveness of even strict state regulations.

REASONABLE POLICIES

[Three] core public health concepts are (1) prevention is preferable to treatment, (2) alterations in the environment are more likely to be effective than attempts to change individual behaviors, and (3) multiple strategies directed toward different risk factors are necessary to solve the problem. These principles can be used to structure programs to prevent firearm deaths and injuries.

—E. C. Powell, K. M. Sheehan, and K. K. Christoffel

Many policies that have nothing directly to do with guns could reduce firearm injuries in the United States. For example, policies aimed at preventing and treating depression and mental illness could reduce suicide attempts by all methods, including firearms. Policies that improve parenting skills, channel anger, or reduce racism and injustice could help prevent all kinds of violence, including gun violence. Policies that reduce alcohol and drug problems can help prevent injuries of all sorts, including both intentional and unintentional gunshot injuries. Policies focusing directly on firearms may be categorized in various ways. Policies may be divided into governmental versus nongovernmental (e.g., actions taken by churches and professional medical societies). Within governmental policies, there are actions taken by federal, state, or municipal authorities. Some governmental policies ban certain products or conduct; other governmental policies attempt to change behavior through education or incentives (e.g., taxes or subsidies). Some governmental action is directed at the demand side of the market, some at the supply side. Government action in the gun arena may be designed to restrict access to some products for almost all citizens (e.g., machine guns, plastic guns); other policies are designed to restrict access to some groups (e.g., minors, felons). Some policies focus on manufacturers, some on distributors, some on owners, some on gun use. Some policies target the gun, some the ammunition.

However they are categorized, there are scores of reasonable policies that could reduce U.S. firearm injuries while keeping almost all of the recreational and self-defense benefits of firearms. Many of these policies were discussed in previous chapters. This section highlights those policies that may reduce our firearms problem and are acceptable to the large majority of Americans. This approach is consistent with the underlying assumptions of the 1994 Task Force on Gun Violence of the American Bar Association (ABA):

> While the ABA has steadfastly recognized the traditions of gun owner-ship for sporting purposes and for self-defense, there is nothing incon-sistent with those traditions in requiring guns to carry safety features to protect children, or in requiring firearms dealers to operate bona fide businesses, or in requiring licenses and education of handgun owners. Personal responsibility and accountability for safety and protection of others must be required of every firearms dealer, every hunter and every parent who maintains a firearm in their home. (American Bar Association Task Force 1994)

At the nongovernmental level, schools, community organizations, medical professionals, the media, private companies, and others can play an impor-tant role in reducing firearm violence. Education is needed, perhaps through local parent-teacher associations, particularly concerning children and guns. Two pressing topics are gun storage practices and teaching parents routinely to inquire about possible access to firearms when their children are invited to friends' houses.

Medical professionals can influence their patients to improve their gun safety I.Q. In one study, almost three-quarters of gun-owning parents said they were very likely to follow a pediatrician's recommendations regarding the safe storage of firearms (Webster et al. 1992).

Hollywood can also do its part by modeling nonviolent nongun behavior and safe gun practices. Television shows helped spread the idea of a desig-nated driver and have promoted seat belt use by having the shows' role mod-els buckle up. With this in mind, public health injury-control experts have been meeting with members of Hollywood's creative community to explore ways the medium can promote safe and responsible gun ownership and use (*Hollywood Reporter* 1999).

Private companies that ship firearms need to be more vigilant. Gun thefts sometimes rely on someone working inside a packaging center. In 1999, United Parcel Service changed its gun shipping policy to reduce theft. All gun shipments must now be sent by overnight airmail rather than by ground transportation. This policy reduces transit time and the number of people who handle the package, thus reducing the likelihood of theft (Wolcott 1999).

In terms of governmental policy, a crucial first step is to create a new agency or provide an existing agency with the power to regulate firearms as a consumer product (Sugarmann and Rand 1994; Freed, Vernick, and Hargarten 1998). The agency should create and maintain a national violent death data system (a surveillance system) that provides information on the circumstances and weapon for every fatality, along with a sample of nonfatal firearm injuries. The agency should make that information readily available and provide funds for social scientists, criminologists, and other expert researchers interested in reducing firearm violence and firearm injuries. For the first time, comprehensive data would be available to guide and evaluate firearm policy.

The agency should also investigate in-depth a sample of gun injuries. When an airplane crashes, the National Transportation Safety Board investigates what went wrong so that future tragedies can be prevented. By contrast, when a gun tragedy occurs, little is done to explore what happened and thereby prevent the next catastrophe. This needs to be changed. For a sample of firearm injuries, a team of behavioral, engineering, and policy experts should systematically investigate the facts and circumstances surrounding the incidents and recommend changes that could prevent future firearm injuries (Rosenbloom 1998).

The agency should have the power to require safety and crime-fighting characteristics on all firearms manufactured or sold in the United States. For example, guns should not fire when dropped and should be made childproof (a toddler should not be able to fire any gun). Pistols should have magazine safeties that prevent firing once the clip has been removed. The agency should have the power to ensure that every gun has a unique identifier, that the serial number is virtually impossible to obliterate, and that bullets can be readily traced to a particular gun. The agency should have the funds to promote research on personalized or "smart guns" and on less lethal ammunition and weapons.

The agency should have the power to ban from regular civilian use certain products that are not needed for protection and endanger the public. As bazookas, machine guns, and plastic guns have been banned, so probably should caseless ammunition and .50-caliber bullets. Except perhaps for bona fide collectors, the agency should prohibit the manufacture, possession, and sale of silencers, short-barreled shotguns, large capacity ammunition magazines, and "gadget" guns that are difficult for metal detectors to identify or are disguised as innocuous items such as key chains, cigarette lighters, or pens. The agency should also have jurisdiction over firearm-related products, such as laser sights, trigger activators, and ammunition. The agency should also have the power to prevent the introduction into the civilian market of new firearm products that are more lethal, more concealable, or more conducive to crime than current firearms.

The key point is not to prescribe exactly what the agency would or should do but to create such an agency and invest it with the resources and power—including standard setting, recall, and research capability—for making reasonable decisions about firearms. The power to determine the side-impact performance standards for automobiles resides with a regulatory agency, as does the power to decide whether or not to ban three-wheeled all-terrain vehicles (while allowing the safer four-wheeled models). Similarly, each specific rule regulating the firearm as a product should go through an administrative rather than a legislative process.

To reduce criminal gun use, all gun sales and other nonfamily transfers should be required to go through licensed dealers. In addition, the dealers should make such sales only from their licensed retail premises—not from their home kitchens, garages, or automobile trunks. These simple requirements will help eliminate the enormous secondary-market loophole that currently makes it ridiculously easy for juveniles, criminals, and terrorists to obtain firearms at flea markets and gun shows and through friends.

Licensed dealers should be under greater scrutiny from both the manufacturers and the government. The Bureau of Alcohol, Tobacco, and Firearms should have the ability to bring felony suits against rogue dealers and make unannounced visits at the bureau's discretion. Background checks should be required for all gun store employees. All firearm thefts should be reported.

To reduce gunrunning, there should be a national law prohibiting the sale of more than one handgun per month to any single individual. Police should routinely trace all crime guns, as is done in drug enforcement, to help identify and prosecute illegal sellers.

At the level of the individual gun user, gun possession should be banned for those convicted of violent crimes—misdemeanors as well as felonies. A national waiting period for gun purchases should be reenacted to reduce homicides and suicides resulting from momentary impulses. The legal age for gun ownership should be raised: just as the national minimum legal drinking age is twenty-one, so too should the legal age for possessing a handgun be twenty-one (although a lower age for long guns is probably reasonable).

To reduce criminal access to firearms, there should be licensing of gun owners and registration of guns. Licensing and registration are currently required of automobile owners and do not limit the availability of motor vehicles. Licensing and registration of guns are policies used by most other high-income countries as part of their overall regulation of firearms. Some twenty U.S. states already have licensing and/or registration requirements (National Rifle Association 2003).

A licensing system will reduce gunrunning from states with lax gun controls to states with stringent gun controls. A national handgun license card will make it more difficult for gunrunners to obtain fake identification documents and tougher for violent persons to use temporary residences in other states to buy guns they could not purchase in their home states. To obtain a handgun license, the individual should pass a fingerprint-based background check and complete an approved handgun safety course.

Registration of guns will allow all legal firearm transfers to be tracked. Current gun tracing typically provides information only about the initial retail sale. A registration system will make it difficult for an individual to act as a straw purchaser (someone with a clean record who buys guns for a criminal). Registration records will make it possible to identify straw buyers, gunrunners, and rogue dealers.

Gun ownership, possession, and carrying entail responsibilities. To prevent theft, accidents, and suicide, some countries require that guns be stored unloaded and locked, with the ammunition kept separately. Just as swimming pool owners are liable for misadventures if they do not reasonably restrict access, so should gun owners be held liable for juvenile misuse when guns are stored inappropriately. Some scholars argue for strict liability for gun owners to encourage safe storage and other responsible behaviors (LaFollette 2000). Others suggest that just as liability insurance is typically mandated for automobile owners, gun owners might also be required to purchase liability coverage for injuries caused by their firearms (Saltman 1994).

Drinking is legal and driving is legal, but we have wisely made it illegal to drink and drive, even if the driver has not broken any other law. Similarly we should make the combination of heavy drinking and gun carrying illegal. Gun-carrying laws should give police discretion to prohibit gun carrying by persons they believe to be dangerous to the community.

Because of the external costs imposed on society by gun availability, the tax on the retail sales of guns and ammunition should be increased. The revenue should be earmarked to help underwrite the direct costs of gun injuries (e.g., medical care) and gun-related regulatory activities (e.g., surveillance, licensing).

Many creative police tactics and community activities should be used to reduce gun violence. A recent U.S. Department of Justice publication describes sixty different "promising strategies"—innovative local programs designed to reduce gun violence. (U.S. Department of Justice, OJJDP 1999). For example, in 1994, Rhode Island established the nation's first stand-alone Gun Court to increase the speed of disposition and level and certainty of punishment. In Detroit, a court-based intervention program requires gun violence education for gun-toting youths as a condition of their bond.

In some communities, police have created special teams that target illegal gun traffickers (Charleston, West Virginia), scofflaw dealers (Oakland, California), and violent career criminals (Charlotte, North Carolina). Memphis has created a Weapon Watch hotline that allows students anonymously to report fellow students who bring firearms to school. In Baton Rouge, police-probation teams implement intensive, regular home visits to monitor probation compliance. Various other campaigns are designed to promote safe gun storage, change truant youths' attitudes about guns and violence, and prevent at-risk youths from becoming involved with gangs.

Many other policies merit attention. Voluntary gun buyback programs, for example, have a minimal effect on street gun violence but could reduce gun accidents, suicides, and the use of firearms in domestic disputes. Firearm advertising probably should be monitored more closely; for example, in the 1990s, many ads deceptively implied that handguns in the home were protective for children, wives, and family members in general (Vernick, Teret, and Webster 1997). This list is not comprehensive. It merely indicates some of the many policies that, when combined, can effectively decrease firearm crime and injuries.

PUBLIC HEALTH SURVEILLANCE

> The first step in addressing any public health problem is collecting the data that help you describe and understand the extent and nature of the problem. This requires systematic surveillance.
>
> —T. Christoffel and S. S. Gallagher

In criminal justice parlance, *surveillance* is the term for monitoring the behavior of suspicious individuals. The public health meaning of *surveillance* is quite different—it refers to the systematic and continuing collection of health data essential for determining the nature of the problem, suggesting effective interventions, and providing the information for policy evaluation.

Although some data on firearm fatalities are available from death certificates—the vital statistics system (e.g., on age and gender of victims)—and from crime databases (e.g., on victim-perpetrator relationship), the United States does not have an adequate surveillance system for firearm injury, intentional injury, or injury generally. National data are not systematically collected on the circumstances of unintentional gunshot fatalities, the circumstances of firearm suicides, or the circumstances of nonfatal firearm injuries (unless reported to the police). National data are also not systematically collected on the characteristics of the firearm for any type of firearm injury.

The enormous benefits that can be provided by a national injury surveillance system are well known. Studies using motor vehicle surveillance data (e.g., from the Fatality Analysis Reporting System for all fatal crashes and from the National Accident Sampling System and the Crash Outcome Data Evaluation System for nonfatal collisions) have established the effects of driver behavior, vehicle characteristics, and environmental conditions on collision frequency and severity. Such data have permitted the scientific evaluation of a wide variety of interventions, including drunk-driver legislation, child restraint laws, mandatory-belt-use laws, revised speed limits, vehicle crash survivability standards, motorcycle helmet laws, vehicle inspection laws, minimum drinking age laws, driver education programs, driver licensing restrictions, no-fault automobile insurance, and right-turn-on-red laws (Azrael et al. 2003). Recently, the surveillance data have been used to evaluate the effectiveness of driver- and passenger-side air bags, resulting in the promotion of rear seating of children, the depowering of air bags, and regulation that allows the disconnection of air bag systems (Segui-Gomez 2000).

In contrast to discussions about U.S. motor vehicle policy, debates about firearm policy are driven more by rhetoric than by fact, since comprehensive, national information about firearm injuries does not exist. We do not know, for example, whether there are temporal trends in the proportion of gun-related deaths from small, cheap handguns, whether adolescents preferentially use certain types of guns to commit suicide, or whether there are particular characteristics common to the guns that are involved in unintended childhood shootings. A comprehensive firearms surveillance system could answer questions like these, plus provide crucial data for the evaluation of child-protection laws, assault weapons bans, one-gun-per-month laws, and so on (Teret, Wintemute, and Beilenson 1992; Teret 1996; Barber et al. 2000).

An initial step toward the creation of a national firearm injury surveillance system occurred in 1994, when CDC funding led to the development or enhancement of more than half a dozen firearm surveillance systems, primarily at state health departments (Ikeda, Mercy, and Teret 1998). Unfortunately, lobbying by the National Rifle Association led to cuts in the appropriations for this activity, and federal funding for the system was withdrawn in 1997.

As a result, most cities and states lack firearm injury surveillance systems, those that exist are usually rudimentary, and the data collected are not completely comparable across jurisdictions. Nonetheless, states and localities that do have surveillance systems (drawing on more sources than vital statistics and police-collected uniform crime report data) have provided information that would not otherwise have been available (Barber et al. 2000), such as the following:

1. The Massachusetts Department of Public Health surveillance system collects information about all injuries caused by firearms and knives, using emergency department, hospital, and other data. The system has revealed that in rural Massachusetts, pellet gun injuries to children are common; they often require emergency department visits and are sometimes very serious. It has also shown that the dramatic decline in gun violence in Boston in the mid-1990s that followed innovative initiatives by the police and others—called the Boston miracle and widely cited as a model for other cities trying to reduce youth gun violence—may not have resulted entirely from the initiatives; the surveillance system documents substantial declines in firearm injuries in other large Massachusetts cities without such policy initiatives.

2. Begun in the mid-1990s, the Medical College of Wisconsin's firearm surveillance system was one of the first to link firearm fatality reports from medical examiners, police, and crime labs. It has revealed that five specific

gun makes account for almost 50 percent of the fatalities in the Milwaukee area. Yet these makes accounted for only 6 percent of the guns turned in during the city's buyback program. The buyback program may have had some beneficial effects, including reducing accidents and suicides, but it did not help rid the streets of the weapons most commonly used in fatal criminal shootings.

The Wisconsin system revealed that the Clinton crime bill of September 1994, which targeted nineteen specific types of guns, may have had little short-term effect. In the Milwaukee area, guns of these types were involved in 9 percent of homicides in the three years before the bill. In the three years after its passage, these types of guns were still involved in 9 percent of homicides.

3. A trauma center in Maine has linked emergency medical service, emergency department, and hospital data for the entire state. It has revealed that in 20 percent of gunshot-wound cases, the time between notification of the emergency medical service and arrival at the appropriate hospital is longer than sixty minutes, the "golden hour" for survival. An improved, integrated trauma system could reduce the time and save lives.

These rudimentary existing systems show the great promise of a national firearm injury surveillance system for informing rational gun policy. Contrary to some skeptics' claims, such a system would not only make plain avenues of effective gun policy but also reveal existing measures that do not work and should be eliminated. To help realize this promise, six foundations—Soros, Joyce, MacArthur, Annie E. Casey, Atlantic Philanthropies, and Packard—funded the Harvard Injury Control Research Center to become the coordinating center for firearm surveillance. The center promotes local and state surveillance efforts and works to ensure that consistent and comparable data are collected over time. Working with the Medical College of Wisconsin and other institutions, the Harvard center began a national pilot program in 1998.

As of the beginning of 2003, fifteen sites from around the nation are part of the pilot project. A 120-page coding manual was created to describe the exact data and definitions of all variables to be collected. Consistent and comparable data are being assembled not only on firearm injuries but also on all suicides and homicides. In addition, the Harvard center is collaborating with leaders of state child fatality review teams from around the country to help create a uniform set of data elements to fit with the violent-death reporting system (Azrael, Barber, and Mercy 2001). Creating a unified national system takes more time and funding than foundations can supply, and a federal agency needs to be the ultimate national coordinator.

In the short run, there is much additional work that can be done to improve surveillance. More states should mandate external-cause-of-injury coding (formerly e-coding) at hospitals and emergency rooms. That means that data will be collected not only according to the body part injured but on the cause of the injury (e.g., Did a head injury result from being hit unintentionally by a baseball or intentionally by a bullet?). Such coding is currently mandated in fewer than half of U.S. states.

City and state health departments should receive funding to develop or expand firearm surveillance systems (Marwick 1999) or, even better, violence or total injury surveillance systems. These systems should link data from a variety of sources, including emergency medical services (e.g., ambulance reports), medical examiner reports, emergency department and hospital data, police data, crime lab data, and gun tracing information. The data (without identifiers) should be readily available to outside researchers.

In the long run the goal is to create a good surveillance system for all injuries, including drownings, falls, and fires. An intermediate step is to create a data system for all violent deaths that will include all firearm fatalities. The creation of such a system—a National Violent Death Reporting System—is now the focus of the pilot program's efforts (Azrael, Barber, and Mercy 2001).

No additional data need be collected for a National Violent Death Reporting System. The information already being collected by medical examiners, crime labs, vital statistics, police, and others just needs to be assembled together in a consistent way. The system has been endorsed by many organizations and is included as recommendations in the surgeon general's 2001 Suicide Reduction Plan (Surgeon General 2001) and the Institute of Medicine's report on reducing suicide (Goldsmith et al. 2002). The federal government appropriated $1.5 million to the CDC for 2002 to begin work on this system at the national level; with increased funding for 2003, CDC is now supporting thirteen state health departments for initial collection efforts. It is estimated that twenty million dollars is required for a complete system, a small amount given the size of the problem.

Data alone, of course, are not enough. Funding is also required—from universities, foundations, the government, and others—for unbiased scientific analysis of the data and for firearms research and evaluation generally. Analysis of the surveillance data can help indicate the type of policies that are needed and can be used to determine whether the policies are effective.

SUMMARY

U.S. gun laws are weaker than those of every other industrialized nation. For example, unlike other high-income countries, we do not have national requirements for firearms training, licensing, registration, or safe storage. Our patchwork regulatory system has had some apparent successes—for example, reducing (but not always eliminating) the problems that could be caused by machine guns, sawed-off shotguns, silencers, plastic handguns, and cop-killer bullets. But many more initiatives are needed to reduce our gun problems.

The most important step is to create a federal agency with the power to regulate firearms as a consumer product. The agency should engage in a multitude of activities, including creating a surveillance (data) system of all violent deaths and other gun injuries, funding research, mandating tamperproof and unique serial numbers for firearms, banning gadget guns, requiring magazine safeties on pistols, and so on. To eliminate the current loophole regarding background checks, all firearm transfers should be required to go through licensed dealers, who would face stronger government oversight.

A good data system is crucial. The public health approach to injury prevention consists of answering four questions: What is the problem? What are the causes? What works to prevent this problem? And how do you get these programs implemented? To answer the first question, one needs to know what any good reporter would ask: Who? What? Where? When? How? Many cases need to be examined to answer these questions and to look for patterns. That first step is the essence of public health surveillance (Rosenberg and Hammond 1998).

"You don't have to know where you are to be there. But you do have to know where you are to get somewhere else" (Foege 1996b, xxv). A first step in addressing the epidemic of motor-vehicle-related crashes during the 1960s was to start tracking all fatal motor vehicle crashes and collecting and analyzing detailed information about the circumstances and outcomes of each crash. This science-based public health approach to preventing injuries saved hundreds of thousands of lives without significantly affecting the availability of cars. The goal of improved and enhanced data collection on our firearm problem is one that deserves support from participants on all sides of the public policy debate.

> Since 1980, there have been only 137 polio cases in the United States while an estimated 120,000 Americans are injured or killed every year by firearms. Yet government does a better job of tracking polio. That's appalling and must change if this country is going to effectively and fairly address the problem posed by misuse of firearms. (*Milwaukee Journal-Sentinel* 1999)

The vast majority of Americans favor creating a good data system, as they favor almost all the policies outlined in this chapter. Such policies would substantially reduce (but not eliminate) our firearm injury problem without limiting the availability of firearms for regular citizens. We need to change social norms, and we need the political will to act. We should no longer accept our high levels of lethal violence as an inevitable by-product of a free American society.

CONCLUSION

Good ideas are not automatically accepted. They must be driven into practice with courageous patience.

—Admiral Hyman Rickover

The United States has more guns in civilian hands than any other industrialized nation. We have far more handguns per capita, and a gun is easily obtainable by virtually anyone who wants one. Our crime and violence rates are comparable to other developed countries; what distinguishes the United States is our rate of lethal violence, most of which involves guns.

During the 1990s, ninety people a day were killed with guns in the United States, and another three hundred were wounded. Guns were also used in the commission of about three thousand crimes per day. Firearms violence is a major public health problem in the United States.

The public health approach, so successful in reducing the burden of infectious disease and the risks and dangers of many everyday products, can also be used to reduce gun violence. The public health approach is scientific, emphasizes prevention, focuses on the community as a whole, and encourages multidisciplinary and multifaceted research and action.

While the gun lobby wants only to punish the "criminal," the public health approach emphasizes that it is not cost-effective to direct policy exclusively at the individual product user. Good policy also needs to focus on the manufacture and distribution of the product and the environment of product use. It is unrealistic to expect every individual to behave appropriately and responsibly on every occasion. To prevent injuries, it is more effective to build a system that makes it easier for people to act properly, more difficult to make errors, and less likely for serious injury to occur when people behave improperly, inappropriately, or illegally.

People should be held accountable for their actions. Such responsibility pertains not only to the behavior of gun users but also to the conduct of gun owners, gun carriers, gun manufacturers, gun distributors, public officials, and other decision makers. However, the goal of public health is not to find fault but to prevent injury and death.

The threat of punishment can deter criminals, and incarceration can help prevent them from harming members of society; criminal justice (like tort law) is part of the prevention package. But it is only one part. Instead of looking exclusively at the pathologies of the hundreds of thousands of perpetrators and victims of firearm violence and injuries each year, public health tries to understand why these events occur with regularity year after year and to determine how best to break the cycle of violence and injuries.

To reduce the problem of gun violence, public health not only urges multiple strategies but also recognizes the importance of mobilizing many partners. Public health understands the need to involve the entire community and sees roles for many groups, such as educational institutions, religious organizations, medical associations, and the media. The public health approach also broadens the discussion of firearms policy from an exclusive criminal justice orientation to one concerned with all firearm injuries—including suicides and unintentional gun deaths. The entry of public health practitioners into the field of firearm injury control brings new data sources (e.g., hospital data), new types of statistical analyses (e.g., odds ratios), new research designs (e.g., case-control studies), and new organizations and interest groups (e.g., the American Academy of Pediatrics). It also brings an increased spirit of science, pragmatism, and optimism.

The public health approach is not about banning guns. It is about creating policies that will prevent violence and injuries. In the late 1990s, Massachusetts Attorney General Scott Harshbarger unveiled the first consumer protection regulations in America designed to promote handgun safety. Harshbarger used his office's consumer protection powers to require safety warnings, childproofing, and other safety features for handguns (Massachusetts Attorney General 1997). However, these requirements hold only for firearms sold in Massachusetts.

Action is needed at the federal level. The crucial first step is to create an agency that has the power to regulate firearms as a consumer product. Like the National Highway Traffic Safety Administration, which requires cars to have seat belts, collapsible steering columns, and shatterproof windshields, the firearms agency could require that firearms are childproof, that pistols have magazine safeties, and that serial numbers be tamper resistant. The agency should probably ban certain products from regular civilian use, such as caseless ammunition and .50-caliber bullets. It should require recalls on defectively designed firearms. It is crucial for this federal agency to have the power to make reasoned policies and the ability to respond quickly to changes in technology and the marketplace.

The regulatory agency should actively promote new technology that will make society safer. For example, "smart" or personalized guns that cannot be fired except by authorized users can help prevent unintentional injuries of children and adolescents and limit criminal use of stolen guns. Advances in the technology of less lethal firearms—such as electric stun phasers, tranquilizer guns, or bean-bag guns—could mean that police, civilian, and even criminal shootings would be less likely to result in death or serious injury.

The agency should ensure the creation of a national firearm injury surveillance system and each year should investigate in depth a large sample of shootings. It should make the data available to researchers and provide funding for research.

To reduce criminal gun use, there should be licensing of gun owners and registration of handguns, as is common in other high-income countries. A one-gun-per-month law should be created at the national level to reduce gunrunning. To eliminate the secondary-sales loopholes, all gun transfers should be required to go through licensed dealers, with attendant background checks on purchasers. Licensed dealers should face greater scrutiny from government regulators.

The public health approach has had measurable success in helping to reduce the societal burdens imposed by many products, including tobacco and motor vehicles. A key to public health successes is to change social norms—at one time, for example, spitting on the subway was acceptable and smoking was sophisticated. Just as these norms have changed, it is time now to change the norm that placidly accepts lethal violence as a normal part of American life. Fortunately, it is becoming increasingly understood that among high-income countries, gun violence is a uniquely American public health problem and that a public health approach can be effective in reducing these injuries and deaths.

APPENDIX A   METHODOLOGY

THE GUN-HOMICIDE CONNECTION

1. Case-Control and Ecological Studies

The gold standard among study designs is the experimental or interventional randomized control trial. The goal is typically to evaluate the effects of an exposure or a treatment for a disease or condition. Randomization of assignment of subjects to different exposure or treatment groups tends, on average, to balance the groups on other factors that could influence the outcome. All else being equal, the randomized control trial is more likely than any other to give the correct answer about whether the treatment works or the exposure is causally related to the outcome (Rothman 1986; Koepsell 2001).

By contrast, in nonexperimental or observational studies, the investigator has no control over which subjects are exposed and which are not. In most circumstances, limitations imposed by society, ethics, and cost restrict epidemiologic research to nonexperimental studies (Rothman 1986; Koepsell 2001). Virtually all firearm studies have been nonexperimental studies.

One type of nonexperimental study is the case-control study. "The sophisticated use and understanding of case-control studies is the most outstanding methodologic development of modern epidemiology" (Rothman 1986, 62). A major advantage of the case-control study design is that it is efficient for the study of rare outcomes (e.g., suicide or homicide), especially where exposure is common (e.g., to guns in the United States) (Cummings, Koepsell, and Roberts 2001).

In case-control studies, the investigator begins by identifying a group of individuals known to have the outcome of interest (the cases) and compares them to a group of individuals known not to have the outcome (the controls). The controls must be people who would have been counted as cases if they had the outcome of interest (Cummings, Koepsell, and Roberts 2001; Koepsell 2001).

Epidemiologists have used case-control studies to examine risk factors for many injuries, including suicide and homicide (Cummings, Koepsell, and Roberts 2001). Like all study designs, case-control studies have various limitations. Three of the potential weaknesses in case-control studies of guns and violent death are measurement error (e.g., the possibility of recall bias), confounding, and reverse causation.

In many but not all (e.g., Cummings, Koepsell, Grossman, Savarino, and Thompson 1997) of the case-control studies of homicide (or suicide) and guns, case and control families are asked about the presence of guns in the home. After a gun homicide (and particularly a gun suicide) occurs in the home, it is likely that all adults will know about the presence of a firearm. The relationship between guns and homicide (or suicide) could be overstated if guns in control households are underascertained while guns in case households are more accurately estimated (Kleck 1997b).

The first case-control study of guns and homicide (Kellermann et al. 1993) and an early case-control study of guns and adolescent suicide (Brent et al. 1991) have been criticized in this regard (Kleck 1997b). The Kellermann study found that 36 percent of case households contained handguns, compared to 23 percent of control households. The Brent study found that 55 percent of case households contained handguns (72 percent contained firearms), compared to 20 percent of control households (37 percent contained firearms). These large differences suggest that the size of the underascertainment problem, at least by itself, is not important enough to eliminate the differences found in firearm availability between case and control households. (Kleck's tables 8.2c and d make no sense.)

A central problem for all epidemiologic studies is the possibility of confounding. The goal of the case-control study is to estimate the association between an exposure (e.g., guns) and an outcome (e.g., homicide). Confounding occurs when the estimate is erroneous because of failure to account for a third factor that is associated with both the exposure and the outcome (Cummings, Koepsell, and Roberts 2001). In case-control studies of guns and homicide, for example, one can imagine many potential confounders (e.g., aggressive behavior) and question the extent to which the distorting effect of potential confounders has been adequately accounted for in the reported associations.

The Kellermann et al. (1993) study has been criticized on the grounds of possible confounding. Gary Kleck (1997b, 244), for example, argues that A. L. Kellermann and coauthors "failed to control for whether subjects were drug dealers or members of street gangs, persons who are both much more likely to own guns and far more likely to become victims of homicide." However, Kellermann did control for many potential risk factors, including illicit drug use, prior arrests, and household members hit or hurt in fights in the home. The study—for better or worse—examined only homicides occurring in the home, whereas drug dealers and street gang members are most likely to die in the streets. The study found that virtually all the increased risk of a gun in the home resulted from homicide by family members or intimate acquaintances—not from shootouts between drug dealers or gangs but domestic homicides. And the increased risk caused by guns in the home was greater for women than for men (Bailey et al. 1997).

A related potential threat to the validity of a case-control study is the possibility of reverse causation: it is plausible, for example, that guns do not put people at higher risk but instead that persons at higher risk for homicide are more likely to own or acquire firearms. It is sometimes difficult to decide the direction of primary causation in an association of guns and homicide. Looking at disaggregate findings may provide some insight. For example, Kellermann et al. (1993) found that gun-owning households were not at higher risk for nongun homicide—and we might well expect that people at risk for nongun homicide would be just as likely to obtain firearms as those at risk for gun homicide.

The Kellermann et al. (1993) article has the virtue of highlighting its own limitations and attempting, where possible, to address them. It does not address them perfectly, by any means: "If, for example, people who keep guns in their homes are more psychologically prone to violence than people who do not, this could explain the link between gun ownership and homicide in the home. Although we examine several behavioral markers of violence and aggression and included two in our final logistic regression, psychological confounding of this sort is difficult to control for" (Kellermann et al. 1993, 1089).

A few case-control studies cannot completely settle an important issue, such as the relationship between gun prevalence and violent death. For example, the first case-control studies that linked smoking and lung cancer were quite controversial; only after more than a dozen studies did a scientific consensus emerge. However, while the mechanism by which smoking causes cancer is still not completely understood, the method by which gun availability might increase homicide is clear.

A prime hypothesis linking gun availability and homicide outside the home is not so much that one's own gun affects the risk of death—though it might increase or reduce it—but that the firearms of others (i.e., the perpetrators) increase the likelihood of being murdered on the street. In this instance, instead of a case-control study, an ecological study may be more germane.

Ecologic or group-level studies are nonexperimental studies in which the units of analysis are groups (e.g., states) rather than individuals. Ecologic studies are common when evaluating the effect of a law or policy. Threats to the validity of an ecologic study not only include measurement error, confounding, and reverse causation but also the possibility of ecological fallacy.

Ecological fallacy occurs when an investigator incorrectly interprets group-level associations as reflecting individual-level relationships. For example, a classic injury-related example of ecologic bias comes from the work of nineteenth-century sociologist Emile Durkheim. Suicide in Prussian provinces in the nineteenth century was highly positively associated with the proportion of Protestants in each province. However, that did not mean that Protestants were committing suicide at substantially higher rates. Many suicides in predominantly Protestant provinces were in fact committed by non-Protestants (Hingson et al. 2001).

The potential for the ecological fallacy is probably less for a study examining the relationship between firearms and violent death than, say, a study examining the relationship between poverty and violent death. For example, if higher-poverty areas have more homicides, we don't know from that fact alone whether the people who were the victims or the perpetrators of homicide were poor. However, if studies show, as they do, that people living in gun-dense areas have higher homicide rates (because of higher gun homicide rates), we do know that a gun was linked with each gun homicide death. While we do not know if the people who were victims or perpetrators of homicide had guns in their homes, we do know for sure that the perpetrators somehow gained access to firearms.

2. Time-Series Analyses

Most time-series analyses that examine the gun-homicide connection have been ecological studies. Unfortunately, these studies often have substantial limitations. First, measures of gun ownership levels are imprecise and changes, particularly at the national level, occur very slowly because guns are highly durable—the size of the gun stock is largely determined by past acquisitions. Taken together, these facts mean that researchers do not really know the extent to which gun ownership has been increasing or decreasing from one year to the next.

Second, changes in homicide rates over time have been difficult to model. Homicide rates are cyclical, but we currently lack sufficient understanding of these waves to accurately model them. Thus we have a poor model, with a badly measured key explanatory variable (gun ownership levels). Therefore, little faith can be put in the results of national ecological time-series analyses; indeed, it is not surprising that many time-series analyses of the United States find no significant relationship between gun ownership levels and homicide (Kleck 1984, 1997b; Magaddino and Medoff 1984). Nonetheless, some studies do find a significant relationship—that more guns are associated with more murders (Phillips, Votey, and Howell 1976; Kleck 1979). And studies of areas in Detroit have consistently found a significant relationship between gun levels and homicide (Newton and Zimring 1969; Fisher 1976; McDowall 1991).

3. Controlling for Urbanization

A key element in case-control, cohort, and ecological studies is accounting for possible important confounders that influence the relationship between the variable of interest (firearm availability) and the outcome (homicide). An important first step is to compare likes to likes. For case-control studies of homicide, that usually means matching on age, gender, and neighborhood, at a minimum. For international studies it means comparing high-income countries to other high-income countries, thus helping to hold constant many socioeconomic variables. In U.S. ecological studies, it means comparing states to states, cities to cities, and rural areas to rural areas (Hepburn and Hemenway 2003).

Compared to suburbs or rural areas, cities in the United States have higher rates of all types of crime, including homicide (U.S. Department of Justice, Bureau of Justice Statistics 2000). Many factors account for the higher urban crime rates, including concentrations of poverty, poor housing and bad schools, immigration, many encounters with strangers, and the relative ease of organizing youth street gangs. By contrast, more families in rural areas have firearms because of the relative importance of hunting, shooting, and killing varmints.

One case-control study of homicide offenders (Kleck and Hogan 1999) failed to match on or otherwise control for neighborhood or even urban versus rural residence, making it more likely to find a spurious negative association between gun prevalence and crime.

A cross-sectional study of Illinois regions and counties shows the importance of controlling for the effects of urbanization. Bordua (1986) examined homicide in Illinois's nine regions and 102 counties. The author found that the rate of firearm ownership in both region and county analyses were negatively associated with all measures of violent crime, including homicide. However, he initially failed to control for important confounders, including urbanization. Instead of comparing Cook County (Chicago) with downstate rural counties, the more relevant comparison is among the rural counties or among suburban areas. In a step in this direction, the author performed multivariate analyses, controlling for urbanization and population density as well as other factors. In these analyses, the results showed no significant association between the rate of firearm ownership and homicide.

A recent cohort study (Merrill 2002) pooled data from two national surveys to determine the likelihood of violent death for adults over a one-year period. While the study controlled for gender, income, education, and other factors, it did not control for urbanization. Thus, not surprisingly, it found that a gun in the home was associated with a decreased risk for homicide (but an increased risk for both suicide and accidental gun death). For even a suggestion of cause and effect, the study needed to compare rural residents with guns to rural residents without guns and urban residents with guns to urban residents without guns, which it could not do. A study using similar data found that a gun in the home was associated with a higher risk of homicide, after controlling for other factors (Wiebe 2003b).

4. Reverse Causation

Increased accessibility to guns may lead to more lethal violence, but more lethal violence may also induce more people to acquire guns. Theoretically, a positive relationship between gun levels and homicide could imply a relationship in either or both directions (as well as no causal relationship). Consider an ecological study examining the gun prevalence–homicide connection.

The hypothesized effect of gun prevalence on homicide is primarily that the availability of guns in any year affects the homicide rate in that year. In terms of timing, the possible reverse effect of homicide on gun prevalence is not as straightforward and is far more difficult to model accurately. Firearms are highly durable products. The availability of firearms today is determined largely by past decisions concerning firearms purchases. Current homicide rates may have some influence on the decision to purchase a firearm, but they have little impact on the overall stock of firearms in a community. Past homicide rates as well as many other past factors may have affected past acquisitions, which largely determine current household gun prevalence. Making the relationship even more complicated, this year's purchase decision is affected by the prior firearm purchase decisions of the household; if one already has a handgun for protection, purchasing another one may be less important, and the purchase of another gun has no effect on the percentage of households with at least one firearm. Also important is the fact that consumers may acquire firearms for expected future needs. For example, whether an individual decides to purchase a firearm for protection may depend on whether this year's high homicide rate is seen as a trend or merely as an aberration.

A good model of the effects of homicide on current levels of household gun ownership might want to include consumer knowledge about homicide rates, consumer expectations about the future, and past acquisition decisions. The research that has tried to model the two-way relationship between guns and homicide typically has not done an adequate job on the complex influence of homicide on the current availability of firearms.

A statistical technique designed to try to account for the possibility of two-way causation is two-stage least squares. In the first stage, there is an attempt to estimate the level of gun ownership were there no effect of homicide on gun levels; in the second stage, those estimates of gun ownership are regressed against the homicide rate. Many pitfalls exist in this statistical approach. One large statistical analysis of gun levels and homicide rates appears to have a number of very serious problems, making the reported results of little value.

A cross-sectional study of 170 large U.S. cities in 1980 tried to analyze the effects of gun prevalence on homicide rates (Kleck and Patterson 1993). The authors concluded that homicide rates affect gun prevalence but that gun prevalence does not affect homicide rates. Problems exist with the study at the theoretical level (e.g., as explained earlier, the correct relationship is that the homicide rate in one year should primarily affect the change in gun ownership rates the next year rather than the proposed relationship that the homicide rate in one year affects the total firearm ownership level that same year). But the most serious deficiencies are in the empirical analysis.

The first stage of the two-stage least-squares analysis is crucial, providing an estimate of the gun levels that would have existed had there been no effect of homicide on gun ownership. If that estimate is not accurate, the second-level analysis cannot be accepted as valid. The first stage requires an instrumental variable, which must meet three criteria: it has to be (1) strongly correlated with gun availability; (2) have no direct effect on homicide; and (3) have no correlation with other factors that are not in the model but are correlated with homicide (e.g., political tastes for anticrime measures). The instrument variables used in the analysis do not meet these requirements. National Rifle Association (NRA) membership, gun magazine subscriptions, and liberalism are used as the instrumental variables but are probably only weakly related to gun availability in cities, and these variables are likely to be related to city size and regional attitudes that are correlated with homicide and policies toward homicide. Some statistical tests are available to determine whether the necessary conditions for instrumental variables are met. These tests do not appear to have been run.

There are other statistical problems with Kleck and Patterson's study. All control variables included in the second-stage analysis should also be included in the first stage, yet some are not (e.g., divorce rate, inverse of the population); homicide should not be included in the first stage, yet it seems to have been included. The authors also examine gun laws' effects on homicide yet do not use two-stage methods to control for the fact that gun laws, like gun prevalence, are likely to cause and be caused by local area homicide rates.

Many of the policies Kleck and Patterson examine are relatively minor ones (e.g., prohibiting gun possession by the mentally ill or by alcoholics, state licenses for gun dealers) with expected minor effects. The authors fail to provide power tests to show how big the effect of an individual gun policy would need to be to expect statistically significant findings. Lack of power in the analysis means that null findings (lack of statistical significance) have little policy relevance.

A review of Kleck and Patterson's analysis by criminologists R. D. Alba and S. F. Messner (1995, 397) takes into account only some of these problems but still concludes, "In short, Kleck's analysis of the effect of gun ownership on city crime rates is seriously flawed by ambiguous measurement of a key construct and by severe model misspecification. These flaws appear to render moot Kleck's conclusion[s]."

5. International Studies

Across nations, what is the association between guns and homicide? A book by Kleck (1997b, 254) contains a paragraph describing the results of a simple correlation. Kleck takes data from Krug, Powell, and Dahlberg (1998) and compares the homicide rate in thirty-six nations with the gun ownership rate.

A major problem is that the thirty-six nations are not all high-income countries as defined by the World Bank. The sample contains ten nonindustrialized nations, including Brazil, Mexico, and Estonia, each with very high homicide rates. Social scientists are taught that it is generally inappropriate to include high-income and other countries in the same analysis because their different social, political, and economic structures can confound the associations of interest.

A second problem concerns the quality of the data: Krug, Powell, and Dahlberg warn that "the data need to be viewed with some caution. . . . The sensitivity and specificity of the surveillance systems may differ from country to country" (1998, 220). Problems with data accuracy are particularly acute for the non-high-income nations. Inaccurate measures generally make it less likely that an analysis will find the true relationship between the variables.

Still, the correlation between gun ownership levels and homicide is positive (.27) and significant at $p < .06$. Nonetheless, Kleck strongly concludes that "there is no significant (at the five percent level) association between gun ownership levels and the total homicide rate in the largest sample of nations available to study this topic" (1997b, 254).

D. D. Polsby and D. B. Kates Jr. use Kleck's analysis to claim that

homicide and gun homicide compared to [legal] gun ownership figures from thirty-six nations shows no correlation; lower rates of legal firearm ownership did not coincide with lower rates of homicide or gun homicide; neither did higher legal ownership rates coincide with higher rates of homicide. (1998, 983)

This statement is incorrect on many counts. Kleck doesn't examine gun homicides, he has no measure of legal gun ownership, and his results actually show a positive correlation between gun ownership and homicide—lower rates of gun ownership correspond to lower rates of homicide (statistically significant at the .06 level). Furthermore, when the data are analyzed looking only at the twenty-six high-income nations, a strong and significant association exists between gun ownership levels and homicide (Hemenway and Miller 2000).

M. Killias et al. (2001) examine the relationship between gun prevalence and homicide for twenty-one nations, three of which do not have high incomes (e.g., Estonia) and find no significant association. However, when the analysis is confined to the eighteen high-income nations, the association between gun prevalence and homicide is strong and statistically significant. Cross-national comparisons have many problems, but for high-income nations, there is an extremely strong and significant association between gun ownership levels and total homicide rates.

What about two-nation comparisons? In a study comparing Canadian provinces with adjacent U.S. states, B. S. Centerwall (1991) claims that the homicide rates in the two countries are similar. But it turns out that the rates are not at all similar. Centerwall did not report the fact that our overall homicide rate for these states is three times the rate for the Canadian provinces—primarily because of our high homicide rates in such northern cities as New York, Detroit, and Seattle compared to such Canadian cities as Montreal, Toronto, and Vancouver. The United States has more guns per capita (particularly more handguns) and higher rates of gun homicide and overall homicide, especially in urban areas.

In a recent book, historian Joyce Malcolm (2002, 253) claims, "In England, fewer guns have meant more crime. In America more guns have meant less crime." Her claim rests on her assertions that (1) homicide and other violent crimes in England decreased between 1500 and 1953, while the number of firearms in private hands increased; and (2) in the past two decades, gun availability fell in England and crime increased, while the reverse happened in the United States.

The most important problem with Malcolm's thesis is that she infers cause and effect ("more guns mean less crime") without providing evidence to support this belief (Hemenway 2003b). Many things changed in England between 1500 and 1953, few of which she takes into account. She does not analyze the effects of changes in industrialization, urbanization, poverty, policing, alcohol, or a myriad other important determinants of crime. Nor does she make a good case for the effects of firearms on crime. For example, there were virtually no guns in 1500 when Malcolm says the English homicide rates started falling. While it is true that in 1800 there were more guns, most of these guns seem to have been muskets, which were inaccurate and unreliable, shot one bullet at a time, and took time to reload. Such weapons were not very useful for either crime or self-defense against criminals. Any change in English crime rates between 1500 and 1800 had little to do with guns.

A second problem with Malcolm's argument is that her "facts" are suspect. For example, for England between 1980 and 2000, Malcolm provides no evidence on the change in gun availability, which seems to have been very low throughout the twentieth century. And according to Britain's victimization survey, the probability of becoming a crime victim in Britain recently has been falling, not rising, reaching a twenty-year low in 2001 (Simmons et al. 2002; Leitzel 2003). On the U.S. side, since the early 1990s, both homicide rates and household gun ownership rates have fallen dramatically. In both Britain and the United States in the past decade, fewer guns have been associated with less crime.

A cross-sectional comparison of the United States and England also suggests that guns are part of the problem rather than part of the solution. The English appear to be as violent as Americans but have much lower gun violence and lethal violence rates. While recent victimization surveys find that robbery, assault, burglary, and motor vehicle theft are as high or higher in England, the U.S. homicide rate is typically six times higher (principally because of gun homicides), and a far higher percentage of our robberies involve guns. England–United States comparisons are consistent with the more guns–more homicide association.

6. Nongun Homicide

Cross-sectional ecological studies find a large and statistically significant association between firearm prevalence and firearm homicide. In addition, the studies sometimes find a weaker but significant positive association between firearm prevalence and nonfirearm homicide. This latter finding might indicate omitted-variable bias. For example, areas with more guns may have cultures that are more lethally violent even without guns, and the control variables in the analysis do not sufficiently account for this. However, there are at least four possible reasons why more guns may causally increase nongun homicide.

1. *Retaliation.* If more guns lead to more serious violence, the victims' family, friends, or gang associates may be more likely to seriously retaliate, killing the perpetrator and his friends or gang associates, by any means, gun or nongun.
2. *Court congestion.* If more guns lead to more serious crime, the police and court system may become overtaxed, reducing the probability of apprehending and convicting the correct perpetrator. This reduces the costs of crime to the perpetrator, which can increase the amount and seriousness of criminal behavior.
3. *Reduction in social capital.* When serious crime increases, community trust and interaction fall. Regular citizens become afraid to go out at night, making the streets even less safe. Fear may lead to neighborhood instability as longtime residents decide to move out. The reduction in the social fabric of the community may increase the likelihood of serious crime, including homicide by all methods. Evidence shows that in the United States, states with more guns not only have more homicides but also have lower levels of trust and social interaction (Hemenway et al. 2001).
4. *Changes in social norms.* An increase in gun homicide may increase the social tolerance for lethal violence of all kinds, reducing community responses to high homicide rates.

The fact that areas with more guns have higher nongun homicide rates may also result from reverse causation—higher homicide rates, by any method, lead to more households obtaining guns for protection. Studies have not been able to accurately determine the extent to which the gun-homicide connection comes from reverse causation. However, it is sometimes also claimed that if guns become less available, determined killers will simply substitute other methods of killing. This hypothesis suggests that in areas with fewer guns, after accounting for other factors, there should be more nongun homicides. However, studies typically show either a positive relationship (Miller, Azrael, and Hemenway 2002c) or no relationship (Killias 1993, Hemenway and Miller 2000) rather than a negative relationship between gun prevalence and nongun homicide, which is inconsistent with the claim of substitution.

SELF-DEFENSE GUN USE

Estimates of the number of self-defense gun uses come from self-report surveys. A large potential problem with using this approach is what epidemiologists call the false-positive problem. Misclassification is an important source of bias in virtually all surveys. Incorrect classification comes from a wide variety of causes, including miscoding, misunderstanding, misremembering, misinterpretation of events, mischief, and downright mendacity. All self-report surveys have some problems with inaccuracy (misclassification). For example, respondents substantially overreport seat belt use and often incorrectly report whether and for whom they voted in the last election (Parry and Crossley 1950). People do not report with great accuracy whether they were employed or unemployed during the past year (Akerlof and Yellen 1985). Some people do not report truthfully about such mundane details as their age, height, and weight (Weaver and Swanson 1974). A literature review of the validity of self-report responses characterizes as "quite high" 83–98 percent accuracy rates for answers to questions about possession of an automobile, a home, a driver's license, or a library card (Wentland and Smith 1993). In other words, in very good surveys, responses are inaccurate between 2 and 17 percent of the time.

A figure of 2.5 million self-defense gun uses each year is cited continually in the gun debate. The number comes from a survey by Kleck and Gertz (1995). Two aspects of this survey combine to create a severe false-positive problem. The first is the likelihood of "social desirability" responses (sometimes referred to as personal-presentation bias). The bias occurs as individuals respond to questions in a way that presents themselves in the best possible light. For example, an individual who acquires a gun for protection and then uses it successfully to ward off a criminal is displaying the wisdom of his precautions and his capacity to protect himself. His action is to be commended and admired. In addition, an individual with a good self-defense story presents himself as interesting.

Some positive social-desirability bias might not by itself lead to serious overestimation. However, combined with a second aspect of the survey—the attempt to estimate a rare event—it does. The search for a needle in a haystack has major methodological dangers (Cook, Ludwig, and Hemenway 1997; Hemenway 1997a, 1997b).

For example, assume that the actual incidence of a rare event in the population is 0.2 percent. In a random survey, on average, for every 1,000 respondents, 998 will have a chance to be misclassified as a positive (a false positive). On average, however, only two respondents could be misclassified as a negative (a false negative). In addition, because the survey is trying to estimate the incidence of a rare event, a small percentage bias can lead to extreme overestimation. Say that survey findings are a 1 percentage point overestimate of the true incidence. If the true incidence were 40 percent, estimating it at 41 percent might not be a problem. But if the true incidence were 0.2 percent, measuring it at 1.2 percent would be six times higher than the true rate, and if the true incidence were 0.1 percent, measuring it at 1.1 percent would be a tenfold overestimate. In Kleck and Gertz's (1995) self-defense gun survey, if as few as 1.3 percent of respondents were randomly misclassified, the 2.5 million figure would be thirty-three times higher than the true figure.

Using surveys to estimate rare occurrences, especially occurrences with some positive social-desirability bias, will lead to large overestimates. For example, the NRA reports about three million dues-paying members, or about 1.5 percent of American adults. In national surveys, however, 3–9 percent of respondents regularly claim that they are dues-paying NRA members. Similarly, although *Sports Illustrated* reports that fewer than 3 percent of American households purchase the magazine, in national surveys, 15 percent of respondents claim that they are current subscribers (Hemenway 1997a). In a recent survey, five times as many respondents claim to have been hospitalized for fractures in the past year as are reported in hospital discharge data (Harvard Injury Control Research Center 2001).

Consider the most extreme case, in which the true incidence is 0 percent. In that case, a survey can overestimate but not underestimate the true incidence. In May 1994, ABC News and the *Washington Post* conducted a random-digit-dial telephone survey of more than fifteen hundred adults. One question asked, "Have you yourself ever seen anything that you believe was a spacecraft from another planet?" Ten percent of respondents answered in the affirmative. These 150 individuals were then asked, "Have you personally ever been in contact with aliens from another planet or not?" and 6 percent answered, "Yes." Extrapolating to the U.S. population as a whole, we might conclude that 20 million American adults have seen alien spacecraft and 1.2 million have been in actual contact with beings from other planets.

Doctors testing patients for a rare disease are well aware of the problem of false positives. As one example, consider the Breast Cancer Screening Project conducted by the Health Insurance Plan of greater New York (Hennekens and Buring 1987). In a total of almost sixty-five thousand screening examinations (mammography plus physical exam), more than one thousand women tested "positive" and were followed up with biopsies. As it turned out, 92 percent of these positive tests were false. Yet the result is not an indictment of mammography—indeed, the false-positive rate was only 1.5 percent. But that was sufficient, given the rarity of the true disease, to ensure that most positive results would be false. Any ill-advised attempt to use the mammography results to estimate the actual prevalence of breast cancer among these women would lead to a huge overestimate.

The main way the National Crime Victimization Surveys (NCVS) reduce the false-positive problem is by asking about self-defense gun use only to those respondents who first report that someone tried to commit a crime against them. After all, it is not a genuine self-defense gun use unless it is protecting against an attempted crime. A preemptive strike should not be considered a genuine self-defense use.

It turns out that Kleck and Gertz's estimate of self-defense gun use is more than twenty times higher than the estimates using the NCVS. To preserve the 2.5 million self-defense gun estimate, Kleck and Gertz are forced to claim that nineteen out of every twenty people with a genuine self-defense use do not report it to the NCVS (and virtually no one without a genuine self-defense use in the time frame does report one).

Given the problem of social-desirability response, Kleck and Gertz are also forced to argue that there is little that is positive about self-defense gun use and much that is negative. They claim the reports of self-defense gun use are "distinctly unheroic." "What was most striking about the reported events was their banality" (1997, 1455).

However, to get huge overestimates, the social-desirability bias does not have to be important for most people. Given the rare nature of the event, it just has to be dominant for a few. And all the available evidence indicates that most people perceive self-defense gun use as beneficial, socially desirable, and often heroic. For example, in Kleck and Gertz's survey, more than 46 percent of respondents claimed that their gun use might have saved—or probably would have saved or almost certainly did save—someone from dying. If the respondents' claims are correct, hundreds of thousands of murders a year may have been directly prevented by self-defense gun use.

Progun organizations and advocates—and Kleck and Gertz—see self-defense gun use as a good thing. Every issue of the *American Rifleman* includes a column entitled "The Armed Citizen," with examples of self-defense gun incidents in which "good guys" fend off "bad guys." As Kleck and Gertz write, "To acknowledge high defensive gun use frequency would be to concede the most significant cost of gun prohibition" (1997, 1447).

Kleck and Gertz's self-defense gun users almost always report that they are defending themselves against serious crimes, crimes that should be reported on the NCVS. So Kleck and Gertz imply that much self-defense gun use is deliberately hidden from NCVS surveyors. These authors argue that "most of the reported defensive gun uses involved illegal behavior" (1997, 1455) and that asking about self-defense gun use is equivalent to "requiring respondents to report their own illegal behavior" (1458, 1447).

Kleck and Gertz claim that respondents are acting illegally because the survey "revealed at least seventeen million adults carrying guns for protection in public, only a small fraction of whom have permits allowing them to do this legally" (Kleck 1997b, 209). The authors claim that these respondents would not report this behavior to the Bureau of Census surveyors conducting the NCVS.

But the NCVS never asks directly about respondents' potentially unlawful activity. Admitting to owning, carrying, or using a gun admits nothing about illegal behavior, just as responding that one was the driver in a car crash admits to no illegal behavior. In addition, the NCVS responses are confidential; it would be illegal for the interviewers to provide individual information to the authorities, and there is no evidence that interviewers have ever done so.

Finally, much evidence exists that people being surveyed willingly report minor and not-so-minor criminal behavior, even behavior that has little possibility of positive social-desirability bias. In one of the earliest self-report studies, a suggestive if nonrandom survey of one thousand adult males, 64 percent of respondents effectively admitted to being unarrested felons, having engaged in such activities as grand larceny (13 percent), auto theft (26 percent), assault (49 percent), and burglary (17 percent) (Wallerstein and Wyle 1947). More recent self-report studies find that well over 70 percent of adolescents aged twelve to nineteen admit to having engaged in delinquent behavior for which they could have been arrested (Fagan, Weis, and Cheng 1990). Even prisoners willingly report prior illegal behavior (Wright and Rossi 1986).

In summary, Kleck and Gertz argue that most respondents do not report their self-defense gun use to NCVS interviewers because it was illegal. This claim is not persuasive because (1) it is not clear why the use should be illegal; (2) respondents are not asked about any possible illegality; (3) Census Bureau interviewers are not permitted to report individual information to any authority, and ethical survey researchers on self-defense gun use cannot and will not report such information; (4) there is no evidence that any such information has ever been provided to authorities; (5) no respondent has ever been punished for providing a particular response; and (6) on similar surveys, respondents report all sorts of real crime.

Finally, in a search for rare events, false negatives (i.e., people who report "no" who should have reported "yes") are almost never the issue. Even if 50 percent of those with a genuine self-defense gun use in Kleck and Gertz's survey deliberately lied and answered in the negative, if only one of one hundred true negatives is misclassified, then the 2.5 million figure is still seventeen times too high.

Kleck and Gertz's claim can be put to the test. For example, one implication is that the ratio of gun/nongun self-defense use should be higher on the type of survey they did than on the NCVS. After all, respondents should not be afraid to report self-defense with a baseball bat to NCVS surveyors. However, this is not the case. Ratios of gun/nongun self-defense uses are similar on the NCVS and on onetime private surveys. Kleck and Gertz's claim about respondents' fear of reporting gun use to the NCVS is not supported by any evidence.

In conclusion, the order-of-magnitude difference between Kleck and Gertz's results and the NCVS results regarding self-defense gun use shows that there must be some differential misreporting/misclassification. Even though the NCVS asks only about serious crimes, the results should be comparable for almost all Kleck and Gertz's respondents' claims that their self-defense gun use was for protection during a serious crime.

Kleck and Gertz do not believe that sixty out of five thousand respondents in their survey might be misclassified, but they are quite willing to claim that more than 95 percent of the individuals who supposedly used their guns in self-defense do not tell census surveyors. If we were to accept Kleck and Gertz's 2.5 million figure as accurate for 1993, then 1,400 of the more than 100,000 adults interviewed in 1993 by the NCVS had a self-defense gun use. However, only about forty report any such use. If we are to believe Kleck and Gertz's results, this pattern of misrepresentation occurs continuously on the semiannual NCVS surveys.

To put it another way, say we believed that either Kleck and Gertz's or the NCVS results were perfectly correct. Let's determine the pattern of misclassification that could have caused the incorrect findings on the other survey. All it would take to make Kleck and Gertz's results compatible with the NCVS would be a random misclassification of 1.3 percent of respondents. However, to make the NCVS compatible with Kleck and Gertz's results would require that 95 percent of the people with genuine self-defense gun uses did not report them and none of the more than one hundred thousand individuals who did not have genuine self-defense gun uses reported one. Which pattern of misclassification seems more likely?

APPENDIXES

GUN CARRYING

How can we determine the appropriateness of a statistical model? Five criteria are: (1) Does it pass the statistical tests designed to determine its accuracy? (2) Are the results robust (or do small changes in the modeling lead to very different results)? (3) Do the disaggregate results make sense? (4) Do results for the control variables make sense? and (5) Does the model make accurate predictions about the future?

A widely cited econometric study of the effects of gun-carrying laws (Lott and Mustard 1997; Lott 1998a) fails all five tests. First, it fails the statistical tests (Heckman and Hotz 1989; Black and Nagin 1998). Second, the results are not robust (Webster, Vernick, and Ludwig 1998; Ludwig 2000; Duggan 2001)—small changes in the model can lead to very different results. Third, the disaggregate results do not make sense. For example, if permissive gun-carrying laws reduce crime, the effect should primarily be seen in a reduction in robberies rather than crimes such as burglary, which is not the case; the beneficial effects should be seen primarily among people who obtain new carry permits—older white males—more than blacks, females, or youth, which again is not the case. Fourth, many of the results for the other control variables do not make sense. For example, the results show both that increasing the rate of unemployment and reducing income will significantly reduce the rate of violent crime. The results indicate that reducing the number of middle-aged and elderly black women (who are rarely either perpetrators or victims of murder) will substantially reduce homicide rates. Indeed, according to the results, a decrease of 1 percentage point in the percentage of the population that is black, female, and aged forty to forty-nine is associated with a 59 percent decrease in homicide (and a 74 percent increase in rape). Fifth, the model does not predict at all well what happened to crime in the following few years (Ayres and Donohue 2003; Donohue 2003).

One problem with the original Lott model is that crime moves in waves, yet his analysis does not include variables that can explain these cycles. For example, his model does not include variables on gangs, drug consumption, community policing, or illegal gun carrying. When he uses a time trend, he uses a linear time trend, which, when crime is increasing, forecasts that crime will continue to increase forever (Hemenway 1998b).

Rates of violent street crime seem to behave like a contagion—like the incidence of measles, tuberculosis, or AIDS. A large homicide wave occurred beginning in the mid-1980s, peaking in 1993. Yet in this same period, homicide rates decreased among those forty and over (with only a small increase for thirty- to thirty-nine-year-olds), and nongun homicide rates decreased for everyone. Virtually all the homicide increase occurred among adolescents and young adults, and all the increased deaths were firearm homicides. The outbreak occurred in the inner cities of major metropolitan areas, spread to other parts of the metropolis, and finally traveled to medium-sized cities. It probably started with the crack epidemic but fed on itself as more guns among youths led other youths to feel the need for guns for protection (Blumstein 1995). Any simple model of crime that does not sufficiently account for its cyclical, contagious nature can produce spurious results.

The Lott model effectively compares rural states (new "shall-issue" states) with urban states between 1985 and 1993. The urban states were experiencing a great cyclical increase in crime during that period; the rural states were not. Unlike other criminologists, Lott effectively attributes that difference not to the advent of the crack cocaine epidemic but to gun-carrying laws. Expanding Lott's analysis to include 1993–97 or 1993–99, periods when crime went down in urban areas faster than in rural areas, it appears that, in most states, permissive gun-carrying laws increased homicide rates (Donohue 2003; Hepburn et al. 2003; Ayres and Donohue 2003b). An excellent in-depth critique of Lott's study can be found on Tim Lambert's Web page: http://www.cse.unsw. edu.au/~lambert/guns/lott/onepage.html (Lambert 2003a).

Lott and Landes (1999; see also Lott 2003) have another model that finds that permissive gun-carrying laws reduce the number of people shot in multiple-victim public shootings by 90 percent. This result should not be taken seriously. One problem is the model does not account for the fact that the changes in state carrying laws were in part the result of newsworthy mass shootings or for the well-known statistical phenomenon called regression to the mean (Ludwig 1999).

Lott and Landes's model examines a specific and rare event: a multiple-shooting incident in which at least two people were shot in a public place (specifically, a church, business, bar, street, government building, public transit, place of employment, park, health care facility, mall, or restaurant), a shooting that made the news, did not involve a gang (e.g., drive-by shootings), and did not involve organized crime, professional hits, serial killings, or shootings that were the by-product of another crime (e.g., a robbery or drug deal).

These events occur exceedingly infrequently. In the nineteen years analyzed by Lott and Landes (1977–95), many states (e.g., South Dakota,

Delaware, Nevada, Tennessee) had no such events. In the peak year (1993), which was also the peak of total gun homicides in the United States, eighty-seven people were killed in such shootings. This number of fatalities was 50 percent higher than the number killed in such shootings in the second-highest year during this period. Those eighty-seven people represented less than 0.5 percent of all the gun homicide deaths for 1993.

Consider a very unusual event—e.g., Worcester, Massachusetts, gets hit by a deadly hurricane. The city council meets and decides to chant before each meeting so that the wind will not return. If the council does this, when one compares that year to the next year, the number of hurricanes hitting Worcester will undoubtedly decrease. Attributing the reduction to the chanting would be silly.

Many states in the late 1980s and early 1990s changed from "may issue" to "shall issue" carrying laws. Proponents of such laws often used a newsworthy multiple shooting as an argument for their passage. For example, after the 1995 multiple-victim shooting in Texas that claimed the life of pop music star Selena, Texas State Representative Ron Wilson noted that he "wished Selena had a gun. . . . Had Selena had a license to carry a gun, then maybe the other woman would have been dead instead" (Walt and Tuell 1995). While such arguments may be misguided, they have carried weight in state legislatures.

Wyoming had a multiple-victim shooting in 1993 (it had only one other in the previous sixteen years). In 1994 it passed a shall-issue law, and, presto, there were no multiple-victim shootings in 1994 or 1995—as there had been none in 1977, 1978, 1979, 1980, 1981, 1982, 1983, 1984, 1985, 1986, 1987, 1989, 1990, 1991, or 1992. Montana had three multiple-victim shootings in 1990. It had not had any such shootings in the thirteen previous years, from 1977 to 1989. In 1991 it passed a shall-issue law, and, presto, it had no multiple-victim shootings during the next five years. Maine had one multiple-victim shooting in nineteen years, 1985, the year it passed its law (Ludwig 1999).

The pattern is the same in states that did not pass permissive carry laws. Alaska has had three multiple-victim shootings, one in 1979 and two in 1983. In 1983 it did not pass a gun-carry law, and, presto, in the next twelve years it had no such shootings. Oklahoma had two multiple-victim shootings in 1986 and one in 1987. It did not pass a permissive gun-carrying law, and it had no shootings in the next eight years. What we have is simply a reversion back to the expected—in this case zero—trend (Ludwig 1999).

Sometimes it takes a couple of years after the shootings before the legislature acts (in Texas, the 1991 Luby's shootings were still being invoked in the mid-1990s as a main reason for passing permissive carrying laws). Before-after comparisons will still be the same. If the Worcester city council doesn't start chanting until two years after the hurricane, an analysis comparing before and after will still find one hurricane before the chants started and none after.

The modeling problem faced by Lott and Landes is a common one in econometrics, endogeneity—the problem of reverse causation, in this case that the passage of the carrying laws are in part a consequence of the events they are intended to affect (multiple shootings). Lott and Landes's model does not sufficiently account for this reverse causation, and thus no claims can be made about their results (Ludwig 1999).

A recent, more careful, and more appropriate statistical analysis of the impact of concealed-carry laws on rampage shootings found "virtually no support for the hypothesis that the laws increase or reduce the number of mass public shootings" (Duwe, Kovandzic, and Moody 2002, 271).

ACCURACY

A good scientist needs to use reliable data and appropriate models and to present findings fairly and accurately. All scientists make mistakes, but one widely cited gun proponent, John Lott Jr., all too often presents inaccurate information, uses inappropriate data and models, and obtains questionable results. He then publicizes them extensively.

In an interview with *Reason* magazine, Lott says,

> My guess is that if you go out and ask people, how many gun deaths involve children under age 5, or under age 10, in the United States, they're going to say thousands. When you tell them that in 1996 there were 17 gun deaths for children under age 5 in the United States and 44 for children under age 10, they're just astounded. (Sullum and Lynch 2000, 40)

The people to whom he tells that information should be astounded. In 1996 there were actually 88 firearm deaths of children aged zero to four (the first time in the 1990s that the number fell below 100), and there were 183 firearm deaths for children between zero and nine (the first time in the 1990s that number fell below 200); for children between zero and fourteen, the number of firearm deaths totaled 693 (Centers for Disease Control and Prevention 2003b).

In his book *More Guns, Less Crime,* Lott says, "The entire number of accidental handgun deaths in the United States in 1988 was only 200" and uses statistical analysis to examine the effects of gun-carrying laws on these accidental gunshot injuries (1998a, 54, 112). Actually, there were more than 1,500 unintentional gun fatalities in 1988; one estimate is that more than 42 percent were by handguns. Kleck (1997b) estimates that 632 accidental handgun deaths occurred that year.

Lott (1998a, 19) asserts, "Over the last decade, gun ownership has been growing for virtually all demographic groups." Yet national surveys of the entire population indicate a substantial decrease in the percentage of U.S. households with firearms from 1986 to 1996 (Kleck 1997b) and from 1996 to 2001 (Smith 2001).

Lott (1998a, 3) says, "If national surveys are correct, 98 percent of the time that people use guns defensively, they merely have to brandish a weapon to break off an attack." He repeats this claim in numerous interviews. What national surveys actually show is that between 21 and 67 percent of respondents report firing their guns during self-defense gun uses (Duncan 2000). And the surveys do not show that all self-defense brandishings are sufficient "to break off an attack."

Lott has repeatedly changed his story about the source of the 98 percent figure. He now claims (Lott 2000) he conducted a survey over three months in 1997, but he has been unable to present any credible evidence that he conducted the survey. Lott made the 98 percent claim on February 6, 1997, well before his purported survey could have been complete. And the mysterious survey was not large enough to provide precise estimates of the percentage of self-defense gun users who merely brandished their firearms (Lambert 2003b).

The Lott episode is just one incident in a seemingly inexorable trend toward eliminating professionally competent research from discussions of social policy or overwhelming it with junk science. If that trend is not halted, the life blood of democracy itself will dry up. The people cannot make sensible choices without reliable information. (Duncan 2003)

In his book *The Bias against Guns* (2003), Lott writes, "The few existing studies that test for the impact of gun control laws on total suicide use purely cross-sectional level data, and find no significant relationship" (143). But articles by Lester and Murrell (1982, 1986), Medoff and Magaddino (1983), Boor and Bair (1990), Yang and Lester (1991), Loftin et al. (1991), and Carrington and Moyer (1994) all find a significant negative relationship between gun control laws and suicide rates; there are also review articles that summarize the literature on guns and suicide (e.g., Miller and Hemenway 1999; Brent 2001).

Lott (2003) writes about one Harvard Injury Control Research Center article and gets it completely wrong. We show that across regions and states, where there are higher levels of firearm ownership, there are more suicides, more homicides, and more accidental (gun) deaths of children (and adults, males, and females), holding various factors constant, including poverty, urbanization, educational levels (alcohol consumption and nonlethal violent crime) (Miller, Azrael, and Hemenway, 2001, 2002a, 2002b, 2002c, 2002d). About the study of five- to fourteen-year-olds, Lott writes,

> The biggest problem is how the study measures what gun ownership rates are. The first two measures used were: 1) the adult firearm homicide and firearm suicide rates and 2) the adult firearm suicide rate, under the assumption that those rates are higher where guns are more common. Unfortunately, juvenile firearm homicide or suicides could be related to those measures for reasons unrelated to gun ownership. Assume two areas have the same gun ownership rates, if one had more adult firearm homicides, is it really surprising that it would also have more juvenile firearm homicides? (316)

While Lott's logic is correct, he seems not to have read our study. We did not use either of these measures for gun ownership rates and know of no one who ever has. We do use a variety of measures, including one that we carefully validate as the best measure (Azrael, Cook, and Miller 2004); all the measures show a strong positive relationship between gun prevalence and homicide rates, suicide rates, and rates of accidental gun deaths.

Lott proceeds to use the National Opinion Research Center (NORC) survey data to measure household gun ownership rates, apparently for each state for each year (Lott 2003, 255). Yet the NORC survey cannot legitimately be used in this manner. The survey is not designed to give a representative sample for even one of the fifty states. For example, in North Dakota, all the survey respondents come from one county, and it is the same county in virtually every survey. More important, even if the survey were representative for states, it is far too small to give a reasonable estimate each year for the least populous states. Until recently, there were only about fifteen hundred respondents, or an average of thirty per state; in North Dakota, perhaps ten people were surveyed (conversation with Tom Smith, NORC, 2003).

Lott not only uses questionable measures of gun ownership but also inappropriately adds forty-four explanatory variables to his state-level analysis, an analysis that is largely cross-sectional ($n = 50$) (it is largely cross-sectional since gun ownership rates change very slowly over time, and the best measures of gun ownership probably have confidence intervals wider than the yearly changes). Lott's approach virtually ensures that whatever the true relationship between guns and death, his analysis will not find them.

State laws on gun shows or assault weapons should have only a small impact on crime rates. Yet Lott (2003) produces models that find enormous impacts. For example, Lott's analyses indicate that the impact from closing the state gun show "loophole" was a 72 percent reduction in Indiana's violent crime rate and a 102 percent reduction in Indiana's auto theft rate, while the effect on New York was to increase the violent crime rate by 83 percent and the auto theft rate by 34 percent. According to Lott's model, the impact of banning assault weapons in Hawaii was that the state's violent crime rate increased 55 percent and its robbery rate rose 95 percent. By contrast, the assault weapons ban reduced Maryland's auto theft rate by 57 percent. Of course, none of these incredible things happened. Indiana certainly did not experience what would have been a crime miracle—a negative car theft rate, which would mean thieves returning cars—following the closing of its gun show loophole. Lott's results are just one piece of evidence that his models are misspecified and should not be accepted as valid.

Lott (2003) also has a model to determine the effects of state safe storage laws. The earliest date a state law went into effect was in October 1989 in Florida. Lott uses a 1994 poll that asked about gun storage to determine the effect of the laws. His results "indicate that states with safe storage laws had higher rates at which households left guns loaded and unlocked but that the rate fell the longer that the law was in effect. Six years [sic] after adoption of the law, states with safe storage laws have a lower percentage of homes with loaded, locked guns than do states without those laws" (175). Yet in 1994, when the data were collected, only one state had experienced the law for five years, and none had done so for six years.

High-profile mass shootings in Australia and Scotland in the mid-1990s led to the enactment of stronger gun control measures in those countries, and Lott states that these laws caused crime to increase (Lott 2002). However, an evaluation of these laws concludes, "In general it seems that both the Australian and the British ban-buybacks did not increase crime, and they may even have contributed to some short-term postban declines in criminal activity" (Leitzel 2003, 153; Reuter and Mouzos 2003).

In his analyses, Lott usually uses complicated econometrics. For readers to accept the results requires complete faith in Lott's integrity, faith that he will always use the best available data, conduct careful and competent research, and make accurate claims that are no stronger than the findings support. Lott does not merit such faith.

APPENDIX B   FAMOUS CIVILIANS
SHOT IN THE UNITED STATES

Homicides

Lyman Bostock (baseball player)
*Sam Cooke (singer)
Ennis Cosby (son of comedian Bill Cosby)
Luke Easter (baseball player)
Medgar Evers (civil rights leader)
Marvin Gaye (singer)
James Garfield (president)
Alexander Hamilton (statesman)
Phil Hartman (actor)
James Butler "Wild Bill" Hickok (U.S. marshal)
James Jordan (father of Michael Jordan)
John F. Kennedy (president)
Robert F. Kennedy (senator)
Martin Luther King Jr. (civil rights leader)
John Lennon (singer/composer)
Abraham Lincoln (president)
Huey Long (senator)
Malcolm X (civil rights leader)
William McKinley (president)
Harvey Milk (member, San Francisco board of supervisors)
George Moscone (San Francisco mayor)
Huey Newton (civil rights leader)
Selena Quintanilla-Perez (singer)
Yetunde Price (sister of Venus and Serena Williams)
Rebecca Schaeffer (actress)
Tupac Shakur (singer)

Herman Tarnower (Scarsdale diet doctor)
Gianni Versace (designer)
Chris Wallace (Notorious B.I.G.) (singer)
Stanford White (architect)

Assaults (survived)

James Brady (presidential press secretary)
Larry Flynt (publisher)
Vernon Jordan (civil rights leader)
Ronald Reagan (president)
Theodore Roosevelt (president)
George Wallace (governor)
Eddie Waitkus (baseball player)
Andy Warhol (artist)

Suicides

Kurt Cobain (singer)
Vince Foster (presidential adviser)
Ernest Hemingway (writer)
Brian Keith (actor)
Donnie Moore (pitcher)
Freddie Prinze Sr. (actor)
+George Reeves (actor)
Will Rogers Jr. (actor)
Del Shannon (singer)
Walter Slezak (actor)
Gig Young (actor)

Unintentionally Wounded

Billy Jurges (shortstop)
Greg LeMond (bicyclist)

Unintentionally Killed

Brandon Lee (actor)

*Sam Cooke's murder was ruled a justifiable homicide
+There is some suspicion that George Reeves was murdered, but his death was ruled a suicide

BIBLIOGRAPHY

ABC News. 1994. *Turning Point*. Transcript 133. October 5.

ABC News/*Washington Post*. 1994. National Poll. May 12–15. Storrs, CT: Roper Center.

ABCnews.com. 1999. Smith and Wesson pledge wins praise: Move seen as bringing sides of gun debate together. October 22.

ABC-TV. 1999. *20/20*. Children and guns. May 21.

Akerlof, G., and J. L. Yellen. 1985. Unemployment through the filter of memory. *Quarterly Journal of Economics* 100:747–73.

Alba, R. D., and S. F. Messner. 1995. "Point Blank" against itself: Evidence and inference about guns, crime, and gun control. *Journal of Quantitative Criminology* 11:391–410.

Albright, T. L., and S. K. Burge. 2003. Improving firearm storage habits: Impact of a brief office counseling by family physicians. *Journal of the American Board of Family Practice* 16:40–46.

Alschuler, A. W. 1997. Two guns, four guns, six guns, more guns: Does arming the public reduce crime? *Valparaiso University Law Review* 31:365–73.

American Academy of Pediatrics. Committee on Adolescence. 1992. Firearms and adolescents. *Pediatrics* 89:784–87.

American Academy of Pediatrics. 1994. *Stop Firearm Injury*. Elk Grove Village, IL: American Academy of Pediatrics.

American Bar Association. 1999. Second Amendment issues. http://www.abanet.org/gunviol/secondamend.html/ (accessed December 2001).

American Bar Association Task Force on Gun Violence. 1994. Report to the House of Delegates. Approved: August.

American Civil Liberties Union (ACLU). 1999. Gun control. http://archive.aclu.org/library/aaguns.html (accessed September 2003).

American College of Physicians. 1998. Firearm injury prevention. *Annals of Internal Medicine* 128:236–41.

Anderson, B. 2002. Instructor shot in accident on gun range. *Advocate*, July 17.

Anderson, J. 2002. Iowan who wanted to surprise fiancé dies in accidental shooting. *Omaha World-Herald*, June 12.

BIBLIOGRAPHY

Anderson, M., J. Kaufman, T. R. Simon, L. Barrois, L. Paulozzi, G. Ryan, R. Hammond, W. Modzeleski, T. Feucht, and L. Potter. 2001. School-associated violent deaths in the United States, 1994–1999. *Journal of the American Medical Association* 286:2695–2702.

Annest, J. L., J. A. Mercy, D. R. Gibson, and G. W. Ryan. 1995. National estimates of nonfatal firearm-related injuries: Beyond the tip of the iceberg. *Journal of the American Medical Association* 273:1749–54.

Ash, P., A. L. Kellermann, D. Fuqua-Whitley, and A. Johnson. 1996. Gun acquisition and use by juvenile offenders. *Journal of the American Medical Association* 275:1754–58.

Ayoob, M. 1999. Arm teachers to stop school shootings. *Wall Street Journal*, May 21.

Ayres, I., and J. J. Donohue III. 2003a. The latest misfires in support of the "more guns less crime" hypothesis. *Stanford Law Review* 55:1371–86.

Ayres, I., and J. J. Donohue III. 2003b. Shooting down the "more guns less crime" hypothesis. *Stanford Law Review* 55:1193–1312.

Azrael, D., C. Barber, D. Hemenway, and M. Miller. 2003. Data on violent injury. In *Evaluating Gun Policy*, ed. J. Ludwig and P. J. Cook, 412–30. Washington, DC: Brookings Institution.

Azrael, D., C. Barber, and J. Mercy. 2001. Linking data to save lives: Recent progress in establishing a national violent death reporting system. *Harvard Health Policy Review* 2:38–42.

Azrael, D., P. J. Cook, and M. Miller. 2004. State and local prevalence of firearms ownership: Measurement, structure, and trends. *Journal of Quantitative Criminology* 20 (1): 43–62.

Azrael, D., and D. Hemenway. 2000. "In the safety of your own home": Results from a national survey on gun use at home. *Social Science and Medicine* 50:258–91.

Bai, M. 1999. Guns in the crossfire. *Newsweek*, August 2, 38–42.

Bailey, J. E., A. L. Kellermann, G. W. Somes, J. G. Banton, F. P. Rivara, and N. P. Rushforth. 1997. Risk factors for violent death of women in the home. *Archives of Internal Medicine* 157:777–82.

Baker, S. P. 1985. Without guns, do people kill people? *American Journal of Public Health* 75:587–88.

Baker, S. P., B. O'Neil, M. J. Ginsburg, and L. Guohua. 1992. *Injury Fact Book*. New York: Oxford University Press.

Baker, S. P., S. P. Teret, and P. E. Dietz. 1980. Firearms and the public health. *Journal of Public Health Policy* 1:224–29.

Barber, C., D. Hemenway, S. Hargarten, A. Kellermann, D. Azrael, and S. Wilt. 2000. A call to arms for a national surveillance system on firearm injuries. *American Journal of Public Health* 90:1191–93.

Barber, C., D. Hemenway, J. Hochstadt, and D. Azrael. 2002. Underestimates of unintentional firearm fatalities: Comparing Supplementary Homicide Report data with the National Vital Statistics System. *Injury Prevention* 8:252–56.

BIBLIOGRAPHY

Barrett, P. M., and V. O'Connell. 1999. Personal weapon: How a gun company tries to propel itself into the computer age. Colt's safety chip bonds a firearm and its user. *Wall Street Journal,* May 12.

Bayer, R., and J. Colgrove. 2002. Science, politics, and ideology in the campaign against environmental tobacco smoke. *American Journal of Public Health* 92:949–54.

BBC. 1996. Seven slashed in school machete attack. http://news.bbc.co.uk/onthisday/hi/dates/stories/July/8/newsid_2496000/2496685.stm.

Beauchamp, D. E. 1988. *The Health of the Republic: Epidemics, Medicine, and Moralism as Challenges to Democracy.* Philadelphia: Temple University Press.

Beautrais, A. L., P. R. Joyce, and R. T. Mulder. 1996. Access to firearms and the risk of suicide: A case-control study. *Australian and New Zealand Journal of Psychiatry* 30:741–48.

Becker, T. M., L. Olson, and J. Vick. 1993. Children and firearms: A gunshot injury prevention program in New Mexico. *American Journal of Public Health* 83:282–83.

Beeghley, L. 2003. *Homicide: A Sociological Explanation.* New York: Rowman and Littlefield.

Beloit Daily News. 1999. Knight cited for shooting hunting pal. October 22.

Bergstein, J. M., D. Hemenway, B. Kennedy, S. Quaday, and R. Ander. 1996. Guns in young hands: A survey of urban teenagers' attitudes and behaviors related to handgun violence. *Journal of Trauma* 41:794–98.

Berman, A. L., R. Brown, and G. T. Diaz et al. 1998. Consensus statement on youth suicide by firearms. *Archives of Suicide Research* 4:89–94.

Bertrand, M., and S. Mullainathan. 2002. Are Emily and Brendan more employable than Lakisha and Jamal? A field experiment on labor market discrimination. Paper presented at Boston University microeconomics seminar, November 19.

Bethel, A. 1999. Happy hours grow fewer. *Boston Globe,* December 5.

Bhattacharyya, N., C. A. Bethel, D. A. Caniano, S. B. Pillai, S. Deppe, and D. R. Cooney. 1998. The childhood air gun: Serious injuries and surgical interventions. *Pediatric Emergency Care* 14:188–90.

Bijur, P. 1998. A funny thing happened on the way to the meeting: On guns and triggers. *Injury Prevention* 4:77.

Birckmayer, J. 1999. The role of alcohol and firearms in youth suicide and homicide in the United States. Ph.D. diss., Harvard School of Public Health.

Birckmayer, J., and D. Hemenway. 1999. Minimum age drinking laws and youth suicide, 1970 to 1990. *American Journal of Public Health* 89:1365–68.

Birckmayer, J., and D. Hemenway. 2001. Suicide and gun prevalence: Are youth disproportionately affected? *Suicide and Life Threatening Behavior* 31:303–10.

Black, C., and D. Bush. 2000. CNN. Democrats propose Senate gun-control resolution. http://www.cnn.com/2000/ALLPOLITICS/stories/04/14/democrats.guns

Black, D. A., and D. S. Nagin. 1998. Do right-to-carry laws deter violent crime? *Journal of Legal Studies* 27:209–19.

BIBLIOGRAPHY

Blakeman, K. 2000. Japanese couple joins anti-gun fight in U.S. *Honolulu Advertiser,* July 9. http://www.HonoluluAdvertiser.com/.

Blendon, R., J. Young, and D. Hemenway. 1996. The American public and the gun control debate. *Journal of the American Medical Association* 275:1719–23.

Block, C. R., and A. Christakos. 1995. Intimate partner homicide in Chicago over 29 years. *Crime and Delinquency* 41:496–526.

Block, R. 1977. *Violent Crime.* Lexington, MA: Lexington Books.

Block, R. 1993. A cross-national comparison of victims of crime: Victim surveys of twelve countries. *International Review of Victimology* 2:183–207.

Block, R. 1997. Firearms in Canada and eight other Western countries: Selected findings of the 1996 International Crime (victim) Survey. Canadian Firearms Centre Research Report. Document WD1997–4e.

Blumstein, A. 1995. Youth gun violence, guns, and the illicit-drug industry. *Journal of Criminal Law and Criminology* 86:10–36.

Blumstein, A., and D. Cork. 1996. Linking gun availability to youth gun violence. *Law and Contemporary Problems* 59:5–24.

Blumstein, A., and R. Rosenfeld. 1998. Explaining recent trends in U.S. homicide rates. *Journal of Law and Criminology* 88:1175–1216.

Bogus, C. T. 1998. The hidden history of the Second Amendment. *University of California at Davis Law Review* 31:309–11.

Bogus, C. T. 2000. The history and politics of Second Amendment scholarship. In *The Second Amendment in Law and History,* ed. C. T. Bogus, 1–15. New York: New Press.

Boor, M., and J. H. Bair. 1990. Suicide rates, handgun control laws, and sociodemographic variables. *Psychological Reports* 66:923–30.

Bordua, D. J. 1986. Firearms ownership and violent crime: A comparison of Illinois counties. In *The Social Ecology of Crime,* ed. J. Byrne and R. J. Sampson, 156–88. New York: Springer-Verlag.

Bork, R. H. 1996. *Slouching towards Gomorrah: Modern Liberalism and American Decline.* New York: Reagon Books.

Boston Globe. 1994. L.A. girl playing prank on parents is killed by father: After jumping out of closet, she's shot as intruder. November 9.

Boston Globe. 1996. No murder in Texas road shooting. March 21.

Boston Globe. 1997a. Reuters: Senior citizens shoot suspect trying to rob a Florida eatery. September 25.

Boston Globe. 1997b. Two slain in Texas in celebrations. January 2.

Boston Globe. 1998a. Accidental shootings spur makers to work on developing smart guns. June 7.

Boston Globe. 1998b. Boy kills self, avoiding beating. October 24.

Boston Globe. 1998c. GM targets child deaths in trunks. December 17.

Boston Globe. 1998d. Key-chain gun challenges airports. May 7.

Boston Globe. 1999a. Boy, six, kills relative in hunting accident. November 22, 1999.

BIBLIOGRAPHY

Boston Globe. 1999b. California governor signs "toughest" U.S. gun ban. July 20.

Boston Globe. 1999c. Naked swordsman injures ten in church. November 29.

Boston Globe. 1999d. Police say officer shot boy after chase. November 23.

Boston Globe. 1999e. Safety panel tightens rules on bunk beds. December 3.

Boston Globe. 1999f. Store owner dies in mock robbery. December 1.

Boston Globe. 1999g. Teen hurt in school shooting is killed while hunting. October 7, A31.

Braga, A. A., D. M. Kennedy, E. J. Waring, and A. M. Piehl. 2001. Problem-oriented policing, deterrence, and youth violence: An evaluation of Boston's Operation Ceasefire. *Journal of Research in Crime and Delinquency* 38:195–225.

Brandt, A. 1992. The rise and fall of the cigarette: A brief history of the antismoking movement in the United States. In *Advancing Health in Developing Countries,* ed. L. C. Chen, A. Kleinman, and N. C. Ware, 59–77. New York: Auburn House.

Brearley, H. C. 1932. *Homicide in the United States.* Chapel Hill: University of North Carolina Press.

Brent, D. A. 2001. Firearms and suicide. *Annals of the New York Academy of Sciences* 932:225–39.

Brent, D. A., M. Baugher, B. Birmaher, D. Kolko, and J. Bridge. 2000. Compliance with recommendations to remove firearms in families participating in a clinical trial for adolescent depression. *Journal of the American Academy of Child and Adolescent Psychiatry* 39:1220–26.

Brent, D. A., and J. Bridge. 2003. Firearms availability and suicide. *American Behavioral Scientist* 46:1192–1210.

Brent, D. A., J. A. Perper, and C. J. Allman. 1987. Alcohol, firearms, and suicide among youth. Temporal trends in Allegheny County, Pennsylvania, 1960 to 1983. *Journal of the American Medical Association* 257:3369–72.

Brent, D. A., J. A. Perper, C. J. Allman, G. M. Moritz, M. E. Wartella, and J. P. Zelenak. 1991. The presence and accessibility of firearms in the homes of adolescent suicides: A case-control study. *Journal of the American Medical Association* 266:2989–95.

Brent, D. A., J. A. Perper, C. E. Goldstein, D. J. Kolko, M. J. Allan, C. J. Allman, and J. P. Zelenak. 1988. Risk factors for adolescent suicide: A comparison of adolescent suicide victims with suicidal inpatients. *Archives of General Psychiatry* 45:581–88.

Brent, D. A., J. A. Perper, G. Moritz, M. Baugher, and C. Allmann. 1993. Suicide in adolescents with no apparent psychopathology. *Journal of the American Academy of Child and Adolescent Psychiatry* 32:494–500.

Brent, D. A., J. A. Perper, G. Moritz, M. Baugher, J. Schweers, and C. Roth. 1993. Firearms and adolescent suicide: A community case-control study. *American Journal of Diseases of Children* 147:1066–71.

Brent, D. A., J. A. Perper, G. Moritz, M. Baugher, J. Schweers, and C. Roth. 1994. Suicide in affectively ill adolescents: A case-control study. *Journal of Affective Disorders* 31:193–202.

BIBLIOGRAPHY

Brent, D. A., J. A. Perper, G. Moritz, A. Friend, J. Schweers, C. J. Allman, L. McQuiston, M. B. Bolan, C. Roth, and L. Balach. 1993. Adolescent witnesses to a peer suicide. *Journal of the American Academy of Child and Adolescent Psychiatry* 32:1184–88.

Brill, S. 1977. *Firearm Abuse: A Research and Policy Report.* Washington, DC: Police Foundation.

Britt, C. J., D. J. Bordua, and G. Kleck. 1996. A reassessment of the D.C. gun law: Some cautionary notes on the use of interrupted time series designs for policy impact assessment. *Law and Society Review* 30:361–80.

Brown, L. M. 2002. Suicidal risk factors with an elderly population: Standards of care practices. Ph.D. diss., Pacific Graduate School of Psychology.

Browne, A. 1987. *When Battered Women Kill.* New York: Free Press.

Browne, A. 2001. Violence in the lives of homeless and incarcerated women. Lecture at the Harvard School of Public Health, March.

Browne, A., and E. Lichter. 2001. Imprisonment in the United States. *Encyclopedia of Women and Gender,* 1:611–23. London: Academic Press.

Browne, R. C. 1999a. Racial difference in support for gun control. In Racial and Gender Differences in Attitude toward and experiences with violence and gun ownership, Ph.D. diss., Harvard School of Public Health, Department of Health Policy and Management.

Browne, R. C. 1999b. Racial differences in youth gun ownership and victimization. In Racial and Gender Differences in Attitude toward and experiences with violence and gun ownership, Ph.D. diss., Harvard School of Public Health, Department of Health Policy and Management.

Bruun, K., G. Edwards, and M. Lumio et al. 1975. *Alcohol Control Policies in Public Health Perspective.* Helsinki: Finnish Foundation for Alcohol Studies.

Bukstein, O. G., D. A. Brent, J. A. Perper, G. Moritz, M. Baugher, J. Schweers, C. Roth, and L. Balach. 1993. Risk factors for completed suicide among adolescents with a lifetime history of substance abuse: A case-control study. *Acta Psychiatrica Scandinavia* 88:403–8.

Bunn, F., T. Collier, C. Frost, K. Ker, I. Roberts, and R. Wentz. 2003. Traffic calming for the prevention of road traffic injuries: systematic review and meta-analysis. *Injury Prevention* 9:200–204.

Bureau of Alcohol, Tobacco, and Firearms (ATF). Department of the Treasury. 1990. *Commerce in Firearms in the United States.* Washington, DC.

Bureau of Alcohol, Tobacco, and Firearms. Department of the Treasury. 1997. *Youth Crime Gun Interdiction Initiative. Crime Gun Trace Analysis Reports: The Illegal Youth Firearms Market in Seventeen Communities.* Washington, DC.

Bureau of Alcohol, Tobacco, and Firearms. Department of the Treasury. 1999. *Youth Crime Gun Interdiction Initiative. Crime Gun Trace Analysis Reports: The Illegal Youth Firearms Market in Twenty-seven Communities.* Washington, DC.

BIBLIOGRAPHY

Bureau of Justice Statistics. 2000. *Sourcebook of Criminal Justice Statistics.* Washington, DC.

Burnette, S. 1998. Post traumatic stress disorder among firearm assault survivors: Risk and resiliency factors in recovering from violent victimization. Ph.D. diss., University of Pittsburgh. AAT 9837559.

Burney, L. E. 1959. Smoking and lung cancer: A statement of the Public Health Service. *Journal of the American Medical Association* 171:1829–37.

Business Day. 1999. Poor quality guns flood South African market. July 15.

Business Week. 1999. Under fire: Gun-control legislation, litigation, and angry public. Gun makers are feeling the heat. A close-up look at the secretive industry. August 16, pp. 62, 67–68.

Butterfield, F. 1998. New data point blame at gun makers. *New York Times,* November 28.

Butterfield, F. 1999a. Do limits on power and zeal hamper firearms agency? *New York Times,* July 22.

Butterfield, F. 1999b. Instant check on gun buyers has halted 100,000 of them. *New York Times,* September 9.

Butterfield, F. 1999c. Most crime guns are bought, not stolen. *New York Times,* April 30.

Butterfield, F. 1999d. Police chiefs shift strategy, mounting a war on weapons. *New York Times,* September 7.

Butterfield, F. 1999e. Study exposes illegal traffic in new guns. *New York Times,* February 21.

Butterfield, F. 2003. Gun industry ex-official describes bond of silence. *New York Times,* February 4.

Byck, D. L. 1998. The Second Amendment: Do newspapers tell us we have the right to bear arms? Ph.D. diss., Harvard School of Public Health.

Callahan, C. M., and F. P. Rivara. 1992. Urban high school youth and handguns: A school-based survey. *Journal of the American Medical Association* 267:3038–42.

Campbell, D. 2001. It's murder in classrooms U.S. teachers are warned; Leading union offers insurance after twenty-nine violent deaths in nine years. Special Report: Gun Violence in America. *Guardian* (UK), July 27.

Campbell, J. C. 1986. Nursing assessment for risk of homicide with battered women. *Advances in Nursing Science* 8:36–51.

Campbell, J. C., J. McFarlane, D. Webster, S. Wilt, C. R. Block, P. Sharps, D. Campbell, C. J. Sachs, and J. Koziol-McLain. 2001. The danger assessment instrument: Modification based on findings from the intimate partner femicide study. Paper presented at the American Society of Criminology conference, Atlanta, Nov. 7–10.

Campbell, J. C., D. Webster, J. Koziol-McLain, et al. 2003. Risk factors for femicide in abusive relationships: results from a multisite case control study. *American Journal of Public Health* 93:1089–97.

BIBLIOGRAPHY

Canadian Department of Justice. Research and Statistics Division. 1999. *Firearm Statistics.*

Canadian Firearms Centre. 1998. Firearms: Canadian/United States Comparison. Government of Canada. http://www.cfc-ccaf.gc.ca/en/research/other_docs/notes/canus/default.asp (accessed September 2003).

Canham, M. 2003. Expert killed in gun-lab accident. *Salt Lake Tribune.* January 3.

Cantor, D. 1989. Substantive implications of longitudinal design features: The National Crime Survey as a case study. In *Panel Surveys,* ed. D. Kasprzyk, G. Duncan, G. Kalton, and M. P. Singh, 25–51. New York: Wiley.

Carrington, P. J., and S. Moyer. 1994. Gun control and suicide in Ontario. *American Journal of Psychiatry* 151:606–8.

Caruso, R. P., D. I. Jara, and K. G. Swan. 1999. Gunshot wounds: Bullet caliber is increasing. *Journal of Trauma* 46:462–65.

Cassel, C. K., E. A. Nelson, T. W. Smith, C. W. Schwab, B. Barlow, and N. E. Gary. 1998. Internists' and surgeons' attitudes toward guns and firearm injury prevention. *Annals of Internal Medicine* 128:224–30.

CBS News (Channel 2000, Los Angeles). 2000. Child, man injured from falling bullets. January 1.

Centers for Disease Control and Prevention (CDC). 1992. Unintentional firearm-related fatalities among children and teenagers: United States 1982–88. *Morbidity and Mortality Weekly Report* (MMWR), June 26, 442–46.

Centers for Disease Control and Prevention. 1996. Mortality Patterns. *Morbidity and Mortality Weekly Report* (MMWR), March 1, 161–64.

Centers for Disease Control and Prevention. 1997a. *Fatal Firearm Injuries in the United States 1962–1994.* Violence Surveillance Summary Series, no. 3.

Centers for Disease Control and Prevention. 1997b. Rates of homicide, suicide, and firearm-related death among children: Twenty-six industrialized countries. *Morbidity and Mortality Weekly Report,* February 7, 101–5.

Centers for Disease Control and Prevention. 1999a. Motor-vehicle safety: A twentieth century public health achievement. *Morbidity and Mortality Weekly Report,* May 14, 369–74. Reprinted in *Journal of the American Medical Association* 281 (1999): 2080–82.

Centers for Disease Control and Prevention. 1999b. *National Vital Statistics Reports* 47 (June 30).

Centers for Disease Control and Prevention. 2000. *National Vital Statistics Report* 48 (July 24).

Centers for Disease Control and Prevention. 2001. National Center for Health Statistics data, 1996. http://wonder.cdc.gov/injury.shtml/ (accessed September 2003).

Centers for Disease Control and Prevention. 2003a. Source of firearms used by students in school-associated violent deaths: United States 1992–1999. *Morbidity and Mortality Weekly Report,* March 7, 169–72.

BIBLIOGRAPHY

Centers for Disease Control and Prevention. 2003b. Web-based Injury Statistics Query and Reporting System (WISQARS). http://www.cdc.gov/ncipc/wisqars/ (accessed February 2003).

Centers for Disease Control and Prevention. 2003c. WISQARS. Injury Mortality Report. http://webapp.cdc.gov/sasweb/ncipc/mortrate.html.

Centerwall, B. S. 1991. Homicide and the prevalence of handguns: Canada and the United States, 1976–1980. *American Journal of Epidemiology* 134:1245–65.

Centerwall, B. S. 1995. Race, socioeconomic status, and domestic homicide. *Journal of the American Medical Association* 273:1755–58.

Chafee, J. H. 1992. It's time to control handguns: The phantom "right to keep and bear arms" carries a high price tag. *Public Welfare* 50:18–21.

Chafetz, M. 1967. Alcoholism prevention and reality. *Quarterly Journal of Studies on Alcohol* 28:345–48.

Chapdelaine, A., E. Samson, and M. D. Kimberly. 1991. Firearm related injuries in Canada: Issues for prevention. *Canadian Medical Association Journal* 145:1217–23.

Chicago Tribune. 1999. State trooper accidentally kills another. March 7.

Christoffel, T., and S. S. Gallagher. 1999. *Injury Prevention and Public Health.* Gaithersburg, MD: Aspen.

Cina, S. J., C. D. Lariscy, S. T. McGown, M. A. Hopkins, J. D. Batts, and S. E. Conrad. 1996. Firearm-related hunting fatalities in North Carolina: Impact of the "hunter orange" law. *Southern Medical Journal* 89:395–96.

Coate, D., and M. Grossman. 1987. Changes in alcoholic beverage prices and legal drinking ages: Effects on youth alcohol use and motor vehicle mortality. *Alcohol Health and Research World* (fall): 22–25.

Coben, J. H., and C. A. Steiner. 2003. Hospitalization for firearm-related injuries in the United States 1997. *American Journal of Preventive Medicine* 24:1–8.

Commonwealth of Massachusetts. Office of the Attorney General. 1996. 940 CMR 16.00: Handgun Sale Regulations.

Conklin, J. E. 1972. *Robbery and the Criminal Justice System.* Philadelphia: Lippincott.

Connor, S. M., and K. L. Wesolowski. 2003. "They're too smart for that": Predicting what children would do in the presence of guns. *Pediatrics* (electronic pages) 111:e109–14.

Contra Costa County Health Services Department. 1995. *Taking Aim at Gun Dealers: Contra Costa's Public Health Approach to Reducing Firearms in the Community.* Pleasant Hill, CA: Prevention Program.

Conwell, Y., P. R. Duberstein, K. Connor, S. Eberly, C. Cox, and E. D. Caine. 2002. Access to firearms and risk for suicide in middle-aged and older adults. *American Journal of Geriatric Psychiatry* 10:407–16.

Cook, P. J. 1979. The effect of gun availability on robbery and robbery murder. In *Policy*

BIBLIOGRAPHY

Studies Review Annual, ed. R. Haveman and B. Zellner, 743–81. Beverly Hills, CA: Sage.

Cook, P. J. 1985. The case of the missing victims: Gunshot woundings in the National Crime Survey. *Journal of Quantitative Criminology* 1:91–102.

Cook, P. J. 1986. The relationship between victim resistance and injury in noncommercial robbery. *Journal of Legal Studies* 15:405–16.

Cook, P. J. 1987. Robbery violence. *Journal of Criminal Law and Criminology* 78:357–76.

Cook, P. J. 1991. The technology of personal violence. In *Crime and Justice: An Annual Review of Research,* ed. M. Tonry, 14:1–72. Chicago: University of Chicago Press.

Cook, P. J. 1996. Letter to the editor. *Society* 33 (6): 6–7.

Cook, P. J., and A. A. Braga. 2001. Comprehensive firearms tracing: Strategic and investigative uses of new data on firearms markets. *Arizona Law Review* 43:277–309.

Cook, P. J., and T. B. Cole. 1996. Strategic thinking about gun markets and violence. *Journal of the American Medical Association* 275:1765–67.

Cook, P. J., B. A. Lawrence, J. Ludwig, and T. R. Miller. 1999. The medical costs of gunshot injuries in the United States. *Journal of the American Medical Association* 282:447–54.

Cook, P. J., and J. A. Leitzel. 1996. Perversity, futility, jeopardy: An economic analysis of the attack on gun control. *Law and Contemporary Problems* 59:91–118.

Cook, P. J., and J. Ludwig. 1996. *Guns in America: Results of a Comprehensive National Survey on Firearms Ownership and Use.* Washington, DC: Police Foundation.

Cook, P. J., and J. Ludwig. 1998. Defensive gun uses: New evidence from a national survey. *Journal of Quantitative Criminology* 14:111–31.

Cook, P. J., and J. Ludwig. 2000. *Gun Violence: The Real Costs.* New York: Oxford University Press.

Cook, P. J., and J. Ludwig. 2003. Guns and burglary. In *Evaluating Gun Policy,* ed. J. Ludwig and P. J. Cook, 74–107. Washington, DC: Brookings Institution.

Cook, P. J., J. Ludwig, and D. Hemenway. 1997. The gun debate's new mythical number: How many defensive uses per year? *Journal of Policy Analysis and Management* 16:463–69.

Cook, P. J., S. Molliconi, and T. B. Cole. 1995. Regulating gun markets. *Journal of Criminal Law and Criminology* 86:59–92.

Cook, P. J., and M. Moore. 1999. Guns, gun control, and homicide: A review of research and public policy. In *Homicide: A Sourcebook of Social Research,* ed. M. D. Smith and M. A. Zahn, 277–96. Thousand Oaks, CA: Sage.

Cork, D. 1999. Examining space-time interaction in city-level homicide data: Crack markets and the diffusion of guns among youth. *Journal of Quantitative Criminology* 15:379–406.

Cotton, P. 1992. Gun-associated violence increasingly viewed as a public health challenge. *Journal of the American Medical Association* 267:1171–74.

Council of Economic Advisors for the President's Initiative on Race. 1998. *Changing*

BIBLIOGRAPHY

America: Indicators of Social and Economic Well-being by Race and Hispanic Origin. Washington, DC: Council of Economic Advisors for the President's Initiative on Race.

Courtwright, D. T. 1996. *Violent Land.* Cambridge, MA: Harvard University Press.

Craig, T. 2000. Mistake blamed in shooting of brother: Police say man, sixty-nine, apparently thought intruder was entering; Victim critically injured. *Baltimore Sun,* November 17.

Cramer, C. E. 1995. The racist roots of gun control. *Kansas Journal of Law and Public Policy* (winter): 17–25.

Crandall, R., H. Gruenspecht, T. Keeler, and L. Lave. 1986. *Regulating the Automobile.* Washington, DC: Brookings Institution.

Cukier, W. 1998. Firearm regulation: Canada in the international context. *Chronic Diseases in Canada* 19:25–34.

Cukier, W., and S. Shropshire. 2000. Domestic gun markets: The licit-illicit links. In *Running Guns: The Global Black Market in Small Arms,* ed. L. Lumpe, 105–26. London: Zed Books.

Cummings, P., D. C. Grossman, F. P. Rivara, and T. D. Koepsell. 1997. State gun safe storage laws and child mortality due to firearms. *Journal of the American Medical Association* 278:1084–86.

Cummings, P., T. D. Koepsell, D. C. Grossman, J. Savarino, and R. S. Thompson. 1997. The association between the purchase of a handgun and homicide or suicide. *American Journal of Public Health* 87:974–78.

Cummings, P., T. D. Koepsell, and I. Roberts. 2001. Case-control studies in injury research. In *Injury Control: A Guide to Research and Program Evaluation,* ed. F. P. Rivara, P. Cummings, T. D. Koepsell, D. C. Grossman, and R. V. Maier, 139–56. New York: Cambridge University Press.

Dade County Grand Jury. 1997. *Guns and Children: A Call for Great Adult Responsibility.* Final Report of the Dade County Grand Jury, filed May 28. Circuit Court of the Eleventh Judicial Circuit of Florida in and for the County of Dade. Circuit Judge Presiding: Judith L. Kreeger.

Dahl, D. 2003. Decline in hunting changing national gun debate. Co/Motion Gun violence News Research Center. www.jointogether.org. January 3. (Accessed September 2003.)

Daley, R. M. 1998a. Good riddance to public enemy No. 1. *Chicago Tribune,* December 13.

Daley, R. M. 1998b. Gun industry floods Chicago with illegal weapons city and county charge in landmark $433 million lawsuit. Mayor's press release. November 12.

Darity, W. A. Jr., and P. L. Mason. 1998. Evidence on discrimination in employment: Codes of color, codes of gender. *Journal of Economic Perspectives* 12:63–90.

Davidoff, F. 1998. Reframing gun violence. *Annals of Internal Medicine* 128:234–35.

Davidson, L. L., M. S. Durkin, L. Kuhn, P. O'Connor, B. Barlow, and M. C. Heagarty.

BIBLIOGRAPHY

1994. The impact of the Safe Kids/Healthy Neighbors Injury Prevention Program in Harlem, 1988 through 1991. *American Journal of Public Health* 84:580–86.

Davis, J. A., and T. W. Smith. 1994. General Social Surveys 1972–1994. Chicago, IL: National Opinion Research Center. Machine-readable data file.

DeConde, A. 2001. *Gun Violence in America: The Struggle for Control.* Boston: Northeastern University Press.

DeHaven, H. 1942. Mechanical analysis of survival in falls from heights of fifty to one hundred and fifty feet. *War Medicine* 2:586–96.

DeVivo, M. J. 1997. Causes and costs of spinal cord injury in the United States. *Spinal Cord* 35:809–13.

Dezhbakhsh, H., and P. H. Rubin. 1998. Lives saved or lives lost? The effects of concealed-handgun laws on crime. *American Economic Review* 88:468–74.

DeZee, M. R. 1983. Gun control legislation: Impact and ideology. *Law and Policy Quarterly* 5:367–79.

Diaz, T. 1999. *Making a Killing: The Business of Guns in America.* New York: New Press.

Diaz, T. 2001a. *Unintended Consequences: Pro-handgun Experts Prove That Handguns Are a Dangerous Choice for Self-Defense.* Washington, DC: Violence Policy Center.

Diaz, T. 2001b. *Voting from the Rooftops: How the Gun Industry Armed Osama bin Laden, Other Foreign and Domestic Terrorists, and Common Criminals with .50 Caliber Sniper Rifles.* Washington, DC: Violence Policy Center.

Dillon, J. 2001. "Angry young man" shot two in the back, others indiscriminately. *San Diego Tribune,* March 6.

Dionne, E. J. Jr. 1999. America: A nation of killers. *San Francisco Chronicle,* September 20.

Dodge, G. G., T. H. Cogbill, G. J. Miller, J. Landercasper, and P. J. Strutt. 1994. Gunshot wounds: Ten-year experience of a rural referral trauma center. *American Surgeon* 60:401–4.

Dolins, J. C., and K. K. Christoffel. 1994. Reducing violent injuries: Priorities for pediatrician advocacy. *Pediatrics* 94:638–51.

Donenfeld, T. 1999. Analysis of the Crime Gun Trace Analysis Reports: The illegal youth firearms market in twenty-seven communities. Student paper, Harvard Injury Control Research Center.

Donohue, J. 2003. The impact of concealed-carry laws. In *Evaluating Gun Policy,* ed. J. Ludwig and P. J. Cook, 287–325. Washington, DC: Brookings Institution.

Dorf, M. C. 2000. What does the Second Amendment mean today? *Chicago-Kent Law Review* 76:291–348.

Dowd, M. D., L. R. Schwartz, L. Thomas, and Z. Surprenant. 1999. Preventing firearm injury in children: A grassroots speaker's bureau. Paper presented at the American Public Health Association meeting, November 8–10, Chicago.

Dreeben, O. 2001. Health status of African Americans. *Journal of Health and Social Policy* 14:1–17.

BIBLIOGRAPHY

Duggan, M. 2001. More guns, more crime. *Journal of Political Economy* 109:1086–1114.

Duncan, O. D. 2000. Gun use surveys: In numbers we trust? *Criminologist* 25 (1): 1–7.

Duncan, O. D., and J. R. Lott Jr. 2003. On defensive gun use statistics. http://www.cse .unsw.edu.au/~lambert/guns/duncan3.html/ (accessed April 2003).

DuRant, R. H., D. P. Krowchuk, S. Kreiter, S. H. Sinal, and C. R. Woods. 1999. Weapon carrying on school property among middle school students. *Archives of Pediatric Adolescent Medicine* 153:21–26.

Durkin, M. S., L. Kuhn, L. L. Davidson, D. Laraque, and B. Barlow. 1996. Epidemiology and prevention of severe assault and gun injuries to children in an urban community. *Journal of Trauma* 41:667–73.

Durkin, M. S., S. Olsen, B. Barlow, A. Virella, and E. S. Connoly Jr. 1998. The epidemiology of urban pediatric neurological trauma: Evaluation of and implications for injury prevention programs. *Neurosurgery* 42:300–310.

Duwe, G., T. Kovandzic, and C. E. Moody. 2002. The impact of right-to-carry concealed firearm laws on mass public shootings. *Homicide Studies* 6:271–96.

Dwyer, W. F. 1996. Quoted in R. Kluger, *Ashes to Ashes: America's Hundred-Year Cigarette War, the Public Health, and the Unabashed Triumph of Philip Morris* (New York: Knopf, 1996), 468.

Eastman, J. W. 1981. "Doctor's orders": The American medical profession and the origins of automobile design for crash protection, 1930–1955. *Bulletin of the History of Medicine* 55:407–24.

Economist. 1994. Guns in America. March 26.

Economist. 1998. When lawsuits make policy. November 21.

Edsall, T. B. 1999. Missouri voters defeat ballot measure to allow concealed handguns. *Washington Post*, April 7.

Edwards, G. 1997. Alcohol policy and the public good. *Addiction* 92 (supplement 1): S73–79.

Edwards, G., P. Anderson, and T. F. Babor et al. 1994. *Alcohol Policy and the Public Good.* Oxford: Oxford University Press.

Egan, T. 1998. School shootings haunt U.S. psyche. *International Herald Tribune*, June 15, p. 2.

Emory, U. 1904. *The Military Policy of the United States.* Washington, DC: U.S. Government Printing Office.

Environmental Working Group and Violence Policy Center. 2001. *Poisonous Pastime: The Health Risks of Shooting Ranges and Lead to Children, Families, and the Environment.* Washington, DC.

Esler, G. 1998. Logic which makes guns safe but shopping trolleys lethal. *Scotsman* (Edinburgh), November 30.

Evans, L. 1991. *Traffic Safety and the Driver.* New York: Van Nostrand Reinhold.

Evans, R. G., M. L. Barer, and T. R. Marmor, eds. 1994. *Why Are Some People Healthy*

BIBLIOGRAPHY

and Others Not? The Determinants of Health of Populations. New York: Aldine de Gruyter.

Fagan, J., J. G. Weis, and Y. T. Cheng. 1990. Delinquency and substance abuse among inner city students. *Journal of Drug Issues* 20:351–402.

Farah, M. M., H. K. Simon, and A. L. Kellermann. 1999. Firearms in the home: Parental perceptions. *Pediatrics* 104:1059–63.

Fedorowycz, O. 2001. Homicide in Canada 2000. Canadian Centre for Justice Statistics, Statistics Canada—Catalogue no. 85–002-XIE, vol. 21, no. 9.

Fee, E. 1987. *Disease and Discovery: A History of the Johns Hopkins School of Hygiene and Public Health.* Baltimore: Johns Hopkins University Press.

Finkelman, P. 2000. "A well regulated militia": The Second Amendment in historical perspective. *Chicago-Kent Law Review* 76:195–236.

Fisher, J. C. 1976. Homicide in Detroit: The role of firearms. *Criminology* 14:387–400.

Fitzsimon, C. 1998. Editorial, Gun restrictions are long overdue. *Raleigh-Durham Triangle Business Journal,* December 7.

Foege, W. 1996a. Closing remarks from the Haddon Memorial plenary session. *Injury Prevention* 2:175–77.

Foege, W. H. 1996b. Foreword. In *The Global Burden of Disease,* ed. C. J. L. Murray and A.D. Lopez, xxv–xxvi. Cambridge, MA: Harvard University Press.

Fortgang, E. 1999. How they got the guns. *Rolling Stone,* June 10, 51–53.

Foster, B. J. (Michigan Coalition for Responsible Gun Owners). 2000. Editorial, Effective education and enforcement remain best in stopping gun abuse. *Detroit News,* March 5.

Fox, B. 2001. DA: School shooter used dad's gun. AP: Santee, CA. *York News-Times,* March.

Fox News/Reuters. 2000. Most U.S. states lack basic gun control laws, says survey. April 14. See www.texansforgunsafety.org/articles/archives/press.htm #04/14/00.

Frattaroli, S., D. W. Webster, and S. P. Teret. 2002. Unintentional gun injuries, firearm design, and prevention: What we know, what we need to know, and what can be done. *Journal of Urban Health* 79:49–59.

Freed, L. H., J. S. Vernick, and S. W. Hargarten. 1998. Prevention of firearm-related injuries and deaths among youth: A product oriented approach. *Pediatric Clinics of North America* 45:427–38.

Freed, L. H., D. W. Webster, J. Longwell, J. Carrese, and M. H. Wilson. 2001. Factors preventing gun acquisition and carrying among incarcerated adolescent males. *Archives of Pediatric Adolescent Medicine* 155:335–41.

Freeman, T. W., V. Roca, and T. Kimbrell. 2003. A survey of gun collection and use among three groups of veteran patients admitted to veterans affairs hospital treatment programs. *Southern Medical Journal* 96:240–43.

Frey, J. 1999. Recoil: Tom Diaz loved guns, but a lot of little reasons changed his mind. *Washington Post,* May 4.

BIBLIOGRAPHY

Frolik, J. 1999. A gunshot in the dark shatters a family. *Cleveland Live,* December 26.

Funk, T. M. 1995. Gun control and economic discrimination: The melting-point case-in-point. *Journal of Criminal Law and Criminology* 85: 764–806.

Gabor, T. 1994. *The Impact of the Availability of Firearms on Violent Crime, Suicide, and Accidental Death with Special Reference to the Canadian Situation.* Ottawa: Department of Justice.

Gabor, T., M. Baril, M. Cusson, D. Elie, M. LeBlanc, and A. Normandeau. 1987. *Armed Robbery: Cops, Robbers, and Victims.* Springfield, IL: Charles C. Thomas.

Gallagher, S. S., E. Pittel, M. Vriniotis, and D. Azrael. 2002. Psychiatrists' knowledge, attitudes, and practices concerning firearm-related suicide risk assessment. Paper presented at the Sixth World Injury Prevention Conference, Quebec, May 11–13.

Galloway, J. 2002. Antique pistol goes off as it's handed to Barr. *Atlanta Journal Constitution,* August 7.

Gallup Poll. 2000. The gun issue: Women and the "million mom march." National survey of 1,031 adults, May 5–7.

Garavaglia, L. A., and C. G. Worman. 1984. *Firearms of the American West: 1803–1865.* Albuquerque: University of New Mexico Press.

Gazmararian, J. A., S. Lazorick, A. M. Spitz, T. J. Ballard, L. E. Saltzman, and J. S. Marks. 1996. Prevalence of violence against pregnant women. *Journal of the American Medical Association* 275:1915–20.

Geisel, M. S., R. Roll, and R. S. Wettick. 1969. The effectiveness of state and local regulations of handguns. *Duke University Law Journal* 4:647–76.

Gilbert, D. 2000. Hamilton College Youth and Guns Poll. Department of Sociology, Hamilton College, Clinton, NY.

Gill, A. S. C. 1999. Factors predictive of pediatric post traumatic stress disorder one year post traumatic injury. M.S. Texas Women's University. AAT 13949908.

Gilmore, R. S. 1992. Another branch of manly sport: American rifle games 1840–1900. In *Hard at Play: Leisure in America, 1840–1940,* ed. K. Grover, 93–111. Amherst: University of Massachusetts Press.

Gist, R., and Q. B. Welch. 1989. Certification change versus actual behavior change in teenage suicide rates, 1955–1979. *Suicide and Life Threatening Behavior* 19:277–88.

Glock Corporation. 2002. Basic firearm safety rules. Available at http://www.glock.com/safety_rules.htm (accessed September 2003).

Goldberg, B. W., E. R. von Borstel, L. K. Dennis, and E. Wall. 1995. Firearm injury risk among primary care patients. *Journal of Family Practice* 41:158–62.

Goldberg, R. 2000. First grader fatally shoots classmate. *Chicago Sun Times,* February 29.

Goldsmith, S. K., T. C. Pellmar, A. M. Kleinman, and W. E. Bunney. 2002. *Reducing Suicide: A National Imperative.* Institute of Medicine Report. Washington, DC: National Academy Press.

Goldstein, R. B., D. W. Black, A. Nasrallah, and G. Winokur. 1991. The prediction of suicide: Sensitivity, specificity, and predictive value of a multivariate model applied to suicide among 1906 patients with affective disorders. *Archives of General Psychiatry* 48:418–22.

Goodman, R. A., J. A. Mercy, F. Loya, M. L. Rosenberg, J. C. Smith, N. H. Allen, L. Vargas, and R. Kolts. 1986. Alcohol use and interpersonal violence: Alcohol detected in homicide victims. *American Journal of Public Health* 76:144–49.

Gould, S. J. 1997. *Questioning the Millennium: A Rationalist's Guide to a Precisely Arbitrary Countdown.* New York: Harmony Books.

Graham, J. D. 1993. Injuries from traffic crashes: Meeting the challenge. *Annual Review of Public Health* 14:515–43.

Green, G. S. 1987. Citizen gun ownership and crime deterrence: Theory, research, and policy. *Criminology* 25:63–81.

Greenspan, A. I., and A. L. Kellermann. 2002. Physical and psychological outcomes eight months after serious gunshot injury. *Journal of Trauma* 53:709–16.

Grossfeld, S. 1999. Not gun shy. *Boston Globe,* June 27, p. F3.

Grossman, D. C., K. Mang, and F. P. Rivara. 1995. Firearm injury prevention counseling by pediatricians and family physicians. *Archives of Pediatric Adolescent Medicine* 149:973–77.

Grossman, D. C., D. T. Reay, and S. A. Baker. 1999. Self-inflicted and unintentional firearm injuries among children and adolescents: The source of the firearm. *Archives of Pediatric Adolescent Medicine* 153:875–78.

Gruber, I. D. 2002. Of arms and men: Arming America and military history. *William and Mary Quarterly* 59:217–22.

Gunnell, D., and S. Frankel. 1994. Prevention of suicide: Aspirations and evidence. *British Medical Journal* 308:1227–33.

Haddon, W. Jr. 1972. A logical framework for categorizing highway safety phenomena and activity. *Journal of Trauma* 12:197–207.

Haddon, W. Jr. 1970. On the escape of tigers: An ecologic note. *Technology Review* 72:44–48.

Haines, H. H. 1997. Nominal medicalization and scientific legitimacy in the public health approach to violence. Paper presented to the Society for the Study of Social Problems, Toronto, August.

Halpern, T., and B. Levin. 1996. *The Limits of Dissent: The Constitutional Status of Armed Civilian Militias.* Amherst, MA: Aletheia Press.

Handgun Control. 1999. Ten national law enforcement groups call on Congress to close the "gun show loophole." Media release. October 21.

Hannibal Courier-Post. 1999. Missouri pro sports teams opposing right to carry arms. March 26.

Hardy, M. S. 1999. Very young guns. Op-Ed. *New York Times.* May 14.

Hardy, M. S. 2002. Teaching firearm safety to children: Failure of a program. *Journal of Deviant Behavior Pediatrics* 23:71–76.

BIBLIOGRAPHY

Hardy, M. S., F. D. Armstrong, B. L. Martin, and K. N. Strawn. 1996. A firearm safety program for children: They just can't say no. *Journal of Deviant Behavior Pediatrics* 17:216–21.

Harrie, D. 1999. LDS leaders toughen stand against guns. *Salt Lake City Tribune,* May 16.

Harvard Injury Control Research Center (HICRC). 2001. *Analysis of 1999 National Survey.* Harvard Injury Control Research Center.

Hastings, J. E., and L. K. Hamberger. 1988. Personality characteristics of spouse abusers: A controlled comparison. *Violence and Victims* 3:31–48.

Haught, K., D. Grossman, and F. Connell. 1995. Parents' attitudes toward firearm injury prevention counseling in urban pediatric clinics. *Pediatrics* 96:649–53.

Hayes, D. N., and D. Hemenway. 1999. Age-within-school-class and adolescent gun carrying. *Pediatrics* (electronic pages) 103:e64.

Hayeslip, D. W., and A. Preszler. 1993. *National Institute of Justice Initiative on Less-than-Lethal Weapons.* Research in Brief. NCJ 133523. Washington, DC: U.S. Department of Justice, National Institute of Justice.

Heckman, J. J., and V. J. Hotz. 1989. Choosing among alternative non-experimental methods for estimating the impact of social programs: The case of manpower training. *Journal of the American Statistical Association* 84:862–80.

Heins, M., R. Kahn, and J. Bjordnal. 1974. Gunshot wounds in children. *American Journal of Public Health* 64:326–30.

Hellsten, J. J. 1995. Motivation and opportunity: An ecological investigation of U.S. urban suicide, 1970–1990. Ph.D. diss., University of California, Irvine.

Hemenway, D. 1975. *Industrywide Voluntary Product Standards.* Cambridge, MA: Ballinger.

Hemenway, D. 1989. Government procurement leverage. *Journal of Public Health Policy* 10:123–25.

Hemenway, D. 1995. Guns, public health, and public safety. In *Guns and the Constitution: The Myth of Second Amendment Protection for Firearms in America,* ed. D. A. Henigan, E. B. Nicholson, and D. Hemenway, 49–76. Northampton, MA: Aletheia Press.

Hemenway, D. 1997a. The myth of millions of annual self-defense gun uses: A case study of survey overestimates of rare events. *Chance* (American Statistical Association) 10:6–10.

Hemenway, D. 1997b. Survey research and self-defense gun use: An explanation of extreme overestimates. *Journal of Criminal Law and Criminology* 87:1430–45.

Hemenway, D. 1998a. Regulation of firearms. *New England Journal of Medicine* 339:843–45.

Hemenway, D. 1998b. Review of *More Guns, Less Crime: Understanding Crime and Gun Control Laws,* by J. R. Lott Jr. *New England Journal of Medicine* 339:2029–30.

Hemenway, D. 2001. The public health approach to motor vehicles, tobacco, and alcohol, with applications to firearms policy. *Journal of Public Health Policy* 22:381–402.

BIBLIOGRAPHY

Hemenway, D. 2003a. Review of *The Bias against Guns*, by J. R. Lott Jr. Available at: www.hsph.harvard.edu/faculty/Hemenway/book.html (accessed September 2003).

Hemenway, D. 2003b. Review of *Guns and Violence: The English Experience*, by J. L. Malcolm. *Psychology Today* (January/February): 78.

Hemenway, D., and D. Azrael. 1997. Gun use in the United States: Results of a national survey. Report to the National Institute of Justice.

Hemenway, D., and D. Azrael. 2000. The relative frequency of offensive and defensive gun use: Results from a national survey. *Violence and Victims* 15:257–72.

Hemenway, D., D. Azrael, and M. Miller. 2001. U.S. national attitudes concerning gun carrying. *Injury Prevention* 7:282–85.

Hemenway, D., and J. Birckmayer. 1999. The effects of the minimum legal drinking age on youth suicide, drowning, homicide, and aggravated assault. Report to the National Institute for Alcohol Abuse and Alcoholism.

Hemenway, D., B. P. Kennedy, I. Kawachi, and R. D. Putnam. 2001. Firearm prevalence and social capital. *Annals of Epidemiology* 11:484–90.

Hemenway, D., and M. Miller. 2000. Firearm availability and homicide rates across twenty-six high-income countries. *Journal of Trauma* 49:985–88.

Hemenway, D., and M. Miller. 2002. The association of rates of household handgun ownership, lifetime major depression, and serious suicidal thoughts with rates of suicide across U.S. census regions. *Injury Prevention* 8:313–16.

Hemenway, D., and M. Miller. 2003. *Gun Threats against and Self-Defense Gun Use by California Adolescents*. Harvard Injury Control Research Center.

Hemenway, D., M. Miller, and D. Azrael. 2000. Gun use in the United States: Results from two national surveys. *Injury Prevention* 6:263–67.

Hemenway, D., D. Prothrow-Stith, J. M. Bergstein, R. Ander, and B. P. Kennedy. 1996. Gun carrying among adolescents. *Law and Contemporary Problems* 59:39–53.

Hemenway, D., and E. Richardson. 1997. Characteristics of automatic or semiautomatic firearm ownership. *American Journal of Public Health* 87:286–88.

Hemenway, D., T. Shinoda-Tagawa, and M. Miller. 2002. Firearm availability and female homicide victimization across twenty-five populous high-income countries. *Journal of the American Medical Women's Association* 57:1–5.

Hemenway, D., S. J. Solnick, and D. Azrael. 1995a. Firearms and community feelings of safety. *Journal of Criminal Law and Criminology* 86:121–32.

Hemenway, D., S. J. Solnick, and D. Azrael. 1995b. Firearm training and storage. *Journal of the American Medical Association* 273:46–50.

Hemenway, D., and D. Weil. 1990a. Less lethal weapons. *Washington Post,* May 14.

Hemenway, D., and D. Weil 1990b. Phasers on stun: The case for less lethal weapons. *Journal of Policy Analysis and Management* 9:94–98.

Henigan, D. A. 1991. Arms, anarchy, and the Second Amendment. *Valparaiso University Law Review* 26:107–29.

Henigan. D. A., E. B. Nicholson, and D. Hemenway. 1995. *Guns and the Constitution:*

BIBLIOGRAPHY

The Myth of Second Amendment Protection for Firearms in America. Northampton, MA: Aletheia Press.

Hennekens, C. H., and J. E. Buring. 1987. *Epidemiology in Medicine.* Boston: Little, Brown.

Hepburn, L., and D. Hemenway. 2003. Firearm availability and homicide: A review of the literature. *Aggression and Violent Behavior: A Review Journal.* In press.

Hepburn, L., M. Miller, D. Azrael, and D. Hemenway. 2003. Much ado about nothing? The effect of non-discretionary concealed weapon carrying laws on homicide. *Journal of Trauma.* In press.

Heyman, S. J. 2000. Natural rights and the Second Amendment. *Chicago-Kent Law Review* 76:237–90.

Higginbotham, D. 1998. *War and Society in Revolutionary America: The Wider Dimensions of Conflict.* Columbia: University of South Carolina Press.

Hill, J. M. 1997. The impact of liberalized concealed weapon statutes on rates of violent crime. Undergraduate thesis, Duke University.

Hingson, R., J. Howland, T. D. Koepsell, and P. Cummings. 2001. Ecologic studies. In *Injury Control: A Guide to Research and Evaluation,* ed. F. P. Rivara, P. Cummings, T. D. Koepsell, D. C. Grossman, and R. V. Maier, 157–67. New York: Cambridge University Press.

Holder, H. D. 1997. Alcohol use and a safe environment. *Addiction* 92 (supplement 1): S117–20.

Holien, M. 2002. Undersheriff shot leg when finger caught trigger. *Daily Missoulian,* August 6.

Hollywood Reporter. 1999. Hollywood, violence experts try to disarm gun crisis. November 5–7.

Hood, M. V. III, and G. W. Neeley. 2001. Packin' in the hood: Examining assumptions of concealed-handgun carry research. *Social Science Quarterly* 81:523–37.

Horn, A., D. C. Grossman, W. Jones, and L. R. Berger. 2003. Community based program to improve firearm storage practices in rural Alaska. *Injury Prevention* 9:231–34.

Hoskin, A. W. 1999. The impact of firearm availability on national homicide rates: A cross sectional and panel analysis. Ph.D. diss., State University of New York at Albany.

Hosley, W. 1996. *Colt: The Making of an American Legend.* Amherst: University of Massachusetts Press.

Human Rights Watch. 1999. Written statement. United Nations World Conference on Racism, Racial Discrimination, Xenophobia, and All Forms of Discrimination. December 30.

Humphreys, A. 2001. Customs issues alert over Bond-like cellphone gun. *National Post* (Canada), September 1.

Hurt, R. D., and C. R. Robertson. 1998. Prying open the door to tobacco industry's

BIBLIOGRAPHY

secrets about nicotine: The Minnesota tobacco trail. *Journal of the American Medical Association* 280:1173–81.

Huston, T. L., G. Geis, and R. Wright. 1976. The angry samaritans. *Psychology Today,* June, 61–64, 85.

Ide, R. W. III. 1994. Remarks to the National Press Club. April 15.

Ikeda, R. M., R. Gorwitz, S. P. James, K. E. Powell, and J. A. Mercy. 1997. *Fatal Firearm Injuries in the United States 1962–1994.* Atlanta: National Center for Injury Prevention and Control.

Ikeda, R. M., J. A. Mercy, and S. P. Teret, eds. 1998. Firearm-related injury surveillance. Special issue, *American Journal of Preventive Medicine* 15 (supplement 3): 1–126.

Injury Prevention. 1999. News and Notes: New U.S. standard for soccer goals. 5:170.

Injury Prevention Research Unit. 2003. National Injury Query System. University of Otago (N.Z.) http://www.otago.ac.nz/IPRU/statistics/NIQS.html (accessed May 2003).

Institute of Medicine. 1985. *Injury in America: A Continuing Public Health Problem.* Washington, DC: National Academy Press.

Institute of Medicine. 1988. *The Future of Public Health.* Washington, DC: National Academy Press.

Institute of Medicine. 1999. *Reducing the Burden of Injury.* Washington, DC: National Academy Press.

International Hunter Education Association. 1988. Ten commandments of firearm safety. http://www.dfg.ca.gov/ihea/ihea98a.html.

International Hunter Education Association. 2003. Casualty report. http://www.dfg.ca .gov/ihea/ihea98a.html/ (accessed September 2003).

Ismach, R. B., A. Reza, R. Ary, T. R. Sampson, K. Bartolomeos, and A. L. Kellermann. 2003. Unintended shootings in a large metropolitan area: An incident-based analysis. *Annals of Emergency Medicine* 41:10–17.

Jackman, G. A., M. M. Farah, A. L. Kellermann, and H. K. Simon. 2001. Seeing is believing: What do boys do when they find a real gun? *Pediatrics* 107:1247–50.

Jacobs, J. B. 2002. *Can Gun Control Work?* New York: Oxford University Press.

Jamison, K. R. 1999. *Night Falls Fast: Understanding Suicide.* New York: Knopf.

Japan National Police Agency. 1996. Firearms control in Japan. Tokyo.

Joe, S., and M. S. Kaplan. 2002. Firearm-related suicide among young African-American males. *Psychiatric Services* 53:332–34.

Johnson, G. R., E. G. Krug, and L. B. Potter. 2000. Suicide among adolescents and young adults: A cross-national comparison of thirty-four countries. *Suicide and Life Threatening Behavior* 30:74–82.

Johnson, J. M., and B. P. Weiss. 1999. Estimates of gun possessing adults in Los Angeles County. Paper presented at the American Public Health Association meetings, November 8–10, Chicago.

Join Together Online. 1998. International perspectives on US gun laws in Jonesboro's wake. Summary of statement by Wendy Cukier and Rebecca Peters. April 9. http://www.jointogether.org/.

Join Together Online. 1999. Report on campus gun ownership raises concern. July 15. http://www.jointogether.org/.

Join Together Online. 2002. Gun control groups campaign against classified ads. October 24. http://www.jointogether.org/.

Jones, E. D. III. 1981. The District of Columbia's Firearm Control Regulations Act of 1975: The toughest handgun control law in the United States—or is it? *Annals of the American Academy of Political and Social Science* 455:138–49.

Jordan, M. 1997. Guns and the Japanese: A people's fear and fascination. *International Herald Tribune*, March 18.

Kachur, S. P., G. M. Stennies, K. E. Powell, W. Modzeleski, R. Stephens, R. Murphy, M. Kresnow, D. Sleet, and R. Lowry. 1996. School-associated violent deaths in the United States, 1992 to 1994. *Journal of the American Medical Association* 275:1729–33.

Kalbfleisch, J., and F. Rivara. 1989. Principles in injury control: Lessons to be learned from child safety seats. *Pediatric Emergency Care* 5:131–34.

Kansas City Star. 2003. Missouri senate overrides concealed weapons bill veto. September 11.

Karlson, T. A., and S. W. Hargarten. 1997. *Reducing Firearm Injury and Death: A Public Health Sourcebook on Guns.* New Brunswick, NJ: Rutgers University Press.

Kassirer, J. P. 1991. Firearms and the killing threshold. *New England Journal of Medicine* 325:1647–50.

Kassirer, J. P. 1993. Guns in the household. *New England Journal of Medicine* 329:1117–19.

Kates, D. B. Jr. 1983. Handgun prohibition and the original meaning of the Second Amendment. *Michigan Law Review* 82:204–73.

Kates, D. B. Jr. 1990. Guns, murder, and the Constitution: A realistic assessment of gun control. Policy Briefing. San Francisco: Pacific Research Institute for Public Policy.

Kates, D. B. Jr., H. E. Schaffer, J. K. Lattimer, G. B. Murray, and E. H. Cassem. 1995. Bad medicine: Doctors and guns. In *Guns: Who Should Have Them?* ed. D. Kopel, 233–308. Amherst, NY: Prometheus Books.

Katzenbach, N., R. Clark, E. L. Richardson, E. H. Levi, G. B. Bell, and B. R. Civiletti. 1992. Editorial, It's time to pass the Brady Bill. *Washington Post,* October 3, p. A21.

Keck, N. J., G. R. Istre, D. L. Coury, F. Jordan, and A. P. Eaton. 1988. Characteristics of fatal gunshot wounds in the home in Oklahoma: 1982–83. *American Journal of Diseases of Children* 142:623–26.

Kellermann, A. L. 1997. Comment: Gunsmoke—changing public attitudes toward smoking and firearms. *American Journal of Public Health* 87:910–13.

Kellermann, A. L., and S. Heron. 1999. Firearms and family violence. *Emergency Medicine Clinics of North America* 17:699–716.

Kellermann, A. L., R. K. Lee, J. A. Mercy, and J. Banton. 1991. The epidemiologic basis for the prevention of firearm injuries. *Annual Review of Public Health* 12:17–40.

BIBLIOGRAPHY

Kellermann, A. L., and J. A. Mercy. 1992. Men, women, and murder: Gender-specific differences in rates of fatal violence and victimization. *Journal of Trauma* 33:1–5.

Kellermann, A. L., and D. T. Reay. 1986. Protection or peril? An analysis of firearm-related deaths in the home. *New England Journal of Medicine* 314:1557–60.

Kellermann, A. L., F. P. Rivara, N. B. Rushforth, J. G. Banton, D. T. Reay, J. T. Francisco, A. B. Locci, J. Prodzinski, B. B. Hackman, and G. Somes. 1993. Gun ownership as a risk factor for homicide in the home. *New England Journal of Medicine* 329:1084–91.

Kellermann, A. L., F. P. Rivara, G. Somes, D. T. Reay, J. T. Francisco, J. G. Banton, J. Prodzinski, C. Fligner, and B. B. Hackman. 1992. Suicide in the home in relation to gun ownership. *New England Journal of Medicine* 327:467–72.

Kellermann A. L., G. Somes, F. P. Rivara, R. K. Lee, and J. G. Banton. 1998. Injuries and deaths due to firearms in the home. *Journal of Trauma* 42:263–67.

Kellermann, A. L., L. Westphal, L. Fischer, and B. Harvard. 1995. Weapon involvement in home invasion crimes. *Journal of the American Medical Association* 273:1759–62.

Kendell, R. E. 1995. Alcohol policy and the public good. *Addiction* 90:181–203.

Kennedy, D. M. 1994. Can we keep guns away from kids? *American Prospect* 18 (summer): 74–80.

Kennedy, D. M. 1999. Reacting to violence, but Boston proves something can be done. *Washington Post*, May 23, p. B3.

Kennedy, D. M., A. M. Piehl, and A. A. Braga. 1996. Youth violence in Boston: Gun markets, serious youth offenders, and a use-reduction strategy. *Law and Contemporary Problems* 59:147–96.

Kennett, L., and J. L. Anderson. 1975. *The Gun in America: The Origin of a National Dilemma.* Westport, CT: Greenwood Press.

Killias, M. 1993. International correlations between gun ownership and rates of homicide and suicide. *Canadian Medical Association Journal* 148:1721–25.

Killias, M., J. Van Kesteren, and M. Rindlisbacher. 2001. Guns, violent crime, and suicide in twenty-one countries. *Canadian Journal of Criminology* 156:429–48.

Kirschner, E. S. 2000. A survey of primary care physicians' assessment and treatment of depressed older adults with suicidal depression. Ph.D. diss., Pacific Graduate School of Psychology.

Kleck, G. 1979. Capital punishment, gun ownership, and homicide. *American Journal of Sociology* 84:882–910.

Kleck, G. 1984. The relationship between gun ownership levels and rates of violence in the United States. In *Firearms and Violence: Issues of Public Policy,* ed. D. B. Kates, 99–135. Cambridge, MA: Ballinger.

Kleck, G. 1988. Crime control through private use of armed force. *Social Problems* 35:1–21.

Kleck, G. 1991. *Point Blank: Guns and Violence in America.* Hawthorne, NY: Aldine de Gruyter.

BIBLIOGRAPHY

Kleck, G. 1994. Should you own a gun? Interview by G. Witkin. *U.S. News and World Report*, August 15.

Kleck, G. 1997a. Struggling against "common sense": The pluses and minuses of gun control. *The World and I*, 121 (2): 287–99.

Kleck, G. 1997b. *Targeting Guns: Firearms and Their Control*. Hawthorne, NY: Aldine de Gruyter.

Kleck, G. 1998. What are the risks and benefits of keeping a gun in the home? *Journal of the American Medical Association* 280 (5): 473–75.

Kleck, G., and M. Gertz. 1995. Armed resistance to crime: The prevalence and nature of self-defense with a gun. *Journal of Criminal Law and Criminology* 86:150–87.

Kleck, G., and M. Gertz. 1997. The illegitimacy of one-sided speculation: Getting the defensive gun use estimates down. *Journal of Criminal Law and Criminology* 87:1446–61.

Kleck, G., and M. Hogan. 1999. A national case control study of homicide offending and gun ownership. *Social Problems* 46:275–93.

Kleck G., and D. B. Kates. 2001. *Armed: New Perspectives on Gun Control*. Amherst, NY: Prometheus.

Kleck, G., and K. McElrath. 1991. The effects of weaponry on human violence. *Social Forces* 69:669–92.

Kleck, G., and E. B. Patterson. 1993. The impact of gun control and gun ownership levels on violence rates. *Journal of Quantitative Criminology* 9:249–87.

Koepsell, T. D. 2001. Selecting a study design for injury research. In *Injury Control: A Guide to Research and Program Evaluation*, ed. F. P. Rivara, P. Cummings, and T. D. Koepsell, 89–103. New York: Cambridge University Press.

Kohn, A. A. 2000. Shooters: The moral world of gun enthusiasts. Ph.D. diss., University of California, San Francisco.

Koop, C. E., and G. D. Lundberg. 1992. Violence in America: A public health emergency; Time to bite the bullet back. *Journal of the American Medical Association* 267:3075–76.

Kopel, D. B. 1988. Trust the people: The case against gun control. Policy Analysis. Cato Institute.

Kopel, D. B. 1992. *The Samurai, the Mountie, and the Cowboy: Should America Adopt the Gun Controls of Other Democracies?* Buffalo, NY: Prometheus Books.

Kopel, D. B. 1993. The violence of gun control. *Policy Review* 63 (winter): 1–8.

Kovandzic, T. V., and T. B. Marvell. 2003. Right-to-carry concealed handguns and violent crime: crime control through gun decontrol? *Criminology and Public Policy* 2:363–96.

Kreitman, N. 1986. Alcohol consumption and the prevention paradox. *British Journal of Addiction* 81:353–63.

Krug, E. G., J. A. Mercy, L. L. Dahlberg, and K. E. Powell. 1998. Firearm- and non-firearm-related homicide among children. *Homicide Studies* 2:83–95.

Krug, E. G., K. E. Powell, and L. L. Dahlberg. 1998. Firearm-related deaths in the United

States and thirty-five other high-and upper-middle-income countries. *International Journal of Epidemiology* 27:214–21.

LaFollette, H. 2000. Gun control. *Ethics* 110:263–81.

Lambert, M. T., and P. S. Silva. 1998. An update on the impact of gun control legislation on suicide. *Psychiatric Quarterly* 69:127–34.

Lambert, T. 2003a. Do more guns cause less crime? http://www.cse.unsw.edu.au/~lambert/guns/lott/onepage.html/ (accessed April 2003).

Lambert, T. 2003b. Mysterious Lott survey. http://www.cse.unsw.edu.au/~lambert/guns/lott98update.html/ (accessed April 2003).

Landau, S. F. 2002. Violence in Israeli society: Its relation to social stress. In *Studies in Contemporary Jewry*. Vol. 18, *Jews and Violence: Images, Ideologies, Realities*, ed. P. Y. Medding, 126–48. New York: Oxford University Press.

Landes, W. M. 1978. An economic study of U.S. aircraft hijacking, 1961–1976. *Journal of Law and Economics* 21:1–31.

Lane, R. 1999. Murder in America: A historian's perspective. *Crime and Justice: A Review of Research* 25:191–224.

Langan, P. A., and D. P. Farrington. 1998. Crime and justice in the United States and England and Wales, 1981–1996. NCJ 173402. Bureau of Justice Statistics.

Langley, M. 2001. *"A .22 for Christmas": How the Gun Industry Designs and Markets Firearms for Children and Youth*. Washington, DC: Violence Policy Center.

Lantz, P. M., P. D. Jacobson, K. F. Warner, J. Wasserman, H. A. Pollack, J. Berson, and A. Ahlstrom. 2000. Investing in youth tobacco control: A review of smoking prevention and control strategies. *Tobacco Control* 9:47–63.

LaPierre, W. 1994. *Guns, Crime, and Freedom*. Washington, DC: Regnery.

LaPierre, W. 2002. Speech at NRA Annual Meeting, May 3. http://www.nraila.org/speeches.asp/ (accessed July 2002).

Laraque, D., B. Barlow, M. Durkin, and M. Heagarty. 1995. Injury prevention in an urban setting: Challenges and successes. *Bulletin of the New York Academy of Medicine* 72:16–30.

Larson, E. 1993a. Ruger gun often fires if dropped, but firm sees no need for recall. *Wall Street Journal*, June 24, p. A1.

Larson, E. 1993b. The story of a gun: The maker, the dealer, the murdered—inside the out-of-control world of American firearms. *Atlantic*, January, 48–78.

Larson, E. 1999. Squeezing out the bad guys. *Time Magazine*, August 9, 32–36.

Lawrie, L., and J. Kuesters. 1999. Schoolyard killers: Exploring the incidents in Jonesboro, Pearl, West Paducah, and Springfield. Student paper, Harvard Injury Control Research Center.

Lebowitz, L. 2002. Suspected terrorists held without bond in Broward County. *Miami Herald*, May 28.

Lederman, D. L. 1994. Weapons on campus? Officials warn that colleges are not immune from the scourge of handguns. *Chronicle of Higher Education*, March 9, A33–34.

Lee, R. K., R. J. Waxweiler, J. G. Dobbins, and T. Paschetag. 1991. Incidence rates of firearm injuries in Galveston, Texas, 1979–1981. *American Journal of Epidemiology* 134:511–21.

Leenaars, A. A., and D. Lester. 1997. The effects of gun control on the accidental death rate from firearms in Canada. *Journal of Safety Research* 28:119–22.

Leenaars, A. A., F. Moksony, D. Lester, and S. Wenckstern. 2003. The impact of gun control (Bill C-51) on suicide in Canada. *Death Studies* 27:103–24.

Leitzel, J. 2003. Comment: Australia: A massive buyback of low-risk guns. In *Evaluating Gun Policy*, ed. J. Ludwig and P. J. Cook, 145–53. Washington, DC: Brookings Institution.

Lester, D. 1987. Availability of guns and the likelihood of suicide. *Sociology and Social Research* 71:287–288.

Lester, D. 1988. Firearm availability and the incidence of suicide and homicide. *Acta Psychiatrica Belgica* 88:387–93.

Lester, D. 1989. Gun ownership and suicide in the United States. *Psychological Medicine* 19:519–21.

Lester, D. 1990a. The availability of firearms and the use of firearms for suicide: A study of twenty countries. *Acta Psychiatrica Scandinavia* 81:146–47.

Lester, D. 1990b. Relationship between firearm availability and primary and secondary murder. *Psychological Reports* 67:490.

Lester, D. 1993. Firearm availability and accidental deaths from firearms. *Journal of Safety Research* 24:167–69.

Lester, D. 1999. Gun deaths in children and guns in the home. *European Journal of Psychiatry* 13:157–59.

Lester, D., and A. Leenaars. 1993. Suicide rates in Canada before and after the tightening firearm control laws. *Psychological Reports* 72:787–90.

Lester, D., and A. Leenaars. 1994. Gun control and rates of firearms violence in Canada and the United States: A comment. *Canadian Journal of Criminology* 36:463–64.

Lester, D., and M. E. Murrell. 1981. The influence of gun control laws on the incidence of accidents with guns: A preliminary study. *Accident Analysis and Prevention* 13:357–59.

Lester, D., and M. E. Murrell. 1982. The preventive effect of strict gun control laws on suicide and homicide. *Suicide and Life Threatening Behavior* 12:131–40.

Lester, D. , and M. E. Murrell. 1986. The influence of gun control laws on personal violence. *Journal of Community Psychology* 14:315–18.

Levine, H. G., and C. Reinarman. 1991. From Prohibition to regulation: Lessons from alcohol policy for drug policy. *Milbank Quarterly* 69:461–94.

Levinson, S. 1989. The embarrassing Second Amendment. *Yale Law Journal* 99:637–59.

BIBLIOGRAPHY

Lindgren, J., and J. L. Heather. 2002. Counting guns in early America. *William and Mary Law Review* 43 (5): 1777–1843.

Lipman, H. 1997. Survey suggests race has role in gun attitude. *Albany Times Union,* October 26.

Lipschitz, A. 1995. Suicide prevention in young adults (age 18–30). *Suicide and Life Threatening Behavior* 25:155–70.

Litman, R. E., T. J. Curphey, E. S. Schneidman, N. L. Faberow, and N. Tabachnick. 1963. Investigations of equivocal suicide. *Journal of the American Medical Association* 184:924–29.

Locy, T. 1994. Deadly force law itself under fire. *Boston Globe,* April 18.

Loftin, C., D. McDowall, B. Wiersema, and C. J. Talbert. 1991. Effects of restrictive licensing of handguns on homicide and suicide in the District of Columbia. *New England Journal of Medicine* 325:1615–20.

Los Angeles Times. 1997. Lorcin: Firm's saga of lawyers, guns, and money in Southland. December 27.

Lott, J. R. Jr. 1998a. *More Guns, Less Crime: Understanding Crime and Gun Control Laws.* Chicago: University of Chicago Press.

Lott, J. R. Jr. 1998b. The real lesson of the school shootings. *Wall Street Journal,* March 27.

Lott, J. R. Jr. 2000. Reply to Otis Dudley Duncan. *Criminologist.* 25 (5): 1–6.

Lott, J. R. Jr. 2002. Gun control misfires in Europe. *Wall Street Journal,* April 30.

Lott, J. R. Jr. 2003. *The Bias against Guns.* Washington, DC: Regnery Press.

Lott, J. R. Jr., and W. M. Landes. 1999. Multiple victim public shootings, bombings, and right-to-carry concealed handgun laws. Law and Economics Working Paper 73, University of Chicago Law School.

Lott, J. R. Jr., and D. B. Mustard. 1997. Crime, deterrence, and right-to-carry concealed handguns. *Journal of Legal Studies* 26:1–68.

Lott, J. R. Jr., and J. E. Whitley. 2001. Safe-storage gun laws: Accidental deaths, suicides, and crime. *Journal of Law and Economics* 44:659–89.

Louisville (KY) Courier-Journal. 2001. Bullying, American Style. June 3.

Ludwig, J. 1998. Concealed-gun-carrying laws and violent crime: Evidence from state panel data. *International Review of Law and Economics* 18:239–54.

Ludwig, J. 1999. Gun carrying and multiple victim homicide. Paper presented at the American Enterprise Institute conference Washington, DC, May 14.

Ludwig, J. 2000. Gun self-defense and deterrence. *Crime and Justice: A Review of Research* 27:363–417.

Ludwig, J. 1999. Gun self-defense and deterrence. Draft. Georgetown Public Policy Institute. May 25. Cited with permission of author.

Ludwig, J., and P. J. Cook. 2000. Homicide and suicide rates associated with implementation of the Brady Handgun Violence Prevention Act. *Journal of the American Medical Association* 284:585–91.

BIBLIOGRAPHY

Ludwig, J., P. J. Cook, and T. W. Smith. 1998. The gender gap in reporting household gun ownership. *American Journal of Public Health* 88:1715–18.

Luster, T., and S. M. Oh. 2001. Correlates of male adolescents carrying handguns among their peers. *Journal of Marriage and the Family* 63:714–26.

MacLennan, C. A. 1988. From accident to crash: The auto industry and the politics of injury. *Medical Anthropology Quarterly* 2/3:233–50.

Magaddino, J. P., and M. H. Medoff. 1984. An empirical analysis of federal and state firearm control laws. In *Firearms and Violence: Issues of Public Policy,* ed. D. Kates, 225–58. Cambridge, MA: Ballinger.

Magnuson, E. 1989. Do guns save lives? Not as often as the NRA says. *Time.* August 21, pp. 25–26.

Main, G. L. 2002. Many things forgotten: The use of probate records in arming America. *William and Mary Quarterly* 59:211–16.

Malcolm, J. 1994. *To Keep and Bear Arms: The Origins of an Anglo-American Right.* Cambridge, MA: Harvard University Press.

Malcolm, J. 2002. *Guns and Violence: The English Experience.* Cambridge, MA: Harvard University Press.

Males, M. 1991. Teen suicide and changing cause-of-death certification, 1953–1987. *Suicide and Life Threatening Behavior* 21:245–59.

Maltz, M. D., and J. Targonski. 2002. A note on the use of county-level UCR data. *Journal of Quantitative Criminology* 18:297–318.

Maltz, M. D., and J. Targonski. 2003. Measurement and other errors in county-level UCR data: A reply to Lott and Whitley. *Journal of Quantitative Criminology* 19:199–206.

Markush, R., and A. Bartolucci. 1984. Firearms and suicide in the United States. *American Journal of Public Health* 64:123–27.

Marwick, C. 1999. HELP network says firearms data gap makes reducing gun injuries more difficult. *Journal of the American Medical Association* 281:784–85.

Massachusetts Attorney General. 1997. Harshbarger bans sale of "Saturday Night Specials"; issues regulations on gun childproofing and serial numbers. News release. June 4. See http://www.state.ma.us/dph/bhsre/isplisp.html.

Massachusetts Weapons Related Injury Surveillance System. 1996. Victims of violence-related gunshot and sharp instrument wounds, 1994. Massachusetts Department of Public Health.

May, J. P., D. Hemenway, and A. Hall. 2002. Do criminals go to the hospital after being shot? *Injury Prevention* 8:236–38.

May, J. P., D. Hemenway, R. Oen, and K. R. Pitts. 2000a. Medical care solicitation by criminals with gunshot wounds: A survey of Washington D.C. jail detainees. *Journal of Trauma* 48:130–32.

May, J. P., D. Hemenway, R. Oen, and K. R. Pitts. 2000b. When criminals are shot: A survey of Washington D.C. jail detainees. *Medscape General Medicine* (June 28). http://www.medscape.com/.

Mayer, J. D. 1979. Emergency medical service: Delays, response time, and survival. *Medical Care* 17:818–27.

Mayhew, P., and J. J. M. van Dijk. 1997. *Criminal Victimization in Eleven Industrialized Countries: Key Findings from the International Crime Victimization Surveys.* London: Information and Publications Group.

Mayron, R., R. S. Long, and E. Ruiz. 1984. The 911 emergency telephone number: Impact on emergency medical systems access in a metropolitan area. *American Journal of Emergency Medicine* 2:491–93.

McBride, J. 1999. Store's sign brags of top rank for selling guns tied to crime. Owners say they're making light of adverse publicity; DA, police chief not amused. *Milwaukee Journal Sentinel*, November 29.

McDowall, D. 1991. Firearm availability and homicide rates in Detroit, 1951–1986. *Social Forces* 69:1085–99.

McDowall, D., A. J. Lizotte, and B. Wiersema. 1991. General deterrence through civilian gun ownership: An evaluation of the quasi-experimental evidence. *Criminology* 29:541–59.

McDowall, D., C. Loftin, and S. Presser. 2000. Measuring civilian defensive firearm use: A methodological experiment. *Journal of Quantitative Criminology* 16:1–19.

McDowall, D., C. Loftin, and B. Wiersema. 1995. Easing concealed firearms laws: Effects on homicides in three states. *Journal of Criminal Law and Criminology* 86:193–206.

McDowall, D., and B. Wiersema. 1994. The incidence of defensive firearm use by US crime victims, 1987 through 1990. *American Journal of Public Health* 84:1982–84.

McDowall, D., B. Wiersema, and C. Loftin. 1989. Did mandatory firearm ownership in Kennesaw really prevent burglary? *Sociology and Social Research* 74:48–51.

McDowall, D., B. Wiersema, and C. Loftin. 1996. Using quasi-experiments to evaluate firearm laws: Comment on Britt et al.'s reassessment of the D.C. gun law. *Law and Society Review* 30:381–91.

McFarlane, J., K. Soeken, J. Campbell, B. Parker, S. Reel, and C. Silva. 1998. Severity of abuse to pregnant women and associated gun access to the perpetrator. *Public Health Nursing* 15:201–6.

McGinnis, J. M., and W. H. Foege. 1993. Actual causes of death in the United States. *Journal of the American Medical Association* 270:2207–12.

McGuire, A. 1990. *Dogs of War: Raising Alcohol Taxes in California.* Video. San Francisco: Trauma Foundation, San Francisco General Hospital.

McGuire, A. 1992. The case of the fire safe cigarette: The synergism between state and federal legislation. In *Political Approaches to Injury Control at the State Level,* ed. A. B. Bergman, 79–87. Seattle: University of Washington Press.

McKanna, C. V. Jr. 1995. Alcohol, handguns, and homicide in the American west: A tale of three counties, 1880–1920. *Western Historical Quarterly* 26:455–82.

McKeown, R. E., K. L. Jackson, and R. F. Valois. 1998. The frequency and correlates of violent behaviors in a statewide sample of high school students. *Family and Community Health* 20:38–53.

McKinley, W. O., J. S. Johns, and J. J. Musgrove. 1999. Clinical presentations, medical complications, and functional outcomes of individuals with gunshot wound–induced spinal cord injury. *American Journal of Physical Medicine and Rehabilitation* 78:102–7.

McNabb, S. J. N., T. A. Farley, K. E. Powell, W. R. Rolka, and J. M. Horan. 1996. Correlates of gun carrying among adolescents in South Louisiana. *American Journal of Preventive Medicine* 12:96–102.

Medoff, M. H., and J. P. Magaddino. 1983. Suicide and firearm control laws. *Evaluation Review* 7:357–72.

Meier, B. 1999a. Local governments attack gun industry with civil lawsuits. *New York Times*, July 22.

Meier, B. 1999b. Tracing twisted path of pistol used in California killing. *New York Times*, August 14.

Mercury News. 2003. L.A. police arrest one suspect, identify two in school shooting. MercuryNews.com, September 26.

Mercy, J. A., and V. N. Houk. 1988. Firearm injuries: A call for science. *New England Journal of Medicine* 319:1283–85.

Mercy, J. A., and M. L. Rosenberg. 1998. Preventing firearm violence in and around schools. In *Violence in American Schools: A New Perspective,* ed. D. S. Elliot, B. A. Hamburg, and K. R. Williams, 159–87. Cambridge: Cambridge University Press.

Merkle, D. 1999. Little personal activism in support of gun control. ABCNEWS.com, September 8.

Merrill, V. C. 2002. Gun-in-home as a risk factor in firearm-related mortality: A historical prospective cohort study of United States deaths, 1993. Ph.D. diss., Environmental Health Science and Policy, University of California, Irvine.

Miller, M., D. Azrael, and D. Hemenway. 2000. Community firearms, community fear. *Epidemiology* 11:709–14.

Miller, M., D. Azrael, and D. Hemenway. 2001. Firearm availability and unintentional firearm deaths. *Accident Analysis and Prevention* 33:477–84.

Miller, M., D. Azrael, and D. Hemenway. 2002a. Firearm availability and unintentional firearm deaths, suicide, and homicide among 5–14 year olds. *Journal of Trauma* 52:267–75.

Miller, M., D. Azrael, and D. Hemenway. 2002b. Firearm availability and unintentional firearm deaths, suicide, and homicide among women. *Journal of Urban Health* 79:26–38.

Miller, M., D. Azrael, and D. Hemenway. 2002c. Household firearm ownership levels and homicide across U.S. states and regions, 1988–1997. *American Journal of Public Health* 92:1988–93.

Miller, M., D. Azrael, and D. Hemenway. 2002d. Household firearm ownership levels and suicide across U.S. regions and states, 1988–1997. *Epidemiology* 13:517–24

Miller, M., D. Azrael, and D. Hemenway. 2003. The Epidemiology of Case Fatality Rates. Harvard Injury Control Research Center.

Miller, M., D. Azrael, D. Hemenway, and F. I. Solop. 2002. Road rage in Arizona: Armed and dangerous? *Accident Analysis and Prevention* 34:807–14.

Miller, M., and D. Hemenway. 1999. The relationship between firearms and suicide: A review of the literature. *Aggression and Violent Behavior* 4:59–75.

Miller, M., D. Hemenway, and D. Azrael. 2003. Firearms and suicide in the Northeast. *Journal of Trauma.* In press.

Miller, M., D. Hemenway, and H. Wechsler. 1999. Guns at college. *American Journal of College Health* 48:7–12.

Miller M., D. Hemenway, and H. Wechsler. 2002. Guns and gun threats at college. *Journal of American College Health* 51:57–65.

Milwaukee Journal Sentinel. 1999. Editorial, Another good idea on firearms. February 15.

Minneapolis-St. Paul Star Tribune. 2003. Hero coach halts school shooting. September 26.

Miss Manners column. 1993. Check for shooting irons at the door. *Washington Post,* September 15.

Monchukcalgary, J. 2001. Gun lobby leader to plead guilty to unsafe handling of firearm. January 24. *Calgary Herald.*

Moore, M. H., and D. Gerstein, eds. 1981. *Alcohol and Public Policy: Beyond the Shadow of Prohibition.* Washington, DC: National Academy Press.

Moore, M. H., C. V. Petrie, A. A. Braga, and B. McLaughlin, eds. 2002. *Deadly Lessons: Understanding Lethal School Violence.* Washington, DC: National Academy Press.

Morin, R., and C. Deane. 2000. Poll finds firearm threats common. *Washington Post,* May 14.

Morone, J. A. 1997. Enemies of the people: The moral dimensions to public health. *Journal of Health Politics, Policy, and Law* 22:993–1020.

Morrison, A., and D. H. Stone. 1999. EURORISC Working Group. Unintentional childhood injury mortality in Europe 1984–93: A report from the EURORISC working group. *Injury Prevention* 5:171–76.

Moscicki, E. K. 1995. Epidemiology of suicide behavior. *Suicide and Life Threatening Behavior* 25:22–35.

Mouzos, J. 2001. Homicide in Australia, 1999–2000. Australian Institute of Criminology.

Moxley, R. S. 2000. "I . . . shot my son." *Orange County Weekly,* July 14–20. (Contains complete story of this 1998 accidental shooting.)

Moyer, S., and P. J. Carrington. 1992. *Gun Availability and Firearms Suicide.* Ottawa: Department of Justice.

MSNBC. 1999. Special report: Who's packing heat? Tampa, Florida. February 19.

BIBLIOGRAPHY

MSNBC, KSNT 27. 1999. An experiment with kids and gun safety. Topeka, Kansas. February 24.

Murray, D. R. 1975. Handguns, gun control laws, and firearm violence. *Social Problems* 23:81–92.

Nader, R. 1965. *Unsafe at Any Speed: The Designed-in Dangers of the American Automobile.* New York: Grossman.

NAMI Advocate. 1999. Common misconceptions about suicide. http://www.depres sion.8m.com/misconc.html (accessed October 2003).

Nathanson, C. A. 1999. Social movements as catalysts for policy change: The case of smoking and guns. *Journal of Health Politics, Policy, and Law* 24:421–86.

National Archive of Criminal Justice Data. 1998. National Crime Victimization Survey: 1986–1991, 1992–1995. http://www.icpsr.umich.edu:80/NACJD/.

National Center for Education Statistics. 1998. Indicators of school crime and safety, 1998. nces.ed.gov/pubsearch/pubsinfo.asp?pubid=98251 (accessed October 2003).

National Center for Education Statistics. 1999. Indicators of school crime and safety, 1999. nces.ed.gov/pubsearch/pubsinfo.asp?pubid=1999057 (accessed October 2003).

National Center for Injury Prevention and Control. 1995. *1992: Ten Leading Causes of Death.* Atlanta, GA: Centers for Disease Control and Prevention.

National Committee for Injury Prevention and Control. 1989. *Injury Prevention: Meeting the Challenge.* New York: Oxford University Press.

National Crime Victimization Survey. *Crime Victimization 2001.* Bureau of Justice Statistics.

National Journal's Cloakroom. 1998. Today's national polls. May 27. http://www.nationaljournal.com/.

National Journal's Cloakroom. 1999. Today's national polls. February 23. http://www.nationaljournal.com/.

National Journal. 2000. Today's National Polls. May 15. http://www.nationaljournal.com/members/polltrack/2000/todays/hp000515.htm.

National Rifle Association. 1990. *NRA Home Firearm Safety Course: Course Outline and Lesson Plans.* Fairfax, VA: National Rifle Association.

National Rifle Association. 2002. Factsheet: Firearm Facts. www.nraila.org/Issues FactSheets/Read.aspx? ID=83 (accessed October 2003).

National Rifle Association. 2003. Compendium of state firearm laws. www.nraila.org /media/misc/compendium.htm (accessed September 2003).

National Shooting Sports Foundation. 2002. Education and safety. Available at http://www.nssf.org/ (accessed July 2002).

National Shooting Sports Foundation. N.d. Firearm safety in the home. Brochure.

National Shooting Sports Foundation. Firearms responsibility in the home. Brochure.

National Shooting Sports Foundation. N.d. Handgun guide. Brochure.

Naughton, K., and E. Thomas. 2002. Did Kayla have to die? *Newsweek,* March 13, p. 24.

BIBLIOGRAPHY

Naureckas, S. M. 1995. Children and women's ability to fire handguns. *Archives of Pediatric Adolescent Medicine* 149:1318–22.

Nelson, D. E., J. A. Grant-Worley, K. Powell, J. Mercy, and D. Holzman. 1996. Population estimates of household firearm storage practices and firearm carrying in Oregon. *Journal of the American Medical Association* 275:1744–48.

Newbold, G. 1999. The criminal use of firearms in New Zealand. *Australian and New Zealand Journal of Criminology* 32:61–78.

New Republic. 2003. Easy shot: NRA vs. National Security. January 20, p. 18.

News 14 Carolina. 2003. Teen charged in school shooting. News14Charlotte.com, September 26.

Newswire. 2000a. Jamaican legislators lash U.S. gun export policy. February 25. http://www.clw.org/cat/newswire/nw022500.html.

Newton, G. D., and F. Zimring. 1969. *Firearms and Violence in American Life.* A staff report to the National Commission on the Causes and Prevention of Violence. Washington, DC: U.S. Government Printing Office.

New York Office of Oversight and Investigation. New York City Council. 1994. Guns: A survey of 800 New York City youth.

New York Times. 1995a. Two shot as gun is converted. January 24, sect. A, p. 12, col. 6.

New York Times. 1995b. Can you spot the lethal weapon? July 16.

Nichols, W. D. 1995. Violence on campus: The intruded sanctuary. *FBI Law Enforcement Bulletin* (June): 1–5.

Nickerson, C. 1995. Smugglers called peril to gun laws in Canada. *Boston Globe,* February 27.

Nieves, E. 1995. Two collies rescue NY town from a mess of geese. *International Herald Tribune,* October 23.

Nondahl, D. M., K. J. Cruickshanks, T. L. Wiley, R. Klein, B. E. Klein, and T. S. Tweed. 2000. Recreational firearm use and hearing loss. *Archives of Family Medicine* 9:352–57.

Nordstrom, D. L., C. Zwerling, A. M. Stromquist, L. F. Burmeister, and J. A. Merchant. 2001. Rural population survey of behavioral and demographic risk factors for loaded firearms. *Injury Prevention* 7:112–16.

Novello, A. C., J. Shosky, and R. Froehlke. 1992. From the Surgeon General: A medical response to violence. *Journal of the American Medical Association* 267:3007.

O'Donnell, I., and S. Morrison. 1997. Armed and dangerous? The use of firearms in robbery. *Howard Journal of Criminal Justice* 36:305–20.

Ohsfeldt, R. L., and M. A. Morrisey. 1992. Firearms, firearm injury, and gun control: A critical survey of the literature. *Advances in Health Economics and Health Services Research* 13:65–82.

O'Keefe, G. E., C. J. Jurkovich, M. Copass, and R. V. Maier. 1999. Ten-year trend in survival and resource utilization at a level I trauma center. *Annals of Surgery* 229:409–15.

Olinger, D. 1999a. Following the guns. *Denver Post,* August 1.

Olinger, D. 1999b. Police guns in the hands of criminals. *Denver Post,* September 20.

BIBLIOGRAPHY

Olinger, D., and B. Port. 1993. No questions asked. *St. Petersburg Times,* June 27–July 1.

Olson, D. E., and M. D. Maltz. 2001. Right-to-carry concealed weapon laws and homicide in large U.S. counties: The effect on weapon types, victim characteristics, and victim-offender relationships. *Journal of Law and Economics* 44:747–70.

Ordog, G. J., P. Dornhoffer, G. Ackroyd, J. Wasserberger, M. Bishop, W. Shoemaker, and S. Balasubramanium. 1994. Spent bullets and their injuries: The result of firing weapons into the sky. *Journal of Trauma* 37:1003–6.

Ordog, G. J., J. Wassweberger, I. Schatz, D. Owens-Collins, K. English, and S. Balasubramanium. 1988. Gunshot wounds in children under ten years of age. *American Journal of Diseases in Children* 142:618–22.

Ornato, J. P., E. J. Craren, N. M. Nelson, and K. F. Kimball. 1985. Impact of improved emergency medical services and emergency trauma care on the reduction in mortality from trauma. *Journal of Trauma* 25:575–79.

Orr, A. 1999. U.S. gun buyers dodge controls by shopping online. Reuters. Palo Alto, CA. May 30. http://www.zdnet.com/filters/printerfriendly/0,6061,2267962–2,00 .html.

Overlan, L. 1996. Suicide a weighty issue. *Brookline Tab,* June 18–24, p. 21.

Pacurucu-Castillo, S. 1995. A book which deserves wide diffusion. *Addiction* 90:185–87.

Parry, H. J., and H. M. Crossley. 1950. Validity of responses to survey questionnaires. *Public Opinion Quarterly* 14: 61–80.

Patterson, P. J., and A. H. Holguin. 1990. Firearm-related deaths among children in Texas. *Journal of Texas Medicine* 86:92–96.

PAX. 2002. The ASK campaign. http://www.pax.com/.

Perrin, N. 1979. *Giving up the Gun: Japan's Reversion to the Sword, 1543–1879.* Boston: David Godine.

Peterson, H. L. 1956. *Arms and Armor in Colonial America: 1526–1783.* Harrisburg, PA: Stackpole.

Peterson, L. G., M. Peterson, G. J. O'Shanick, and A. Swann. 1985. Self-inflicted gunshot wounds: Lethality of method versus intent. *American Journal of Psychiatry* 142:228–31.

Peterson, R. D., and L. J. Krivo. 1993. Racial segregation and urban black homicide. *Social Forces* 71:1001–26.

Philipson, T. J., and R. A. Posner. 1996. The economic epidemic of crime. *Journal of Law and Economics* 39:405–33.

Phillips, L., H. L. Votey, and J. Howell. 1976. Handguns and homicide. *Journal of Legal Studies* 5:463–78.

Piehl, A. M., D. M. Kennedy, and A. A. Braga. 2000. Problem solving and youth violence: An evaluation of the Boston gun project. JFK School of Government, Harvard University.

Plassmann, F., and T. N. Tideman. 2001. Does the right to carry concealed handguns deter countable crimes? Only a count analysis can say. *Journal of Law and Economics* 44:771–98.

Podell, S., and D. Archer. 1994. Do legal changes matter? The case of gun control laws. In *Violence and the Law*, ed. M. Costanzo and S. Oskamp, 37–60. London: Sage.

Police Executive Research Forum. 1990. *Handgun Safety Guidelines*. Washington, DC: Police Executive Research Forum.

Polsby, D. D., and D. Brennen. 1995. Taking aim at gun control. Heartland Policy Study. Heartland Institute.

Polsby, D. D., and D. B. Kates Jr. 1998. Causes and correlations of lethal violence in America; American homicide exceptionalism. *University of Colorado Law Review* 69:969–1008.

Pons, P. T., B. Honigman, E. E. Moore, P. Rosen, B. Antuna, and J. Derhocoeur. 1985. Prehospital advanced trauma life support for critical penetrating wounds to the thorax and abdomen. *Journal of Trauma* 25:828–32.

Pooley, E. 1991. Kids with guns. *New York Magazine*, August 5, 21–29.

Powell, E. C., K. M. Sheehan, and K. K. Christoffel. 1996. Firearm violence among youth: Public health strategies for prevention. *Annals of Emergency Medicine* 28:204–12.

Rakove, J. N. 2000. The Second Amendment: The highest stage of originalism. *Chicago-Kent Law Review* 76:103–66.

Rakove, J. N. 2002. Words, deeds, and guns: Arming America and the Second Amendment. *William and Mary Quarterly* 59:205–10.

Raphael, S., and J. Ludwig. 2003. Prison sentence enhancements: The case of Project Exile. In *Evaluating Gun Policy*, ed. J. Ludwig and P. J. Cook, 251–86. Washington, DC: Brookings Institution.

Red Deer Advocate (Medicine Hat, Canada). 1996. Police firearms trainer wounded. December 6, p. A5.

Reed, J. S. 1971. To live—and die—in Dixie: A contribution to the study of southern violence. *Political Science Quarterly* 86:429–43.

Rehm, J., M. J. Ashley, and G. Dubois. 1997. Alcohol and health: Individual and population perspectives. *Addiction* 92 (supplement 1): S109–55.

Reich, K., P. L. Culross, and R. E. Behrman. 2002. Children, youth, and gun violence: Analysis and recommendations. Packard Foundation. *The Future of Children: Children, Youth, and Gun Violence* 12:5–24.

Reiss, A. J., and J. A. Roth, eds. 1993. *Violence: Understanding and Preventing*. Washington, DC: National Academy Press.

Remington Arms Company. 2002. The ten commandments of firearms safety. Available at http://www.remington.com/safety/10comm.htm/ (accessed July 2002).

Rengert, G., and J. Wasilchick. 1985. *Suburban Burglary: A Time and Place for Everything*. Springfield, IL: Charles Thomas; 1985.

Reuter, P., and J. Mouzos. 2003. Australia: A massive buyback of low-risk guns. In *Evaluating Gun Policy*, ed. J. Ludwig and P. J. Cook, 121–56. Washington, DC: Brookings Institution.

BIBLIOGRAPHY

Ribadeneira, T. W. 2000. Can't tame the drivers, tame the streets. *Boston Globe,* May 12.

Rich, C. L., D. Young, and R. C. Fowler. 1986. San Diego suicide study: Young vs old subjects. *Archives of General Psychiatry* 43:577–82.

Rivera, J. 1997. Beanbag round used to disarm suspect: Man wielding knife thankful police didn't use bullets to bring him in. *Baltimore Sun,* September 3.

Roanoke Times (Virginia). Agents target gun sales. February 15.

Roberts, A. R. 1996. Battered women who kill: A comparative study of incarcerated participants with a community sample of battered women. *Journal of Family Violence* 11:291–304.

Robinson, K. D., S. P. Teret, J. S. Vernick, and D. W. Webster. 1996. *Personalized Guns: Reducing Gun Deaths through Design Changes.* Baltimore: Johns Hopkins Center for Gun Policy and Research.

Robinson, M.B. 1999. Kennedy opens gun safety campaign, Common Sense about Kids and Guns. October 7. http://www.kidsandguns.org/study/inthenews.asp?10=94 (accessed October 2003).

Robuck-Mangum, G. 1997. Concealed weapon permit holders in North Carolina: A descriptive study of handgun carrying behaviors. Master's thesis, University of North Carolina, Chapel Hill School of Public Health.

Rodgers, G. B. 1996. The safety effects of child-resistant packaging for oral prescription drugs: Two decades of experience. *Journal of the American Medical Association* 275:1661–65.

Ropp, T. 1959. *War in the Modern World.* Durham, NC: Duke University Press.

Rosenberg, M. L., and R. Hammond. 1998. Surveillance the key to firearm injury prevention. *American Journal of Preventive Medicine* 15 (supplement 3): 1.

Rosenbloom, D. L. 1998. Editorial, US needs gun safety board. *Boston Globe,* June 1.

Rosencrantz, B. G. 1972. *Public Health and the State.* Cambridge, MA: Harvard University Press.

Rosenfeld, R. 1986. Urban crime rates: Effects of inequality, welfare dependency, region, and race. In *The Social Ecology of Crime,* ed. J. M. Byrne and R. J. Sampson, 116–30. New York: Springer-Verlag.

Roth, R. 2002. Guns, gun culture, and homicide: The relationship between firearms, the uses of firearms, and interpersonal violence. *William and Mary Quarterly* 59:223–40.

Rothman, E. F. 2003. *Batterers and Firearms: A Survey from the Massachusetts Batterers Intervention Program.* Harvard Injury Control Research Center.

Rothman, K. J. 1986. *Modern Epidemiology.* Boston: Little, Brown.

Rowland, J., and F. Holtzhauer. 1989. Homicide involving firearms between family, relatives, and friends in Ohio: An offender-based case-control study. *American Journal of Epidemiology* 130:825.

Ruane, M. E. 2001. School safety drills' new mantra: Duck and cower. *Washington Post,* March 31.

Rushforth, N. B., C. S. Hirsch, A. B. Ford, and L. Adelson. 1975. Accidental firearm fatalities in a metropolitan county (1958–1973). *American Journal of Epidemiology* 100:499–505.

Russell, C. P. 1967. *Firearms, Traps, and Tools of the Mountain Men.* New York: Knopf.

Rutledge, R., J. Messick, C. C. Baker, S. Rhyne, J. Butts, A. Meyer, and T. Ricketts. 1992. Multivariate population-based analysis of the association of county trauma centers with per capita county trauma death rates. *Journal of Trauma* 33:29–38.

Saltman, R. B. 1994. Why not mandatory gun insurance? *Washington Post,* January 11, A18.

Saltzman, L. E., J. A. Mercy, P. W. O'Carroll, M. L. Rosenberg, and P. H. Rhodes. 1992. Weapon involvement and injury outcomes in family and intimate assaults. *Journal of the American Medical Association* 267:3043–47.

San Antonio Express-News. 1999. Collector accidentally shot at gun show. February 8.

Sanguino, S. M., M. D. Dowd, S. A. McEnaney, J. Knapp, and R. R. Tanz. 2002. Handgun safety: What do consumers learn from gun dealers? *Archives of Pediatrics and Adolescent Medicine* 156:777–80.

Schaechter, J., I. Duran, J. De Marchena, G. Lemard, and M. E. Villar. 2003. Are "accidental" gun deaths as rare as they seem? A comparison of medical examiner manner of death coding with an intent-based classification approach. *Pediatrics* 111:741–44.

Schrade, B. 2003. Off-duty security guard accidently shoots state employee downtown. *The Tennessean,* February 1.

Schumer, C. E. 1997. The war between the states. Report. 9th Congressional District, New York.

Schwaner, S. L., L. A. Furr, C. L. Negrey, and R. E. Seger. 1999. Who wants a gun license? *Journal of Criminal Justice* 27:1–10.

Schwoerer, L. G. 2000. To hold and bear arms: The English perspective. *Chicago-Kent Law Review* 76:27–60.

Seal, J. 1999. Regulating handguns won't make us safer. *Boston Globe,* August 11.

Segui-Gomez, M. 2000. Driver air bag effectiveness by severity of the crash. *American Journal of Public Health* 90:1575–81.

Seiden, R. H. 1977. Suicide prevention: A public health/public policy approach. *Omega* 8:267–75.

Seitz, S. T. 1972. Firearms, homicide, and gun control effectiveness. *Law and Society Review* 6:595–614.

Sells, C. W., and R. W. Blum. 1996. Morbidity and mortality among U.S. adolescents: An overview of data and trends. *American Journal of Public Health* 86:513–19.

Senturia, Y. D., K. K. Christoffel, and M. Donovan. 1996. Gun storage patterns in US home with children: A pediatric practice-based survey. *Archives of Pediatric Adolescent Medicine* 150:265–69.

Sesame Workshop. 2001. Media release. September 5.

BIBLIOGRAPHY

Shaffer, D., M. Gould, and R. C. Hicks. 1994. Worsening suicide rate in black teenagers. *American Journal of Psychiatry* 151:1810–12.

Shear, M. D., and T. Jackman. 1999. Fairfax police put guns back on the market: Officials plan to end trade-ins of seized weapons. *Washington Post,* September 8, p. A1.

Shelden, C. H. 1955. Prevention: the only cure for head injuries resulting from automobile accidents. *Journal of the American Medical Association* 159:981–86.

Sheley, J. F., and V. E. Brewer. 1995. Possession and carrying of firearms among suburban youth. *Public Health Reports* 110:18–26.

Sheley, J. F., C. J. Brody, J. D. Wright, and M. A. Williams. 1994. Women and handguns: Evidence from national surveys, 1973–1991. *Social Science Research* 23:219–35.

Sheley, J. F., Z. T. McGee, and J. D. Wright. 1992. Gun-related violence in and around inner-city schools. *American Journal of Diseases in Children* 146:677–82.

Sheley, J. F., and J. D. Wright. 1993. *Gun Acquisition and Possession in Selected Juvenile Samples.* Research in Brief. NCJ 145326. Washington, DC: U.S. Department of Justice, National Institute of Justice.

Sheley, J. F., and J. D. Wright. 1995. *In the Line of Fire: Youth, Guns, and Violence in Urban America.* New York: Aldine de Gruyter.

Shenassa, E. D., S. N. Catlin, and S. L. Buka. 2003. Lethality of firearms relative to other suicide methods: A population based study. *Journal of Epidemiology and Community Health* 57:120–24.

Sherman, M. A., K. Burns, J. Ignelzi, J. Raia, V. Lofton, D. Toland, B. Stinson, J. L. Tilley, and T. Coon. 2001. Firearms risk management in psychiatric care. *Psychiatric Services* 52:1057–61.

Shihadeh, E. S., and N. Flynn. 1996. Segregation and crime: The effect of black social isolation on the rates of black urban violence. *Social Forces* 74:1325–52.

Shuck, L. W., M. G. Orgel, and A. V. Vogel. 1980. Self-inflicted gunshot wounds to the face: A review of eighteen cases. *Journal of Trauma* 20:370–77.

Simmons, J. 2002. Crime in England and Wales 2001/2002. http://www.homeoffice.gov.uk/rds/patterns1.html/ (accessed April 2002).

Simon, R., M. Chouinard, and C. Gravel. 1996. Suicide and firearms: Restricting access in Canada. Paper presented at the Seventh Annual Conference, Canadian Association of Suicide Prevention, Toronto, October 16.

Simon, S. 1999. Encouraging kids to pick up a gun. *Los Angeles Times,* September 21.

Simon, T. R., J. L. Richardson, C. W. Dent, C. P. Chou, and B. R. Flay. 1998. Prospective, psychosocial, interpersonal, and behavioral predictors of handgun carrying among adolescents. *American Journal of Public Health* 88:960–63.

Simon, O. R., A. C. Swann, K. E. Powell, L. B. Potter, M. J. Kreshow, and P. W. O'Carroll. 2001. Characteristics of impulsive suicide attempts and attempters. *Suicide and Life Threatening Behavior* 32 (supplement): 49–59.

Sinauer, N., J. L. Annest, and J. A. Mercy. 1996. Unintentional, nonfatal firearm-related injuries. *Journal of the American Medical Association* 275:1740–43.

Singh, G. K., and S. M. Yu. 1996. U.S. childhood mortality, 1950 through 1993: Trends and socioeconomic differentials. *American Journal of Public Health* 86:505–12.

Single, E. 1995. A harm reduction approach for alcohol: Between the line of alcohol policy and the public good. *Addiction* 90:195–98.

Sipress, A. 1999. "Oh my God, I can't believe I shot her": In Alabama, road rage engulfs two women and suburbia. *Washington Post,* November 16.

Skogan, W. 1978. Weapon use in robbery. In *Violent Crime: Historical and Contemporary Issues,* ed. J. A. Inciardi and A. E. Pottieger, 61–73. Beverly Hills, CA: Sage.

Skogan, W. 1990. The national crime survey redesign. *Public Opinion Quarterly* 54:256–72.

Sloan, J. H., F. P. Rivara, D. T. Reay, J. A. Ferris, and A. L. Kellermann. 1990. Firearm regulations and rates of suicide: A comparison of two metropolitan cities. *New England Journal of Medicine* 322:369–73.

Small, M., and K. D. Tetrick. 2001. School violence: An overview. *Juvenile Justice* 8 (1): 3–12. Journal of the U.S. Office of Juvenile Justice and Delinquency Prevention.

Smith, J. L., G. C. Wood, E. J. Lengerich, K. A. Snyder, C. A. Rosenberry, and R. C. Boyd. 2002. Hunting-related shooting incidents in Pennsylvania 1987–1999. Paper presented at the Sixth World Injury Conference, Montreal, May 11–14.

Smith, T. W. 1999. *1998 National Gun Policy Survey of the National Opinion Research Center: Research Findings.* Chicago: National Opinion Research Center.

Smith, T. W. 2001. *2001 National Gun Policy Survey of the National Opinion Research Center: Research Findings.* Chicago: National Opinion Research Center.

Smith, T. W., and R. J. Smith. 1995. Changes in firearms ownership among women, 1980–1994. *Journal of Criminal Law and Criminology* 86:133–49.

Snyder, J. R. 1993. A nation of cowards. *Public Interest* 113:40–55.

Society for Adolescent Medicine. 1998. Adolescents and firearms: Position paper. *Journal of Adolescent Health* 23:117–18.

Sorenson, S. B., and R. A. Berk. 2001. Handgun sales, beer sales, and youth homicide, California, 1972–1993. *Journal of Public Health Policy* 22:182–97.

Sorenson, S. B., and K. A. Vittes. 2003. Buying a handgun for someone else: firearm dealer willingness to sell. *Injury Prevention* 9:147–50.

Sowers, J. R., K. C. Ferdinand, G. L. Bakris, and J. G. Douglas. 2002. Hypertension-related disease in African Americans: Factors underlying disparities in illness and its outcome. *Postgraduate Medicine* 112:24–26.

Spangenberg, K. B., M. T. Wagner, S. Hendrix, and D. L. Bachman. 1999. Firearm presence in households of patients with Alzheimer's disease and related dementias. *Journal of the American Geriatrics Society* 47:1183–86.

Spicer, R. S., and T. R. Miller. 2000. Suicide acts in eight states: Incidence and case fatality rates by demographics and method. *American Journal of Public Health* 90:1885–91.

BIBLIOGRAPHY

Spigner, C. 1998. Race, class, and violence: Research policy implications. *International Journal of Health Services* 28:349–72.

Sporting Arms and Ammunition Manufacturers' Institute. 2002. *Firearm Safety Depends on You*. Riverside, CT: Sporting Arms and Ammunition Manufacturers' Institute.

Steckmesser, K. L. 1965. *The Western Hero in History and Legend*. Norman: University of Oklahoma Press.

Stennies, G., R. Ikeda, S. Leadbetter, B. Houston, and J. Sacks. 1999. Firearm storage practices and children in the home, United States, 1994. *Archives of Pediatric Adolescent Medicine* 153:586–90.

Stewart, M., D. F. Konkle, and T. H. Simpson. 2001. The effect of recreational gunfire noise on hearing in workers exposed to occupational noise. *Ear, Nose, and Throat Journal* 80:32–40.

Stone, L. 1993. In K. Gewertz, Ubiquity of handguns contributes to social ills. *Harvard Gazette*, November 19.

Sugarmann, J., and K. Rand. 1994. *Cease Fire: A Comprehensive Strategy to Reduce Firearms Violence*. Washington, DC: Violence Policy Center.

Sullum, J., and M. W. Lynch. 2000. Cold comfort: Economist John Lott discusses the benefits of guns—and the hazards of pointing them out. *Reason* (January): 34–41.

Surgeon General. 2001. http://www.mentalhealth.org/suicideprevention/ (accessed July 2002).

Suter, E. A. 1994. Guns in the medical literature: A failure of peer review. *Journal of the American Medical Association of Georgia* 83:133–48.

Swahn, M. H., and B. J. Hammig. 2000. Prevalence of youth access to alcohol, guns, illegal drugs, or cigarettes in the home and association with health risk behaviors. *Annals of Epidemiology* 10:452.

Switzerland Embassy (Canberra, Australia). Information Service. 1999. http://www.ssaa.org.au/un/swiss.html/ (accessed December 2001).

Sydney Morning Herald/The Age. 1998. Kennett gun law changes passed. March 27.

Tapper, J. 1999. Coming out shooting. May 2. Available at www.salon.com/news/feature/1999/05/02/nra (accessed September 2003).

Tennessee v. Garner. 1985. 471 U.S. 1, 105 Sup. Ct. 1694, 85 L. Ed. 2nd 1.

Teret, S. P. 1996. The firearm injury reporting system revisited. *Journal of the American Medical Association* 275:70.

Teret, S. P., and D. W. Webster. 1999.Reducing deaths in the United States: Personalized guns would help—and would be achievable. *British Medical Journal* 318:1160–61.

Teret, S. P., D. W. Webster, and J. S. Vernick et al. 1998. Support for new policies to regulate firearms: Results of two national surveys. *New England Journal of Medicine* 339:813–18.

Teret, S. P., and G. J. Wintemute. 1993. Policies to prevent firearm injuries. *Health Affairs* 12:96–108.

BIBLIOGRAPHY

Teret, S. P., G. J. Wintemute, and P. L. Beilenson. 1992. The firearm fatality reporting system: A proposal. *Journal of the American Medical Association* 267:3073–74.

Terris, M. 1967. Epidemiology of cirrhosis of the liver: National mortality data. *American Journal of Public Health* 57:2076–88.

Tesh, S. N. 1990. *Hidden Arguments: Political Ideology and Disease Prevention Policy.* New Brunswick: Rutgers University Press.

Tesoriero, J. M. 1998. A longitudinal study of weapon ownership and use among inner city youth. Ph.D. diss., State University of New York at Albany.

Thomas, P., and J. W. Anderson. 1996. Mexico seeks U.S. help on firearms: Forty-three hundred confiscated weapons are suspected of being smuggled. *International Herald Tribune*, November 6.

Time/CNN. 1995. Poll: Gun owners. May 17–18. Yankelovich Partners.

Tjaden, P., and N. Thoennes. 1998. *Prevalence, Incidence, and Consequences of Violence against Women: Findings from the National Violence against Women Survey.* Research in Brief. NCJ 172837. Washington, DC: U.S. Department of Justice, National Institute of Justice.

Toomey, T. L., and A. C. Wagenaar. 1999. Policy options for prevention: The case of alcohol. *Journal of Public Health Policy* 20:192–213.

Toronto Star. 1996. Grenades, anti-tank mines in massive weapons seizure. December 12.

United Nations. 1998. *International Study on Firearm Regulation.* New York: United Nations.

USA Today. 2001. Gun shows give terrorists easy access to firearms. December 13.

U.S. Code. N.d. Title 18, Section 922.

U.S. Consumer Product Safety Commission. 1996. Saving lives through smart government: Success stories. http:// www.cpsc.gov/cpscpub/pubs/success/index.html/ (accessed September 2003).

U.S. Consumer Product Safety Commission. 1997. Annual Report to Congress.

U.S. Department of Education. 1998. *Report on State Implementation of the Gun-free Schools Act, School Year 1996–97.* http://www.ed.gov/pubs/gunfree/gunfree.pdf (accessed September 2003).

U.S. Department of Health, Education, and Welfare (U.S. DHEW). 1964. *Smoking and Health: Report of the Advisory Committee to the Surgeon General of the Public Health Service.* Public Health Service Publication 1103. Washington, DC: U.S. Government Printing Office.

U.S. Department of Health and Human Services. 1986. *Surgeon General's Workshop on Violence and Public Health, October 1985.* DHHS Publication HRS-D-MC 86–1. Washington, DC: U.S. Department of Health and Human Services.

U.S. Department of Health and Human Services. 1991. *Healthy People 2000: National Health Promotion and Disease Objectives.* PHS-50212. Washington, DC: U.S. Department of Health and Human Services.

BIBLIOGRAPHY

U.S. Department of Justice. Bureau of Justice Statistics. 1995. *Sourcebook of Criminal Justice Statistics.* Washington, DC: U.S. Government Printing Office.

U.S. Department of Justice. Bureau of Justice Statistics. 2000. *Urban, Suburban, and Rural Victimization, 1993–1998.* Washington, DC: U.S. Government Printing Office. Available online at www.ojp.usdaj.gov/bjs/pub/pdf/usrv98.pdf.

U.S. Department of Justice. Federal Bureau of Investigation (FBI). 1993. *Crime in the United States.* Washington, DC: U.S. Department of Justice.

U.S. Department of Justice. Federal Bureau of Investigation (FBI). 1997. *Crime in the United States.* Washington, DC: U.S. Department of Justice. http://www.fbi/gov/ucr/ucr.htm (accessed September 2003).

U.S. Department of Justice. Federal Bureau of Investigation. 1998. *Crime in the United States.* Washington, DC: U.S. Department of Justice. http://www.fbi/gov/ucr/ucr.htm

U.S. Department of Justice. Federal Bureau of Investigation. 1999. *Crime in the United States.* Washington, DC: U.S. Department of Justice. http://www.fbi.gov/ucr/ucr.htm (accessed February 2003).

U.S. Department of Justice. Federal Bureau of Investigation. 2001. *Crime in the United States.* Washington, DC: U.S. Department of Justice. http://www.fbi.gov/ucr/ucr.htm (accessed January 24, 2003).

U.S. Department of Justice. Federal Bureau of Investigation. 2002. *Crime in the United States.* Washington, DC: U.S. Department of Justice. http://www.fbi.gov/ucr/ucr.htm (accessed February 2003).

U.S. Department of Justice. Federal Bureau of Investigation. 2003. *Crime in the United States.* Washington, DC: U.S. Department of Justice. http://www.fbi.gov/ucr/ucr.htm (accessed February 2003).

U.S. Department of Justice. Office of Juvenile Justice and Delinquency Programs (OJJDP). 1996. *Reducing Youth Gun Violence: An Overview of Programs and Initiatives.* Washington, DC: U.S. Department of Justice.

U.S. Department of Justice. Office of Juvenile Justice and Delinquency Programs. 1999. *Promising Strategies to Reduce Gun Violence.* OJJDP Report. Washington, DC: U.S. Department of Justice.

U.S. Departments of Justice and Education. 1998. *Annual Report on School Safety.* Washington, DC: U.S. Department of Justice.

U.S. Departments of Treasury and of Justice. 1999. *Gun Crime in the Age Group 18–20.* Washington, DC: U.S. Department of Treasury.

U.S. General Accounting Office. 1991. *Accidental Shootings: Many Deaths and Injuries Caused by Firearms Could Be Prevented.* Washington, DC: U.S. General Accounting Office.

Uviller, H. R., and W. G. Merkel. 2000. The Second Amendment in context: The case of the vanishing predicate. *Chicago-Kent Law Review* 76:403–600.

Valois, R. F., R. E. McKeown, C. Z. Garrison, and M. L. Vincent. 1995. Correlates of aggressive and violent behaviors among public high school adolescents. *Journal of Adolescent Health* 16:26–34.

Van Alstyne, W. 1994. The Second Amendment and the personal right to arms. *Duke Law Journal* 43:1236–55.

Vance, D. A. 1999. Dry Ridge, KY. Boy, eleven, shoots and kills sister. *Kentucky Post*, February 18.

Van Kesteren, J. N., P. Mayhew, and P. Nieuwbeerta. 2000. Criminal Victimisation in Seventeen Industrialised Countries: Key Findings from the 2000 International Crime Victims Survey. The Hague, Ministry of Justice.

Van Tyne, C. H. 1929. *The War of Independence.* Boston: Houghton-Mifflin.

Vernick, J. S., and L. M. Hepburn. 2003. Description and analysis of state and federal laws affecting firearm manufacture, sale, possession, and use. In *Evaluating Gun Policy: Effects on Crime and Violence,* ed. J. Ludwig and P. J. Cook, 345–402. Washington, DC: Brookings Institution.

Vernick, J. S., Z. F. Meisel, S. P. Teret, J. S. Milne, and S. W. Hargarten. 1999. "I didn't know the gun was loaded": An examination of two safety devices that can reduce the risk of unintentional firearm injuries. *Journal of Public Health Policy* 20:427–40.

Vernick, J. S., M. O'Brien, L. M. Hepburn, and S. B. Johnson. 2002. Estimating the proportion of certain firearm-related deaths preventable by safer guns. Paper presented at the American Public Health Association annual meeting, Philadelphia, November 9–13.

Vernick, J. S., and S. P. Teret. 1993. Firearms and health: The right to be armed with accurate information about the Second Amendment. *American Journal of Public Health* 83:1773–77.

Vernick, J. S., and S. P. Teret. 1999. New courtroom strategies regarding firearms: Tort litigation against firearm manufacturers and constitutional challenges to gun laws. *Houston Law Review* 36:1715–54.

Vernick, J. S., S. P. Teret, and D. W. Webster. 1997. Regulating firearm advertisements that promise home protection: A public health intervention. *Journal of the American Medical Association* 277:1391–97.

Vickers, G. 1958. What sets the goals of public health? *Lancet*, March 22, 599–604.

Vienneau, D. 1998. Ontario big on gun control: Poll shows huge support for firearms registry. *Toronto Star*, March 16.

Vigdor, E. R., and J. A. Mercy. 2003. Disarming batterers: The impact of domestic violence firearm laws. In *Evaluating Gun Policy: Effects on Crime and Violence,* ed. J. Ludwig and P. J. Cook, 157–214. Washington, DC: Brookings Institution.

Violence Policy Center. 1997. *Kids Shooting Kids: Stories from across the Nation of Unintentional Shootings among Children and Youth.* Washington, DC: Violence Policy Center.

Violence Policy Center. 1998. *License to Kill.* Washington, DC: Violence Policy Center.

BIBLIOGRAPHY

Violence Policy Center. 1999. One shot, one kill: Civilian sales of military sniper rifles. http://www.vpc.org/studies/sniper.htm/ (accessed December 2001).

Vobejda, B., and D. B. Ottaway. 1999. The .50 caliber rifle. *Washington Post*, August 17.

Vogel, R. E., and C. Dean. 1986. The effectiveness of a handgun safety education program. *Journal of Police Science Administration* 14:242–49.

Waldmeir, P. 2000. Hunting death should be warning to lawmakers. *Detroit News*, December 4.

Walker, L. E. 1984. *The Battered Woman Syndrome*. New York: Springfield.

Walker, S. 1994. *Sense and Nonsense about Crime and Drugs*. 3d ed. Belmont, CA: Wadsworth.

Waller, J. A., and E. B. Whorton. 1973. Unintentional shootings, highway crashes, and acts of violence. *Accident Analysis and Prevention* 5:351–56.

Waller, P. F. 2002. Challenges in motor vehicle safety. *Annual Review of Public Health* 23:93–113.

Wallerstein, J. S., and C. J. Wyle. 1947. Our law-abiding law-breakers. *Probation* 35:107–12.

Wall Street Journal. 1999. Gun dealer criticizes manufacturers for lax policies. June 24.

Walt, K., and S. C. Tuell. 1995. Shootings push concealed-weapon bill to forefront. *Houston Chronicle*, April 5, p. A1.

Washington Post. 1999. America's private gun market is thriving. July 11.

Weaver, C. N., and T. W. Swanson. 1974. Validity of reported date of birth, salary, and seniority. *Public Opinion Quarterly* 38:69–80.

Webb, W. P. 1931. *The Great Plains*. Boston: Ginn.

Webb, W. P. 1951. *The Great Frontier*. Austin: University of Texas Press.

Webster, D. W., P. S. Gainer, and H. R. Champion. 1993. Weapon carrying among inner-city junior high school students: Defensive behavior and aggressive delinquency. *American Journal of Public Health* 83:1604–8.

Webster, D. W., and M. Starnes. 2000. Reexamining the association between child access prevention gun laws and unintentional shooting deaths of children. *Pediatrics* 106:1466–69.

Webster, D. W., J. S. Vernick, and L. M. Hepburn. 2001. Relationship between licensing, registration, and other gun sales laws and the source of state of crime guns. *Injury Prevention* 7:184–89.

Webster, D. W., J. S. Vernick, and L. M. Hepburn. 2002. Effects of Maryland's law banning "Saturday night special" handguns on homicides. *American Journal of Epidemiology* 155:406–12.

Webster, D. W., J. S. Vernick, and J. Ludwig. 1997. Flawed gun policy research could endanger public safety. *American Journal of Public Health* 87:918–21.

Webster, D. W., J. S. Vernick, and J. Ludwig. 1998. Webster and colleagues respond. *American Journal of Public Health* 88:982–83.

BIBLIOGRAPHY

Webster, D. W., M. E. H. Wilson, A. K. Duggan, and L. C. Pakula. 1992. Parents' beliefs about preventing gun injuries to children. *Pediatrics* 89:908–14

Weil, D. S. 1995. Women and handguns. Ph.D. diss., Harvard School of Public Health.

Weil, D. S., and D. Hemenway. 1992. Loaded guns in the home: An analysis of a national random survey of gun owners. *Journal of the American Medical Association* 267:3033–37.

Weil, D. S., and D. Hemenway. 1993. I am the NRA: An analysis of a national random sample of gun owners. *Violence and Victims* 8:353–65, 377–85.

Weil, D. S., and R. C. Knox. 1996. Effects of limiting handgun purchasing on interstate transfer of firearms. *Journal of the American Medical Association* 275:1759–61.

Weiner, T., and G. Thompson. 2001. Guns smuggled into Mexico aid drug war. *New York Times*, May 18.

Weiss, P. 1994. Why they shoot: A hoplophobe among the gunnies. *New York Times Magazine*, September 11.

Wells, W. 2000. The situational role of firearms in violent encounters. Ph.D. diss., University of Nebraska at Omaha.

Wentland, E. J., and K. W. Smith. 1993. *Survey Responses: An Evaluation of Their Validity*. Boston: Academic Press.

Whisker, J. B. 1997. *The American Colonial Militia*. Lewiston, NY: Edwin Mellon Press.

Wiebe, D. J. 2003a. Firearms in U.S. homes as a risk factor for unintentional gunshot fatality. *Accident Analysis and Prevention* 35:711–16.

Wiebe, D. J. 2003b. Homicide and suicide risks associated with firearms in the home: a national case-control study. *Annals of Emergency Medicine* 41:771–82.

Wilkinson, D. L., and J. Fagan. 1996. The role of firearms in the violence "scripts": The dynamics of gun events among adolescent males. *Law and Contemporary Problems* 59:55–89.

Williams, D. 2000. Under the gun. *Jerusalem Post*, November 22.

Williams, D. C. 1991. Civic republicanism and the citizen militia: The terrifying Second Amendment. *Yale Law Journal* 101:551–615.

Wills, G. 1995. To keep and bear arms. *New York Review of Books*, September 21, 62–73.

Wills, G. 1999. *A Necessary Evil: A History of American Distrust of Government*. New York: Simon & Schuster.

Wills, G. 2000. Spiking the gun myth. Review of *Arming America* by M. A. Bellesiles. *New York Times*, October 10.

Winslow, C. E. A. 1923. *The Evolution and Significance of the Modern Public Health Campaign*. New Haven: Yale University Press.

Winsten, J. A. 1994. Promoting designated drivers: The Harvard alcohol project. *American Journal of Preventive Medicine* 10 (supplement): 11–14.

Wintemute, G. J. 1994. *Ring of Fire: The Handgun Makers of Southern California*. Sacramento, CA: Violence Prevention Research Program.

BIBLIOGRAPHY

Wintemute, G. J. 1996. The relationship between firearm design and firearm violence: Handguns in the 1990s. *Journal of the American Medical Association* 275:1749–53.

Wintemute, G. J. 2003. Gun carrying among male adolescents as a function of gun ownership in the general population. *Annals of Emergency Medicine* 41:428–29.

Wintemute, G. J., C. M. Drake, J. J. Beaumont, M. Wright, and C. A. Parham. 1998. Prior misdemeanor convictions as a risk factor for later violent and firearm-related criminal activity among authorized purchasers of handguns. *Journal of the American Medical Association* 280:2083–87.

Wintemute, G. J., C. A. Parham, J. J. Beaumont, M. Wright, and C. M. Drake. 1999. Mortality among recent purchasers of handguns. *New England Journal of Medicine* 341:1583–89.

Wintemute, G. J., S. P. Teret, and J. F. Kraus. 1987. When children shoot children: Eighty-eight unintended deaths in California. *Journal of the American Medical Association* 257:3107–9.

Wintemute, G. J., M. A. Wright, C. A. Parham, C. M. Drake, and J. J. Beaumont. 1998. Criminal activity and assault-type handguns: A study of young adults. *Annals of Emergency Medicine* 32:44–50.

Wintemute, G. J., M. A. Wright, C. A. Parham, C. M. Drake, and J. J. Beaumont. 1999. Denial of handgun purchase: A description of the affected population and a controlled study of their handgun preferences. *Journal of Criminal Justice* 27:21–31.

Wolcott, H. 1999. UPS is taking aim at gun thefts. *Los Angeles Times,* November 8.

World Health Organization. 1996. *World Health Statistics Annual 1996,* and updated. Online. www3.who.int/whosis/menu.cfm.

Wright, J. D. 1988. Second thoughts about gun control. *Public Interest* 91:23–39.

Wright, J. D. 1995. Ten essential observations on guns in America. *Society* 32 (March/April): 63–68.

Wright, J. D., and P. H. Rossi. 1986. *Armed and Considered Dangerous: A Survey of Felons and Their Firearms.* Hawthorne, NY: Aldine de Gruyter.

Wright, J. D., P. H. Rossi, and K. Daly. 1983. *Under the Gun: Weapons, Crime, and Violence in America.* Hawthorne, NY: Aldine Publishing.

Wright, J. D., J. F. Sheley, and M. D. Smith. 1992. Kids, guns, and killing fields. *Society* 30:84–89.

Wright, M. A., G. J. Wintemute, and F. P. Rivara. 1999. Effectiveness of denial of handgun purchase to persons believed to be at high risk for firearm violence. *American Journal of Public Health* 89:88–90.

Yang, B., and D. Lester. 1991. The effect of gun availability on suicide rates. *Atlantic Economic Review* 19:74.

Young, J. T., D. Hemenway, R. J. Blendon, and J. M. Benson. 1996. The polls: Trends (guns). *Public Opinion Quarterly* 60:634–49.

Zimmerman, D. 1999. CDC fires top gun industry researcher; Studies lag; GOP politics are blamed. *Probe* (David Zimmerman's newsletter on science, media, policy and health), (November): 1, 4–5.

Zimring, F. E. 1968. Is gun control likely to reduce violent killings? *University of Chicago Law Review* 35:721–37.

Zimring, F. E. 1972. The medium is the message: Firearm caliber as a determinant of death from assault. *Journal of Legal Studies* 1:97–123.

Zimring, F. E., and G. Hawkins. 1997a. Concealed handguns: The counterfeit deterrent. *Responsive Community* 7 (2): 46–60.

Zimring, F. E., and G. Hawkins. 1997b. *Crime Is Not the Problem: Lethal Violence in America.* New York: Oxford University Press.

Zimring, F. E., and J. Zuehl. 1986. Victim injury and death in urban robbery: A Chicago study. *Journal of Legal Studies* 15:1–40.

Zwerling, C., C. F. Lynch, and M. Schootman. 1993. The epidemiology of firearm deaths in Iowa, 1980–1990. *American Journal of Preventive Medicine* 9 (supplement 1): 21–25.

Zwerling, C., D. McMillan, and P. J. Cook et al. 1993. Firearm injuries: Public health recommendations. *American Journal of Preventive Medicine* 9 (supplement): 52–55.

NAME INDEX

301

NAME INDEX

NAME INDEX

PLACE INDEX

311

PLACE INDEX

GENERAL INDEX

GENERAL INDEX